Cancer and the Adolescent

Peter Selby

Cancer Medicine Research Unit, St James's University Hospital, Leeds

and

Clifford Bailey

Northern and Yorkshire Research School of Medicine, Leeds

BMJ
Publishing
Group

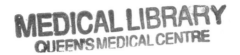
1001131840

© BMJ Publishing Group 1996

First published in 1996
by the BMJ Publishing Group, BMA House, Tavistock Square,
London WC1H 9JR

British Library Cataloguing in Publication Data

A catalogue record for this book is available from the British Library

ISBN 0-7279-0893-6

Typeset by Apek Typesetters Ltd, Nailsea, Bristol
Printed and bound in Great Britain by Latimer Trend Ltd, Plymouth

Contents

Contributors

Clifford Bailey, Professor and Regional Director, Research and Development, Northern and Yorkshire Region Research School of Medicine, Leeds, UK

Ann Barrett, Professor of Clinical Oncology, Beatson Oncology Centre, Western Infirmary, Glasgow, UK

Peter Boyle, Director, Division of Epidemiology and Biostatistics, European Institute of Oncology, Milan, Italy

Ray Cartwright, Professor of Cancer Epidemiology, Leukaemia Research Fund Centre, Leeds, UK

DP Dearnaley, Senior Lecturer and Honorary Consultant in Radiotherapy and Oncology, Royal Marsden Hospital and Institute of Cancer Research, Sutton, Surrey, UK

Jennifer Devlen, Visiting Assistant Professor, Psychology in Palliative Medicine, Department of Anaesthesia, Penn State College of Medicine, Hershey Medical Center, Pennsylvania 17033, USA

Sir Richard Doll, Emeritus Professor of Medicine, Imperial Cancer Research Fund Cancer Studies Unit, Radcliffe Infirmary, Oxford, UK

Christine Eiser, Reader in Health Psychology, Department of Psychology, University of Exeter, Exeter, UK

Margaret Evans, Macmillan Lecturer in Paediatric Oncology Nursing/Macmillan Paediatric Consultant, School of Nursing and Midwifery, The General Hospital, Southampton, UK

Robert J Grimer, Consultant Orthopaedic Oncologist, The Royal Orthopaedic Hospital, Oncology Service, Northfield, Birmingham, UK

Clive Harmer, Head of Radiotherapy Services, Sarcoma Unit, The Royal Marsden Hospital Trust, Fulham Road, London, UK

A Horwich, Professor of Radiotherapy, Royal Marsden Hospital and Institute of Cancer Research, Sutton, Surrey, UK

C Joslin, Yorkshire Cancer Registry, Yorkshire Cancer Organisation, Cookridge Hospital, Leeds, UK

A Kilby, Department of Paediatrics, University College London Medical School, Middlesex Hospital, London, UK

JE Kingston, ICRF Department of Medical Oncology, St Bartholomew's Hospital, London, UK

Sally E Kinsey, Consultant Paediatric Haematologist, St James's University Hospital, Leeds, UK

George Kissen, Hospital Practitioner, Paediatric Oncology, Royal Manchester Children's Hospital, Pendlebury, Manchester, UK

Ian J Lewis, Consultant Paediatric Oncologist, Yorkshire Region Paediatric Oncology Unit, St James's University Hospital, Leeds, UK

TA Lister, Director, ICRF Department of Medical Oncology, St Bartholomew's Hospital, London, UK

JF McCarthy, Department of Oncology, University College, London Medical School, Middlesex Hospital, London, UK

Peter Maguire, CRC Psychological Medicine Group, Stanley House, Christie Hospital, Manchester, UK

Patrick Maisonneuve, Division of Epidemiology and Biostatistics, European Institute of Oncology, Milan, Italy

JS Malpas, ICRF Department of Medical Oncology, St Bartholomew's Hospital, London, UK

John Rees, Department of Haematology, University of Cambridge, MRC Centre, Hills Road, Cambridge, UK

L Rider, Yorkshire Cancer Registry, Yorkshire Cancer Organisation, Cookridge Hospital, Leeds, UK

Peter Selby, Director, Imperial Cancer Research Fund Cancer Medicine Research Unit, University of Leeds, St James's University Hospital, Leeds, UK

SM Shalet, Professor of Endocrinology, Christie Hospital, Wilmslow Road, Manchester, UK

RL Souhami, Professor of Oncology, University College London Medical School, Middlesex Hospital, London, UK

J Whelan, Department of Oncology, University College London Medical School, Middlesex Hospital, London, UK

Foreword

The Teenage Cancer Trust is the first national initiative to appreciate the very special needs of adolescents with cancer.

We are proud that our awareness of these needs has contributed to the First International Conference on Cancer and the Adolescent, held at Weetwood Hall, Leeds, on 12–13 May 1994, and to this book.

The first purpose built Teenager Cancer Trust Unit—designed with young people in mind—was opened in 1990 at the Middlesex Hospital, London and in December 1995 a unit at the Hammersmith Hospital will be opened, followed in 1996 by a unit at the Royal Victoria Infirmary, Newcastle.

It is estimated that ideally 20 Teenage Cancer Trust Units are required throughout the United Kingdom. We are determined to fulfil this need and ensure that every adolescent cancer patient has the opportunity to be treated in a specialist Teenage Cancer Trust Unit.

We see these specialist units as having three main purposes:

- providing an appropriate physical environment for the treatment of adolescents with cancer
- creation of a supportive emotional climate
- enabling cross-fertility of specialties and expertise to advance knowledge in the field.

Physical environment

Although much can be achieved by skilled and dedicated men and women in unsympathetic conditions, treatment in units designed to be 'user-friendly' and sensitive to patients, their families, and staff maximises their efficacy. Appropriate design and great attention to the details of furnishing and equipping from medical, aesthetic and social viewpoints assists in reducing the trauma of 'coming into hospital' and cushions those who have to stay. An optimistic setting enhances and supports the ideology of the medical team.

Emotional climate

A determined philosophy which meets the emotional needs of adolescents, both because of and regardless of their cancer, can provide vital support to teenage patients. Anxiety, lack of confidence and insecurity are all states of mind experienced by young people, and these are further complicated by cancer and its treatment.

Whether recovery is to be complete or temporary, 'now' is very important, particularly for the young, and experiences during the part of their life when suffering from cancer, must be positive too. Inevitably growing up should, indeed must, continue, and all the concerns and queries of the adolescent patients must be satisfied. Parents, extended families, friends and staff require understanding and emotional support both to enable them to strengthen the resolve of adolescent patients to cope with their illness and its treatment, and for their own sake.

Peer group support is an essential part of normal adolescent development. This requirement is even more important for adolescent cancer patients.

Knowledge

It is acknowledged that treatment of cancer is more successful when undertaken by those with the greatest expertise. Treatment of teenage cancers tends to be complex. It follows therefore that the concentration of young cancer patients in specialist Teenage Cancer Trust Units will provide an unprecedented source of experience. This enhanced opportunity for experience and expertise gained will apply not only to doctors and nurses, but to the entire multidisciplinary team involved with our units.

The advancement of knowledge in the field of cancers most affecting adolescents and improved recovery rates are realistic expectations resulting from the provision of specialist, purpose built Teenage Cancer Trust Units.

The First International Conference on Cancer and the Adolescent, and the production of this volume, are significant acknowledgements of the growing awareness of the unique needs of teenage cancer patients which the Teenage Cancer Trust has highlighted.

ADRIAN WHITESON, *Chairman*
MYRNA WHITESON, *Chairman*
Teenage Cancer Trust

Preface

The difficulties of managing cancer in adolescent patients are widely appreciated. Adolescence is associated with psychological changes which are well recognised both in families and by health care professionals who meet these young people, thankfully quite rarely, when they are affected by serious illness. The psychosocial challenge presented by any serious illness is compounded when added to the psychosocial challenge of adolescence itself. In oncology, adolescent patients also represent a major technical challenge. The commoner cancers, leukaemias and lymphomas, melanoma, brain tumours, germ cell tumours, bone sarcomas and soft tissue sarcomas, are in themselves difficult diseases to treat. They are aggressive and life threatening illnesses which require complicated multimodality therapies. However, when these treatments are applied to a high standard, a substantial proportion of patients can be cured. Unfortunately the aftermath of that treatment can include long term disabilities and damaging late effects. In addition to this complexity and these technical demands, cancer in adolescents also includes a very wide range of cancers which are rare in adolescents but common in adult life. A small number of each of the epithelial cancers can be expected to occur in adolescents. This adds a tremendous difficulty for a service aimed at caring for all patients with cancer including adolescents because expertise must be drawn in from many directions in order to ensure that these patients get the right multidisciplinary consultation in the right supportive environment.

Cancers occurring in adolescence may also have particular biological features which merit careful study and may ultimately lead on to improve methods of diagnosis and treatment. The molecular genetics of soft tissue and bone sarcomas, and the special aetiological relationships for rare cancers induced by specific environmental agents such as bladder cancer after cyclophosphamide, or clear cell carcinoma of the vagina after oestrogen treatment of mothers are just a few examples.

These medical and scientific demands are at the moment ill met. Only a minority of adolescent patients with cancer are managed in units with a full range of supportive services with staff especially trained to cope with the additional challenges of oncology in this age group. Understanding of aetiology and biology for cancers in adolescents is still rudimentary and poorly researched.

The purpose of the meeting on which this book is based was to address a wide range of issues from aetiology through treatment to include palliative care and at all stages an appropriate consideration of the psychosocial dimension of these cases. We hope that the meeting and this book will draw attention to the problems and needs of this patient group. We also hope that the work presented here will go some way to indicating appropriate ways of handling these problems and lead on to better outcomes for these young people who are unfortunate enough to get cancer at this sensitive period of their lives.

PETER SELBY
CLIFFORD BAILEY
St James's University Hospital, Leeds

PART I
Epidemiology

1: Epidemiology of cancer in adolescents

PETER BOYLE and PATRICK MAISONNEUVE

Although cancer is a rare disease before middle age, it accounts for a substantial proportion of deaths among children and young adults in industrialised countries. Its study in younger age groups has already yielded important clues about mechanisms of cancer causation and greatly helped the development of effective treatment modalities. In younger persons, there has been more work done in childhood cancer (i.e. under 15 years) than at any other age. The subject of cancer in adolescents has been widely ignored from an epidemiological perspective and there is very little available material specifically relating to adolescent cancer. Indeed, cancer in adolescents appears to be a bit of a desert from the epidemiological point of view despite being more common at ages 10–19 than at ages 0–9, which has been the target of much research activity.

Descriptive epidemiology

There are data available from many sources around the world detailing the incidence of cancer of many forms, organised and presented according to the *International Classification of Diseases*.[1] These data, if the registry is deemed to be of sufficient quality, are routinely published in compendia of cancer incidence statistics according to age class;[2] the classes of age generally employed are 0, 1–4 (or in some instances 0–4), 5–9, 10–14, 15–19, 20–24, and so on.

There is an unfortunate consequence to the use of the *International Classification of Diseases* where cancers other than leukaemias, lymphomas, and melanomas are categorised solely by site of origin. This is very practical for the great majority of cancers recorded in adults, but it presents great problems at the younger ages. Cancers in children and young adults exhibit a great diversity of histological type as well as primary site: in contrast, most cancers found in adults in industrialised countries (e.g. breast, lung, stomach, and large bowel) are hardly ever seen in children.[3] Consequently, it is more appropriate for childhood cancers to be classified according to

3

their histology, and a general classification scheme has been developed for this purpose in which groupings are established for combinations of morphology and topography.[4] The scheme consists of 12 major diagnostic groups: leukaemias, lymphomas, brain and spinal tumours, sympathetic nervous system tumours, retinoblastoma, kidney tumours, liver tumours, bone tumours, soft tissue sarcomas, gonadal and germ cell tumours, epithelial tumours, and other and unspecified malignant neoplasms.

However, *Cancer Incidence in Five Continents*[2] does not make data available for adolescents according to this classification. In order to get a feel for the range and occurrence of cancers in adolescents, it is necessary to make some compromise and adjustment to available data and to re-programme these data as closely as possible to this classification system for childhood cancers.[4] It is useful to pose the question as to whether the epidemiology of cancer in adolescents is similar to that in childhood.

In undertaking this exercise it is also important to define an *adolescent*. For the purposes of the exercise described here it will be taken that 10–19 is the age range of adolescence, recognising that available analytical studies and other publications may choose different age ranges. The selection of typical international populations was made *a priori* on the basis of fulfilment of a number of criteria, principally that the regions needed to be fairly large and to have good cancer registration. Canada, where cancer registration is accomplished by high-quality provincial cancer registries, England and Wales, with regional cancer registration, and the Surveillance, Epidemiology and End Results (SEER) Programme of the United States were chosen for this purpose. The choice was made on *a priori* grounds and without seeing the results from any country or region.

Over the most recent period for which cancer incidence data are available (the 5-year period 1983–87)[2], the average population of Canada was 25 million with an (annual) average of 1 940 000 male adolescents and 1 850 000 female adolescents. During this period, there were 1603 cases of malignant tumours recorded in male adolescents which gave rise to an annual rate of 160 cases per million person-years. In female adolescents, there were 1361 cases recorded with a rate of 143 per million per annum. There was an overall 10% excess in male adolescents: a rate ratio of 1.1.

In contrast to childhood, where the leukaemias are the commonest form of cancer, the group of lymphomas appeared to be the commonest in adolescents: when Hodgkin's disease and non-Hodgkin's lymphoma were combined, the incidence rates were 45.3 and 36.3 per million in male and female adolescents respectively. Leukaemia is also very common as is cancer of the brain and central nervous system (CNS) (Table 1.1). Bone and soft tissue tumours are very common, as they are in younger age groups.

It is of considerable interest, although not easily explicable in aetiological terms, that male adolescents appear to have an excess rate of leukaemias and bone cancers when compared to female adolescents (the rate ratios were both 1.4 indicating a 40% excess risk in males). Similarly, the larger

Table 1.1   Cancer incidence (average rate per 1 000 000 per year) in adolescents (age 10–19) in Canada, 1983–7.

| Cancer type | Male adolescents | | | Female adolescents | | | Rate |
	10–14	15–19	10–19	10–14	15–19	10–19	ratio
Leukaemias	28·0	32·9	30·5	22·7	21·1	21·9	1·4
Hodgkin's disease	17·2	36·7	27·0	9·7	40·6	25·2	1·1
Brain/CNS	23·9	25·6	24·8	22·4	17·4	19·9	1·2
Non-Hodgkin's lymphoma	17·2	18·8	18·0	8·6	12·0	10·3	1·7
Bone	16·3	17·8	17·1	13·1	11·0	12·1	1·4
Soft tissue	6·9	8·9	7·9	7·3	8·7	8·0	1·0
Thyroid	2·4	4·6	3·5	4·8	20·1	12·5	0·3
Malignant melanoma	1·9	6·1	4·0	2·5	13·5	8·0	0·5
Testis	2·2	24·8	13·5	NA	NA	NA	
Ovary	NA	NA	NA	7·3	9·7	8·5	
All cancers	130·1	197·7	163·9	107·9	183·4	145·7	1·1

NA, not applicable.
The rate ratio is the rate in male adolescents divided by that in female adolescents.
Data from Parkin et al.[2]

excess apparent in the incidence rate of non-Hodgkin's lymphomas (rate ratio 1.7) is currently inexplicable and in marked contrast to the similarity of the incidence rates of Hodgkin's disease (rate ratio 1.1).

Thyroid cancer was 3–4 times commoner in female adolescents than in male adolescents: the rate ratio was 0.3. A similar pattern, although not so marked, was also present for malignant melanoma where the rate in female adolescents was the double of the rate in male adolescents (Table 1.1). Testicular cancer was the sixth commonest form of incident cancer in male adolescents (rate 14.9 per million). Ovarian cancer was the seventh commonest form of cancer in adolescent females.

In the SEER Programme data from the United States, only those from whites were used for comparability (Table 1.2). The pattern was very similar to that from Canada with an excess of leukaemias in male adolescents compared to females (again around 1.4). The male excess of non-Hodgkin's lymphoma was more pronounced than in Canada: the rate ratio was 2.4. The female excesses of thyroid cancer and melanoma were visible and similar in magnitude to those found in Canada (Table 1.2).

In England and Wales, the same rate ratio was present for leukaemias as was found in Canada and the SEER data, i.e. 1.4. There was once more a strong excess of non-Hodgkin's lymphoma in male adolescents and similar excesses of thyroid cancer and melanoma in female adolescents as was found in the other regions (Table 1.3). In all regions there was a slight overall excess of cancer in male adolescents.

The situation in the adolescent age range (10–19 years) is different in several important ways from that in children (0–14 years). In children, around one third of all cancers are leukaemias[3] whereas in adolescents the proportion is around one seventh (471/2964). The lymphomas are more important in adolescents, accounting for around one cancer in four (775/2964) compared to one in ten in childhood, and brain and CNS

Table 1.2 Cancer incidence (average rate per 1 000 000 per year) in white adolescents (age 10–19) in the SEER programme 1983–7.

Cancer type	Male adolescents			Female adolescents			Rate ratio
	10–14	15–19	10–19	10–14	15–19	10–19	
Leukaemias	29·4	28·5	29·0	25·5	16·2	20·9	1·4
Hodgkin's disease	15·8	43·7	29·8	14·9	44·6	29·8	1·0
Brain/CNS	20·5	24·0	22·3	20·2	21·5	20·9	1·1
Non-Hodgkin's lymphoma	19·9	20·7	20·3	6·0	10·9	8·5	2·4
Bone	17·4	19·2	18·3	21·3	11·6	16·5	1·1
Soft tissue	5·7	9·0	7·4	7·6	10·6	9·1	0·8
Thyroid	1·6	7·8	4·7	8·9	30·9	19·9	0·2
Malignant melanoma	0·9	10·5	5·7	2·3	16·9	9·6	0·6
Testis	1·6	35·3	18·5	NA	NA	NA	NA
Ovary	NA	NA	NA	6·3	15·3	10·8	NA
All cancers	121·8	220·7	171·3	115·3	206·7	161·0	1·1

NA, not applicable.
The rate ratio is the rate in males divided by that in females.
The SEER program of the National Cancer Institute is a network of cancer registries covering around 12% of the United States population.
Data from Parkin *et al.*

tumours are less important than in childhood accounting for approximately one cancer in seven (423/2964) in adolescents compared to one in four or one in five in childhood.[3] The main embryonal tumours in childhood (neuroblastoma, Wilm's tumour (nephroblastoma), retinoblastoma and hepatoblastoma) are notable by their absence in adolescents and thyroid cancers and malignant melanomas are much more common (Table 1.1).

Although it is incomplete in that the age group 15–19 is missing, some idea of the changing pattern of cancer at younger ages can be observed in data available from the United Kingdom National Childhood Cancer Registry.[3] This is an extremely important and unique resource which has

Table 1.3 Cancer incidence (Average rate per 1 000 000 per year) in adolescents (age 10–19) in England and Wales 1983–7.

Cancer type	Male adolescents			Female adolescents			Rate ratio
	10–14	15–19	10–19	10–14	15–19	10–19	
Leukaemias	25·6	26·8	26·2	20·0	17·6	18·8	1·4
Hodgkin's disease	12·7	29·6	21·2	6·1	28·7	17·4	1·2
Brain/CNS	20·4	15·6	18·0	15·2	14·5	14·9	1·2
Non-Hodgkin's lymphoma	10·9	13·9	12·4	4·1	5·8	5·0	2·5
Bone	10·8	16·8	13·8	12·0	9·7	10·9	1·3
Soft tissue	4·6	7·1	5·9	4·6	5·1	4·9	1·2
Thyroid	0·5	2·1	1·3	2·2	6·1	4·2	0·3
Malignant melanoma	1·5	4·4	3·0	1·6	8·0	4·8	0·6
Testis	0·6	15·6	8·1	NA	NA	NA	NA
Ovary	NA	NA	NA	3·5	8·0	5·8	NA
All cancers	100·4	154·3	127·4	80·3	127·7	104·0	1·2

The rate ratio is the rate in males divided by that in females.
Original data were abstracted from Parkin *et al.*[2]
NA, not applicable.

Table 1.4 Cancer incidence (rates per 1 000 000 person-years) in the United Kingdom by age group (0–14 years)

Diagnostic group	Age group			
	0	1–4	5–9	10–14
Leukaemias	27	65	30	20
Lymphomas	4	7	12	15
Brain and spinal	19	27	25	21
Sympathetic nerve	25	12	3	1
Retinoblastoma	17	7	0	0
Kidney	14	16	4	1
Liver	4	2	1	0
Bone	0	1	4	10
Osteosarcoma	0	0	2	6
Ewing's sarcoma	0	1	2	3
Soft tissue sarcoma	11	8	5	5
Rhabdomyosarcoma	7	6	5	5
Gonadal and germ cell	2	1	1	1
Epithelial	2	1	1	4

been rigorously maintained in the United Kingdom. The peak incidence of leukaemia is in the age range 1–4 and the rate falls by half in the age range 5–9 (Table 1.4). In contrast the lymphomas appear to increase in frequency throughout the entire age period considered. Brain and spinal tumours remain high at each age group although there is an early peak of tumours of the sympathetic nervous system (in the first year of life). Retinoblastoma is relatively common in the first year of life but the incidence has dropped to imperceptible levels by the age of 5 (Table 1.1). Kidney cancers, almost exclusively Wilm's tumours at these ages, peak in the first five years of life and quickly decline thereafter. Bone tumours rise with age, although it would have been instructive to have had some data regarding the major histological types of bone cancer in adolescents. The rates of thyroid cancer and malignant melanoma seen in adolescents, together with the germ cell tumours of the testis and ovary, are markedly different from the relative rarity of these tumours in childhood.

In childhood, cancer is one third more common in boys than in girls,[3] whereas in adolescence the excess has reduced to only one tenth. Why this should be so remains unknown.

Analytical epidemiology

There has been no published aetiological study of cancer restricted to adolescents, although adolescents have been included in some studies of childhood cancer. Observations of familial aggregations of cancers and observed associations with other inherited diseases and congenital anomalies have pointed to a major genetic component in some childhood cancers. The early age peak in incidence and the cell types of origin suggest that important causative factors may operate before birth or even before conception, and studies of possible environmental risk factors have to a large extent focused on exposures in utero rather than on exposures incurred during the lifetime of the subject. The important question is whether the causes of the same forms of cancer are similar in childhood and adolescence. The definitive answer is unknown, although it is difficult to believe at the present time that a particular cancer type has a different aetiology in 9 year olds ("childhood") than in 11 year olds ("adolescents"). The issue really centres around whether cancers which occur early in life (say in the first 2–3 years when genetic factors may be much more important than environmental exposures) arise for different reasons than those which arise later in childhood and adolescence (when the influence of relevant environmental factors may be more dominant). The discussion regarding possible differences in the aetiology of cancer at these younger ages would be more than academic if the aetiology of childhood cancer was well understood: however, despite a relatively large number of epidemiological investigations, hardly anything is known with certainty about the aetiology of childhood cancer.[3]

In the remainder of this chapter, discussion of the aetiology of cancer at younger ages will be briefly reviewed with recent review material referenced and highlighted. The basis of the discussion will be the childhood cancer literature, although wherever there is an opportunity to discuss a form of cancer which is more common in adolescents than in children (such as brain and nervous system tumours) there will be a discussion of the relevance of the most recent findings. The recently published review of Stiller[3] is highly recommended since many of the major issues of childhood cancer epidemiology are discussed in depth there.

General risk factors for cancer of childhood and adolescence

Due in some measure to the rare nature of cancer in childhood, and the consequent difficulty in assembling adequate numbers of cases of even the commonest forms of childhood cancer for an analytical study in all but the largest centres, there have been a number of studies which have investigated the aetiology of childhood cancer as a group. This is problematic: it combines completely different cancers of a variety of cell types and organ systems and assumes that there may be a common aetiological thread.

The most thoroughly understood childhood cancer is retinoblastoma, which has a strong genetic component and in the heritable form is frequently bilateral and is virtually restricted to the early part of life. Retinoblastoma can be explained as a result of two successive mutations as described by Knudson.[5] The pattern of inheritance is autosomal dominant with a high (90%) penetrance. The offspring of survivors of heritable retinoblastoma have themselves a greatly increased risk of retinoblastoma: 44% of a recent series of such offspring (23 out of 52) themselves developed the tumour. Survivors of retinoblastoma also have an elevated risk of developing second primary tumours, particularly osteosarcoma[6 7] although an increased risk of these and other second primary tumours persists well into adulthood.[8] A recent study from the United States, based on 1458 patients followed for a median of 17 years after retinoblastoma diagnosis, noted 305 deaths of which 167 were from retinoblastoma. (Use of death certificates precluded a better definition of bone cancer.) There were 96 deaths from second primary tumours (odds ratio = 30) and 36 from bone cancer (OR = 325).[9] Radiotherapy was also found to further increase the risk of death from a second neoplasm.

A family history of Wilm's tumour (around 1% of cases)[10] and neuroblastoma[11] have been reported, but the proportion of cases is probably low. In the Li–Fraumeni syndrome, members of the same family are at an increased risk for a wide range of cancers including soft tissue sarcomas, adrenocortical carcinoma, breast cancer (particularly at pre-menopausal ages), brain tumours and osteosarcoma.[12] In a study involving follow up of 24 families with this syndrome, the risk of cancer was found to be over 20-fold greater than the general population rates with the risk persisting until the age of 50.[13] Germ line mutations in the p53 tumour suppressor gene on chromosome 17p13 have been identified in all five of a series of Li–Fraumeni families:[14] this suggests that the syndrome could be due to inherited alterations in this gene.

Children with neurofibromatosis (von Recklinghausen's disease, NF-1) have an increased risk for cancer of the brain and spinal tumours (around 40-fold), a risk of optic nerve glioma which has been estimated to be over 1000-fold and an increased risk of soft tissue sarcoma (around 50-fold) especially rhabdomyosarcoma. Virtually all childhood cases of neuro-fibrosarcoma are associated with von Recklinghausen's neurofibromatosis and there is an overall fourfold increased risk of leukaemia, particularly chronic myeloid leukaemia.[15] Various other familial cancer syndromes account for smaller numbers of childhood cancers.[15]

One important distinguishing factor surrounding these genetic cancers is the fact that risk is increased for a variety of different types of cancer. This area of research is very active at present, and important developments are taking place which could potentially provide important insights into our understanding of the mechanisms of carcinogenesis.

Birth characteristics, birthweight, gestational period, and a wide range of other factors have been inconsistently associated with the risk of childhood cancers of various forms.[3] The situation is different for radiation, where the carcinogenic risk of antenatal obstetric irradiation has been established for nearly four decades.[16] For births during 1958–61, the odds ratio for childhood cancer deaths after irradiation in the third trimester was such that exposure to diagnostic rays in utero could have been the cause of 5% of all childhood cancers.[17] This proportion has decreased with the declining use of X-ray examination and its replacement by ultrasound scanning, which on the available evidence does not appear to be associated with an increased risk of cancer.[18] [19]

Childhood leukaemia in the United Kingdom has been linked to domestic radon exposure, although the causal nature of this association has not been demonstrated and the aetiological fraction may be very small.[20] In the United States, mortality from cancer, especially leukaemia, among children in North Carolina was higher in areas where there were higher concentrations of radon in drinking water.[21] The situation should be clarified by the large number of ongoing studies which are addressing this issue.

Reports of associations between electromagnetic fields and childhood cancer are currently the cause of much public concern. The available literature is inconclusive (see Poole and Trichopoulos[22] for a detailed review) and it appears that any risk is unlikely to be large.[3] However, it would be imprudent to dismiss this hypothesis entirely, and detailed studies are underway to shed light on this issue.

Maternal drug exposures during pregnancy have been associated in some studies with an increased risk of several forms of childhood cancer. Drugs taken by children themselves have also been associated with an increased risk of cancer in the child: for example, children treated with chlorambucil (for juvenile rheumatoid arthritis) have been shown to have an excess risk of acute non-lymphoblastic leukaemia (ANLL)[23] and children who received immunosuppressive therapy after heart transplantation have had excesses of Hodgkin's disease.[24] All this is reviewed by Stiller.[3]

Leukaemias and lymphomas

Reports of clusters of childhood leukaemia have raised questions of a possible infective agent involved in the aetiology of leukaemia, particularly in children and, more recently, of the possibility of localised environmental pollution playing a dominant role. Recent research from the United Kingdom supports the hypothesis that a substantial proportion of cases of acute lymphoblastic leukaemia (ALL) in children arise as a rare host response to certain patterns of exposure to common infectious agents—the aberrant response model.[25]

There have been reports of clusters of leukaemia in children throughout this century.[26] Initially these were considered as evidence that acute leukaemia was an infectious disease. The possibility that childhood acute leukaemia was possibly related to viruses was enhanced by observations of viruses as causes of leukaemia in chickens as well as other animal species. This belief continued with reports of clusters until recent times; then it was observed that there were clusters of leukaemia in the vicinity of sources of environmental pollution, in particular ionising radiation, contaminated water, and other fixed environmental hazards. Such associations remain controversial, and causality has not yet been substantially proved, but there is still belief that childhood leukaemia may have an important environmental component.

Recent epidemiological data from the United Kingdom also suggest that population mixing identifies areas where risk of childhood leukaemia is higher: in those communities which were small and tended to be isolated, the influx of large numbers of individuals from cities has been associated with subsequent increases in the risk of childhood leukaemia.[27] It is hypothesised that the arrival of "new" viruses into these somewhat isolated communities has led to a rise in acute leukaemia. Since ALL is a rare disease, unusual host factors or exposure circumstances must be essential aetiological components. Symptoms associated with initial infection must be unremarkable, otherwise there are grounds for thinking that such an association would have been noted already.

Greaves[28] has previously hypothesised that immunological isolation in infancy increases the risk of ALL arising in the childhood peak. With increasing evidence that clustering may be a real characteristic of childhood acute leukaemia, it can now be hypothesised (i) that a specific agent is likely to be involved, and (ii) the same (or related) agent is aetiologically associated with (childhood) leukaemia at other ages. These two can be generalised into a single hypothesis, the aberrant response model. A review of the current literature from this perspective finds considerable support and shows the capacity to unify a number of apparently diverse lines of research into the aetiology of childhood leukaemia, primarily those relating to familial and maternal health, family structure and circumstances, in utero exposures to infection, and past medical history. The model proposed has greater ability than any previous to explain coherently known risk factor associations.

Under the model, a specific (although currently unknown) transmissible agent is causally associated with childhood ALL. For children diagnosed around the childhood peak, primary infection may occur shortly before diagnosis, while for other ages at diagnosis attention is focused on gestational neonatal exposures leading to persistent infection. In this situation also, exposure close to diagnosis may be involved and some reports of temporal clustering would support this. There is no evidence for direct case to case transmission of the (unknown) agent and most studies are consistent with an effect of high-dose exposure occurring in community microepidemics. A most important aspect of this hypothesis is that it is "testable" and this should be an obvious priority in the aetiology of this disease which, although unimportant in the sense that it is not a leading cause of cancer, is very important in that it strikes the youngest and most vulnerable members of society.

The best understood environmental risk factor for leukaemia at young ages is ionising radiation. Among children who survived the atomic bombs in Hiroshima and Nagasaki, an increased risk of leukaemia occurred 1–3 years after exposure, reached a peak 6–7 years after, and declined steadily thereafter.[29] A significant excess of leukaemia was also observed among children in areas of Utah (United States) which received the highest doses of fallout from the Nevada nuclear testing range.[30]

A review of the occurrence of childhood cancer (leukaemia mainly) around nuclear power stations and other nuclear installations concluded that there was no evidence of excess mortality near nuclear installations when all studies from United States, Canada, France and Germany were considered.[31] In the United Kingdom, excesses of childhood leukaemia have been confirmed in areas near the only two nuclear reprocessing plants in the country: at Sellafield[32] and Dounreay[33]. There was a increased risk of childhood leukaemia in Seascale (the village closest to the plant at Sellafield) which was confined to children who were born to mothers who were living there at the time of the birth.[34] An increased rate of leukaemia and other cancers in children was found in an area surrounding two military sites in southern England.[35] A detailed study of mortality (between 1969 and 1978) around 15 nuclear installations, the majority of which were power stations, throughout England and Wales reported significant excess rates of among persons age 0–24 for leukaemia and Hodgkin's disease.[36] Interpretation of this has to be cautioned by the finding of similar excesses in districts near sites where the building of similar installations had been proposed but not yet proceeded with.[37]

Kinlen[38] provided a link between such observations and the infectious nature of childhood leukaemia when he proposed that leukaemia in children is a rare response to a postulated widespread virus infection which may even possibly not produce any detectable symptoms in many individuals who are infected with the virus. Kinlen predicted that leukaemia would be more common in areas where there was a high level of population mixing with the resulting low level of herd immunity: the optimum setting for this would be in remote areas where large influxes of new population occurred over a fairly short period. Using a variety of novel approaches, and employing both incidence and mortality data, Kinlen has provided evidence supporting his initial hypothesis.[27 38 39]

Childhood ALL in the United Kingdom has been demonstrated to have a higher incidence in higher socioeconomic groups.[40] A higher incidence of Hodgkin's disease has been associated with higher socioeconomic status in many studies[41] (it is worth remembering that neuroblastoma may have a higher incidence in lower socioeconomic status groups).[3] MacMahon[42] first called attention to the bimodal nature of the age-incidence curve of Hodgkin's disease with peaks in early adults (20–34 years) and in the elderly (aged 55 and over). He also observed that the disease had a low incidence among young adults in some countries such as Japan and that in developing countries there appeared to be another pattern of occurrence marked by a large male excess.[43] Correa and O'Connor[44] reported distinct patterns in the age-specific incidence of Hodgkin's disease which differed between geographic areas, which they hypothesised to be dependent on the level of urbanisation and economic growth. These observations were important leading to the development of hypotheses on a possible infectious aetiology of Hodgkin's disease.

Recent data (from around the mid-1980s), from an increased number of cancer registries and international populations[2] show distinct differences in age-specific Hodgkin's disease incidence patterns in different geographic areas.[45] In the United States and western Europe, the characteristic pattern of low childhood rates and high young adult rates is still present. In contrast, in populations of central and eastern Europe, the rates in young adults are essentially similar but the rates in children are higher than those in the United States and western Europe. Incidence patterns for South American countries differed from those previously observed with a shift towards patterns observed in more economically developed countries. Analysis of incidence data from earlier sources back to the early 1960s, confirms the original inverse correlation reported by Correa and O'Connor[44] but observes that this association has become weaker over time until there was no correlation between Hodgkin's disease rates in children aged 5–14 years (as well as 0–9 years) and young adults (20–34 years) using the most recent incidence data.[45]

Brain and central nervous system

This is an important form of cancer in adolescents and children which has been examined in a variety of studies including young people up to 20 and sometimes 24 years of age. Although the posterior fossa contains the minority of the brain volume, approximately half of the paediatric tumours arise in that site: these tumours are mainly medulloblastoma, cerebellar and brainstem astrocytomas, and IVth ventricular ependymomas. Half of all paediatric brain tumours are gliomas, with ependymomas and well-differentiated astrocytomas being more frequent than high-grade astrocytomas. Paediatric tumours differ from adult brain tumours in their tendency to be better differentiated and occupy the posterior fossa, but there are also large differences in common tumour types. Meningiomas and acoustic neuromas are rare, while craniopharyngiomas and pineal tumours are proportionately more common, particularly in far Eastern populations. Germ cell tumours, which occur in the midline, are also commoner in the young.[46]

Epidemiological studies of these cancers as a whole have suffered from the lack of reality in the definition of the disease: many studies have included benign and malignant tumours, the histological types have been grouped together and little attention has been paid to the site of the tumour and the age of the patient. A wide variety of potential risk factors for brain and CNS cancers have been proposed, including parental irradiation, previous miscarriages, maternal use of antihistamines, maternal contact with cats or farm animals, genetic factors (such as neurofibromatosis and tuberous sclerosis), socioeconomic status, pesticide exposure, incense, recreational drugs, hair dyes, parental occupation, exposure to infections and fevers, maternal smoking, and paternal smoking.

A major hypothesis was developed during the 1980s regarding the role of potential exposure to N-nitroso compounds (NOC), whether prenatal or postnatal, in the aetiology of brain and CNS in children and young adults. In laboratory animals, maternal exposure to these compounds during pregnancy resulted in the development of nervous system tumours in their offspring.[47] A case-control study in Los Angeles found increased risk associated with disparate factors which had in common postulated exposure to NOC.[48]

There has been a recent flurry of studies published on this hypothesis, with some studies not simply restricted to cancers of the brain and CNS. McCredie *et al.*[49] concluded from a case-control study of childhood brain tumours that analysis of a number of possible sources of exposure to NOC and their precursors provided limited support for the *N*-nitroso hypothesis but recognised that measures of exposure were crude and certainly not exhaustive. In a case-control study of astrocytic glioma in children, a trend was observed for consumption of all cured meats which contained preformed nitrosamines and their precursors (OR=1.7). Risk appeared to be slightly reduced for frequent consumption of vitamin C.[50] In a case-control study of childhood cancer, eating hamburgers one or more times per week was associated with a risk of ALL (OR=2.0) and eating hot dogs one or more times per week was associated with an increased risk of brain tumours (OR=2.1, 95% confidence interval (0.7, 6.1)). The results suggested to the authors a possible adverse effect of dietary nitrites and nitrosamines.[51] A case-control study of leukaemia in children demonstrated an increased risk associated with children's intake of hot dogs (OR=9.5 (1.6,57.6) for 12 or more hot dogs per month) and also fathers' intake of hot dogs (OR=11 (1.2, 98.7) for the highest category of intake). The authors concluded that the results were compatible with the experimental animal literature and the hypothesis that human NOC intake is associated with leukaemia risk.[52]

There are a number of reasons for remaining cautious about this hypothesis. Exposure to NOC and precursors cannot be measured directly in a retrospective study. Potential exposure comes from many possible sources and any questionnaire is generally restricted to questions about 15–20 potential sources. Different studies with different numbers and groups of potential sources present a problem similar to "multiple comparisons" when the data are analysed: each study in effect asks questions about a potentially different subset of potential sources of exposure. The content of NOC obviously varies from one type of exposure to another and even within exposure category: the dose cannot be estimated. The ability to measure this exposure even in a way which could be used in a retrospective study will involve innovative epidemiology and may even be beyond the limits of any questionnaire.

Many of the studies have reported null findings, and many "exposure sources" have been found to have no association in a number of studies. A major effort is required to address this hypothesis adequately in a human study. This is worth doing particularly since much of the attraction surrounding the continuing study of this hypothesis lies in that it closely links laboratory evidence of carcinogenicity with a human target.

Tobacco smoke contains high concentrations of various NOC, especially of nitrosamines which were the first tobacco-specific carcinogens to be identified.[53] The fetus can potentially be exposed to tobacco smoke by two pathways: the mother's active smoke during pregnancy (mainstream smoke) and her passive exposure to her own sidestream smoke and that of the father and others in the home or outside. Sidestream smoke contains high amounts of carcinogenic and cocarcinogenic chemicals, mainly volatile compounds such as nitrogen oxides (NOX) and nitrosamines.[54 45]

Components of cigarette smoke are transported across the placental membrane of women whether by active smoking or as a result of exposure to passive smoking.[56] Bioactivation of procarcinogens to mutagens in human fetal and placental tissues has been demonstrated, as has cigarette smoke induced damage to DNA in human placenta. Cigarette smoke constituents have been shown to be active transplantal carcinogens in animals,[57] and human data suggesting an association with maternal smoking during pregnancy have been reported for all childhood cancers combined,[16] for leukaemia[58] and for brain cancer.[59] An increased risk of brain cancer in children which was not statistically significant was associated with the smoking habit of the father alone during the year prior to the child's birth,[60] and a further study reported an elevated odds ratio of 1.5 for mothers who lived with a smoker during the pregnancy[48] which was not statistically significant. An association with passive smoking and the risk of adult brain tumours was also found in a Japanese prospective study.[61] A feature of the majority of these findings has been that the odds ratios reported were elevated but were not statistically significant in the commonly accepted sense.

Gold et al.[59] reported a five-fold increase in the risk of brain tumours in children associated with maternal smoking during pregnancy: again this study had a small sample size. This finding has not been confirmed by other studies which appear to have a measure of consistency in reporting, similarly to the findings in this study, elevated odds ratios which are not statistically significant.[48 58–60 62–64]

The association with paternal smoking and the risk of childhood brain tumours has tended to be slightly more consistent, although dogged by small odds ratios which are not statistically significant and by an overall lack of confirmatory findings from all studies on the subject, which are all small incidentally. Preston-Martin et al.[48] reported an odds ratio of 1.5 for mothers who lived with a smoker during pregnancy. It may be of interest that Sandler et al.[65] found excess brain cancers among adults to be associated with childhood exposure to fathers' smoking whereas there was no association with exposure to mother's smoking. Filipini et al.[66] make another contribution to what could be described as no more than the suggestion that a father's smoking increases the risk of brain tumour in his offspring.

A curious aspect of these studies has been the inability to find associations with both the smoking habit of the mother and her passive exposure to the smoking of the father during the pregnancy. Although the numbers are small and the confidence limits wide, and the elevated risks are not generally statistically significant, the available studies provide some support of an association with brain tumours in children and the smoking habit of both the mother and the father during the pregnancy.

It is worth reflecting on how strong this suggestion of an association is supported. All previous studies reported may have underestimated the risk of childhood brain tumour associated with maternal cigarette smoking during pregnancy due to potential misclassification of children exposed in utero to the cigarette smoke of the father, other household members, and potentially to work colleagues of the mother. Such misclassification of children as being "unexposed" would lead to an underestimation of the association with maternal smoking. One study[66] differed from most others on this topic by attempting a clearer estimation of "exposed" and "unexposed" since the questionnaire attempted to elicit information on maternal smoking exposure during pregnancy both inside and outside of the home.

The finding finds some support from the available experimental evidence which supports the hypothesis of an association between risk of childhood brain tumour and in utero exposure to cigarette smoke.[57] Sidestream smoke contains more volatile NOX and nitrosamines than active smoke and these substances are potent experimental carcinogens for the fetal nervous system.[54 55 67] The fetus may be more sensitive to the carcinogenic action of NOX and nitrosamines than the adult animal.[68 69] Some recent findings from epidemiological studies lend support to an increased risk of brain tumours and prenatal exposure to NOC compounds.[48 64 70]

Despite all the putative risk factors identified and proposed for cancer of the brain and central nervous system and the proliferation of diverse findings from a variety of small studies comprising different definitions of "cases", there is very little which can be proposed at the present time to increase prospects for the prevention of brain or CNS cancers in children and adolescents.

Soft tissue sarcomas

Soft tissue sarcomas are a heterogeneous group of neoplasms showing different lines of differentiation according to the tissues of origin which include contractile, connective, and supportive tissues, vascular tissue, adipose tissue, and some derived from the neural crest. Rhabdomyosarcoma is the most common soft tissue sarcoma in young adults under the age of 21, accounting for between half and two thirds of all sarcomas in this group.[71] It is a highly malignant tumour and thought to arise from primitive mesenchymal cells committed to develop into striated muscle.[72] It can be found anywhere in the body, including those sites where striated muscles are not normally found.

Rhabdomyosarcoma has been the object of multicentre clinical trials, both national and international, and has been the subject of some limited epidemiological research. An increased incidence of congenital abnormalities, mostly involving the genitourinary system and CNS, have been associated with an increased risk of rhabdomyosarcoma. Rhabdomyosarcoma has been associated with several congenital disorders including neurofibromatosis,[73] Gorlin's syndrome,[74] and the fetal alcohol syndrome.[75] Soft tissue sarcomas in children and young adults have been associated with an excess incidence of breast cancer in the mothers as well as an excess of cancers (breast, glioma) in siblings. This pattern of cancer is consistent with the Li–Fraumeni cancer family syndrome.[76]

Birch et al.[76] analysed 754 first-degree relatives of a population-based series of 177 children with soft tissue sarcoma. Three factors in the index child—age less than 24 months at diagnosis, embryonal rhabdomyosarcoma, and male sex—were associated with high cancer risk in relatives. Developments in molecular biology and genetics will surely clarify the significance of these findings in the coming years and may also increase prospects for prevention.

Bone

Bone cancers constitute approximately 10% of all malignant neoplasms in children and adolescents.[77] Over 95% of all bone cancers in children and adolescents are either osteosarcomas or Ewing's sarcoma, the former being twice as common as the latter.

Osteosarcoma is a malignant tumour originating in bone, consisting of a spindle cell stroma which produces osteoid or immature bone.[78] Although osteosarcoma can occur at any age, 60% of patients are affected during the second decade of life with males being slightly more frequently affected than females. The typical age at presentation, the younger age of females at presentation, and the slight predominance of boys, all suggest a relationship between rapid bone growth and the development of this neoplasm.[79] Additionally there is indirect support for this hypothesis from epidemiology. Fraumeni[80] noted that patients with osteosarcoma are taller than their age peers. Osteosarcoma characteristically occurs at the metaphyseal portion of the most rapidly growing bone in adolescents: the distal femur (around 50%), the proximal tibia (around 25%) and the proximal humerus (around 10%). Everything points to osteosarcoma being most frequent at sites with the greatest increase in length and size of bone and thus it appears that osteosarcoma seems to arise from the malignant transformation of the rapidly proliferating bone forming cell, either as a result of a random event (or events) or induced by viral, chemical, or physical agents.[81] Evidence for genetic predisposition comes mainly from the observations of excess osteosarcoma as a second malignancy among patients with hereditary retinoblastoma (discussed above).

Ewing's sarcoma is a malignant bone tumour histologically composed of small round cells[78] which comprises around 10–15% of all primary bone tumours.[82] Ewing's sarcoma rarely occurs in children below 5 years or in adults over the age of 30 years and has a peak incidence between 10 and 15 years. The disease exhibits a male excess of approximately 50% and is rare in black and Chinese populations.[83] The aetiology is poorly understood.

Discussion

The epidemiology of cancer in adolescents can be characterised as being poorly understood. Indeed, much of the information available exists simply because there is an overlap between the age range covered by childhood and adolescents. It is a big assumption to make that the aetiology of cancer in adolescents is the same as that in childhood cancer since with advancing age it is reasonable to assume that environmental exposure may have a greater role to play than during the first years of life.

The epidemiology of cancer in adolescents requires more attention than it has yet received. Principally, cancer is more common in adolescents than in childhood where there are many studies completed or underway. The limited time for exposure in the study of cancer aetiology in adolescents presents an unusual opportunity for research: it is much easier to recall exposures during the last 10–20 years than making enquiries of 70 year olds about their smoking, drinking, and dietary habits in early life. Given the large excess of non-Hodgkin's lymphoma in male adolescents and the large excess of thyroid cancer and malignant melanoma in female adolescents, these forms of cancer could be very profitably studied in this adolescent age range.

Due to the diverse tumour types and the rare nature of the disease, aetiological studies require international collaboration. This has already occurred to some extent in clinical trials, and should be extended into aetiological studies and assessment of long term complications of treatment and the risk of secondary neoplasm. In view of the nature of the disease, the social and psychological importance of the disease in this age range, it would seem urgent to undertake some of the required studies. Otherwise, an important opportunity to determine the causes of cancer and their mechanisms may be lost.

Acknowledgements

This work was conducted within the framework of support from the Associazione Italiana per la Ricerca sul Cancro (Italian Association for Cancer Research).

1 World Health Organization *International Statistical Classification of Diseases, Injuries and Causes of Death based on the recommendations of the 9th Revision Conference, 1975,* Volumes I and II. Geneva. WHO, 1977.
2 Parkin DM, Muir CS, Whelan S. *et al.,* editors. *Cancer incidence in five continents,* Volume VI. IARC Scientific Publication Number 120, Lyon IARC, 1992.
3 Stiller C. Malignancies. In: Pless IB, editor, *The epidemiology of childhood disorders,* New York: Oxford University Press, 1994; 439–42.

4 Birch JM, Marsden HB. A classification scheme for childhood cancer. *Int J Cancer* 1987; **40**: 620–4.

5 Knudson AG. Mutation and cancer: statistical study of retinoblastoma. *Proc Nat Acad Sci USA* 1971; **68**: 820–3.

6 Schimke R, Lowman J, Cowan G. Retinoblastoma and osteogenic sarcoma in siblings *Cancer* 1974; **34**: 2077–9.

7 Draper GJ, Sanders BM, Kingston JE. Second primary neoplasms in patients with retinoblastoma. *Br J Cancer* 1986; **53**: 661–71.

8 Sanders BM, Jay M, Draper GJ, Roberts EM. Non-ocular cancer in relatives of retinoblastoma patients. *Br J Cancer* 1989; **60**: 358–65.

9 Eng C, Li FP, Abramson DH *et al.* Mortality from second tumours among long-term survivors of retinoblastoma. *J Natl Cancer Inst* 1993; **85**: 1121–8.

10 Breslow N, Beckwirth JB, Ciol M, Sharples K. Age distribution of Wilm's tumour: report from the National Wilm's Tumour Study. *Cancer Res* 1988; **48**: 1653–7.

11 Kushner BH, Gilbert F, Helson L. Familial neuroblastoma: case reports, literature review and etiologic considerations. *Cancer* 1986; **57**: 1887–93.

12. Li FP, Fraumeni JF, Mulvilhill JJ *et al.* A cancer family syndrome in twenty-four kindreds. *Cancer Res* 1988; **48**: 5358–62.

13 Garber JE, Goldstein AM, Kantor AF *et al.* Follow-up of study of twenty-four families with Li-Fraumeni syndrome. *Cancer Res* 1991; **51**: 6094–7.

14 Malkin D, Li FP, Strong L *et al.* Germ line p53 mutations in a familial syndrome of breast cancer, sarcomas and other neoplasm. *Science* 1988; **250**: 1233–8.

15 Narod SA, Stiller C, Lenoir G. An estimate of the heritable fraction of childhood cancer. *Br J Cancer* 1991; **63**: 993–9.

16 Stewart A, Webb J, Hewitt D. A survey of childhood malignancies. *Br Med J* 1958; **1**: 1495–508.

17 Mole R. Childhood cancer after prenatal exposure to diagnostic X-ray examinations in Britain. *Br J Cancer* 1990; **62**: 152–68.

18 Cartwright RA, McKinney PA, Hopton PA *et al.* Ultrasound examinations in pregnancy and childhood cancer. *Lancet* 1984; **2**: 999–1000.

19 Kinnier-Wilson LM, Waterhouse JAH. Obstetric ultrasound and childhood malignancies. *Lancet* 1984; **ii**: 997–9.

20 Muirhead CR, Butland BK, Green BMR, Draper GJ. Childhood leukaemia and natural radiation. *Lancet* 1991; **337**: 503–4.

21 Collmann GW, Loomis DP, Sandler DP. Childhood cancer mortality and radon concentrations in drinking water in North Carolina. *Br J Cancer* 1991; **63**: 626–9.

22 Poole C, Trichopoulos D. Extremely low frequency electric and magnetic fields and cancer. *Cancer Causes Control* 1991; **2**: 267–76.

23 Buriot D, Prieur AM, Lebranchu Y *et al.* Acute leukaemia in three children with chronic juvenile arthritis treated with chlorambucil. *Arch Fr Pediatr* 1979; **36**: 592–8.

24 Michalski A, Radley-Smith R, Crawford D. Non-Hodgkin's lymphoma in a cardiac transplant patient—successful management without chemotherapy. *Med Pediatr Oncol* 1990; **18**: 503–9.

25 Alexander FE. Viruses, clusters and clustering of childhood leukaemia: a new perspective. *Eur J Cancer* 1993; **29A**(10): 1424–3.

26 Boyle P, Walker AM, Alexander FE. Historical review of leukaemia clusters. In: Alexander FE, Boyle P, editors, *Statistical methods in cancer research: the statistical analysis of spatial aggregations of cancer cases.* Lyon IARC, 1996.

27 Kinlen LJ, Hudson CM, Stiller CA. Contacts between adults as evidence for an infective origin of childhood leukaemia: an explanation for the excess near nuclear establishments in West Berkshire. *Br J Cancer* 1991; **64**: 549–54.

28 Greaves MF. Speculations on the cause of childhood acute leukaemia. *Leukaemia* 1988; **2**: 120–5.

29 Shimizu Y, Schull WJ, Kato H. Cancer risk among atomic bomb survivors: the RERF lifespan study. *J Am Med Assoc* 1990; **264**: 601–4.

30 Stevens W, Thomas DC, Lyon JL *et al.* Luekaemia in Utah and radioactive fallout from the Nevada test site. *J Am Med Assoc* 1990; **264**: 585–91.

31 Hill C, Laplanche A. Cancer mortality around nuclear sites. *Eur J Cancer* 1991; **27**: 815–16.

32 Black D. *Investigation of the possible increased incidence of cancer in West Cumbria.* London HMSO, 1984.

33 Committee on Medical Aspects of Radiation in the Environment (COMARE). *Second report: Investigation of the possible increased incidence of leukaemia in young people near Dounreay Nuclear Establishment, Caithness, Scotland.* London HMSO, 1988.

34 Gardner MJ, Hall AJ, Downes S, Terrel JD. Follow-up study of children born to mothers resident in Seascale, West Cumbria (birth cohort). *Br Med J* 1987; **295**: 822–7.

35 Committee on Medical Aspects of Radiation in the Environment (COMARE). *Third report: Report on the incidence of childhood cancer in West Berkshire and North Hampshire area, in which are situated the Atomic Weapons Research Establishment, Aldermaston and the Royal Ordnance Factory, Burghfield.* London HMSO, 1989.

36 Cook-Mozaffari PJ, Darby SC, Doll R *et al.* Geographical variation in mortality from leukaemia and other cancers in England and Wales in relation to proximity to nuclear installations, 1969–1978. *Br J Cancer* 1989; **59**: 476–85.

37 Cook-Mozaffari PJ, Darby SC, Doll R. Cancer near potential sites of nuclear installations. *Lancet* 1989; **2**: 1145–7.

38 Kinlen LJ. Evidence for an infective cause of childhood leukaemia: comparison of a Scottish New Town with nuclear reprocessing sites in Britain. *Lancet* 1988; **ii**: 1323–7.

39 Kinlen LJ, Clarke K, Hudson CM. Evidence from population mixing in British New Towns (1946–1985) of an infective basis for childhood leukaemia. *Lancet* 1990; **336**: 557–82.

40 Draper GJ, Vincent TJ, O'Connor CM, Stiller CA. Socioeconomic factors and variations in incidence rates between County Districts. In: Draper GJ, editor, *The geographical epidemiology of childhood leukaemia and non-Hodgkin lymphoma in Great Britain, 1966–1983.* Studies on Medical and Population Subjects, No. 53. London HMSO, 1991.

41 Alexander FE, Ricketts TJ, McKinney PA, Cartwright RA. Community lifestyle characteristics and incidence of Hodgkin's disease in young people. *Int J Cancer* 1991; **48**: 10–14.

42 MacMahon B. Epidemiologic evidence on the nature of Hodgkin's disease. *Cancer* 1957; **10**: 1045–54.

43 MacMahon B. Epidemiology of Hodgkin's disease. *Cancer Res* 1966; **26**: 1189–200.

44 Correa P, O'Conor GT. Epidemiologic patterns of Hodgkin's disease. *Int J Cancer* 1971; **8**: 192–201.

45 Macfarlane GJ, Evstifeeva T, Boyle P, Grufferman S. International patterns in the occurrence of Hodgkin's disease in children and young adults. *Int J Cancer* 1994; **61**: 165–9.

46 Plowman PN. Tumours of the central nervous system. In: Plowman PN, Pinkerton CR, editors, *Paediatric oncology: clinical practice and controversies.* London: Chapman & Hall Medical, 1992, 240–67.

47 Ivankovich S, Druckrey H. Transplacentare Erzeugung maligner Tumoren des Nervensystems. I. Äthylnitrosoharnstoff (ÄNH) and BD IX-Ratten. *Z. Krebsforsch* 1968; **71**: 320–60.

48 Preston-Martin S, Yu MC, Benton B, Henderson BE. N-nitroso compounds and childhood brain tumours: a case-control study. *Cancer Res* 1982; **42**: 5240–5.

49 McCredie M, Maisonneuve P, Boyle P. Perinatal and early postnatal risks for malignant brain tumours in New South Wales children. *Int J Cancer* 1994; **56**: 11–15.

50 Bunin GR, Kuijen PR, Boesel CP, Buckley JD, Meadows A. Maternal diet and risk of astrocytic glioma in children: a report from the Childrens Cancer Group (United States and Canada). *Cancer Causes and Control* 1994; **5**: 177–87.

51 Sarasua S, Savitz DA. Cured and broiled meat consumption in relation to childhood cancer: Denver, Colorado (United States). *Cancer Causes Control* 1994; **5**: 141–48.

52 Peters JM, Preston-Martin S, London SJ *et al.* Processed meats and risk of childhood leukaemia (California, USA). *Cancer Causes and Control* 1994; **5**: 195–202.

53 United States Surgeon General. *Smoking and health.* Office on Smoking and Health, US Department of Health, Education and Welfare. Washington, DC: US Government Printing Office, 1979.

54 Klus H, Kuhn H. Verteilung verschiedener Tabakrauchbestandteile auf Haupt- und Nebenstromauch (Eine Übersicht). *Beitr Z Tabakforsch Inst* 1982; **11**:229–65.

55 International Agency for Research on Cancer (IARC) Monographs on the Evaluation of the Carcinogenic Risk of Chemicals to Humans. Volume 38, *Tobacco Smoking.* Lyon IARC, 1986.

56 Bottoms SF, Kuhnert BR, Kuhnert PM, Reese AL. Maternal passive smoking and fetal serum thiocyanate levels. *Am J Obstet Gynecol* 1982; **144**: 787–91.

57 Nicolov IG, Chernozemsky IN. Tumors and hyperplastic lesions in Syrian hamster following transplacental and neonatal treatment with cigarette smoke condensate. *J Cancer Res Clin Oncol* 1979; **94**: 249–6.

58 Neutel CL, Buck C. Effect of smoking during pregnancy on the risk of cancer in children. *J Nat Cancer Inst* 1971; **47**: 59–63.

59 Gold E, Gordis L, Tonascia J, Szklo M. Risk factors for brain tumours in children. *Am J Epidemiol* 1979; **109**: 309–19.

60 John EM, Savitz DA, Sandler DP. Prenatal exposure to parents' smoking and childhood cancer. *Am J Epidemiol* 1991; **133**: 123–32.

61 Hirayama T. Cancer mortality in nonsmoking women with smoking husband based on a large-scale cohort study in Japan. *Prev Med* 1984; **13**: 680–90.

62 Strjenfeldt M, Berglund K, Lindsten J, Ludvigsson J. Maternal smoking during pregnancy and risk of childhood cancer. *Lancet* 1986; **i**: 1350–2.

63 Gold E, Leviton A, Lopez R et al. Parental smoking and risk of childhood brain tumours. *Am J Epidemiol* 1993; **137**: 620–8.

64 Howe GR, Burch JD, Chirelli AM et al. An exploratory case-control study of brain tumours in children. *Cancer Res* 1989; **49**: 4349–52.

65 Sandler DP, Everson RB, Wilcox AJ, Browder JP. Cancer risk in adulthood from early life exposure to parents' smoking. *Am J Public health* 1985; **75**: 487–92.

66 Filippini G, Farinotti M, Lovicu G et al. Mother's active and passive smoking during pregnancy and risk of brain tumours in children. *Int J Cancer* 1994; **57**: 769–74.

67 Hoffmann D, Adams JD, Piade JJ, Hecht SS. Chemical studies on tobacco smoke. LXVIII. Analysis of volatile and tobacco-specific nitrosamines in tobacco products. In: Walker EA, Castegnaro M, Griciute L, Börzsönyi M, editors. *N-Nitroso compounds: analysis, formation and occurrence*. IARC Scientific Publication 31. Lyon IARC, 1980, 507–14.

68 Swenberg JA, Koestner A, Wechsler W, Denlinger RH. Quantitative aspects of transplacental tumour induction with ethylnitrosourea in rats. *Cancer Res* 1972; **32**: 2656–60.

69 Druckrey H, Preussmann R, Ivankovic S, Schmähl D. Organotrope carcinogene Wirkungen bei 65 vershiedenen *N*-Nitroso-Verbindungen an BD-ratten. *Z Krebsforsch* 1967; **69**: 103–201.

70 Wilkins JR, Sinks T. Parental occupation and intracranial neoplasms of childhood: results of a case-control interview study. *Am J Epidemiol* 1990; **132**: 275–92.

71 Carli M, Guglielmi M, Sotti G et al. Soft tissue sarcomas. In: Plowman PN, Pinkerton CR, editors, *Paediatric oncology: clinical practice and controversies*. London: Chapman & Hall Medical, 1992, 291–319.

72 Gaiger AM, Soule EH, Newton WA. Pathology of rhabdomyosarcoma: experience of the Intergroup Rhabdomyosarcoma Study, 1972–1978. *Nat Cancer Inst Monograph* 1981; **56**: 19–27.

73 McKeen EA, Bodurtha J, Meadows A et al. Rhabdomyosarcoma complication multiple neurofibromatosis. *J Pediatr* 1978; **93**: 992–3.

74 Beddis IR, Mott MG, Bullimore J. Case report: nasopharyngeal rhabdomyosarcoma and Gorlin's naevoid basal cell carcinoma-syndrome. *Med Pediatr Oncol* 1983; **11**: 178–9.

75 Becker H, Zaunschirm A, Muntean W, Domej W. Alkoholembryopathie und maligner tumor. *Wein Klin Wochenschr* 1982; **94**: 364–5.

76 Birch JM, Hartley AL, Blair V et al. Cancer in the families of children with soft tissue sarcoma. *Cancer* 1990; **66**: 2239–48.

77 Souhami R. Incidence and aetiology of malignant primary bone tumours. *Bailliere's Clin Oncol* 1987; **1**: 1–20.

78 Camponacci M. *Bone and soft tissue tumours*. Berlin, Springer, 1990.

79 Link MP, Eilber F. Osteosarcoma. In: Pizzo PA, Poplack DG, editors. *Principles and Practice of Paediatric Oncology*. Philadelphia: JB Lipincott, 1989, 689–711.

80 Fraumeni JF. Stature and malignant tumours of bone in childhood and adolescence. *Cancer* 1967; **20**: 967–73.

81 Huvos AG. *Bone tumours: diagnosis, treatment and prognosis*. Philadelphia: WH Saunders, 1991.

82 Larsson SE, Lorentzon R. The geographic variation of the incidence of malignant primary bone tumours in Sweden. *J Bone Joint Surg (Am)* 1974; **56**: 592–600.

83 Glass AG, Fraumeni JF. Epidemiology of bone cancer in children. *J Natl Cancer Inst* 1970; **44**: 187–99.

2: Epidemiology of haematological malignancies

RAY CARTWRIGHT

Introduction

Although considerable effort has been directed to the epidemiology of cancers in children, once cancer occurs over the ages of 15 or 18, these malignancies are usually lumped by epidemiologists with older age groups into "adult" categories. It is thus very hard to find details of both the descriptive epidemiology and the risk factors associated with young persons other than children. This is not entirely true for the haematological and lymphoid cancers, however. Overviewing these conditions, it seems likely that some subtypes represent late occurring childhood cancers, others early but rare forms of adult diseases and perhaps some are typical of this age group.

For the purposes of this review, "adolescent" is taken to cover the age range 15–24, but wider age bands are also included because more appropriate age groups do not exist.

The malignancies

Using a specialist register created in 1984 and still continued in parts of England and Wales it can be shown (Table 2.1) that the age band 15–29 produces very low rates for most types of leukaemias and lymphomas.[1] The very rare instances of myeloma and myeloproliferative conditions have been excluded from this table, and the equally rare hairy cell leukaemias, chronic lymphocytic leukaemias, and related conditions are included with the non-Hodgkin's lymphomas.

Some rates decrease with increasing age, such as acute lymphoblastic leukaemia (ALL), while others remain constant, but Hodgkin's disease appears to be increasing. Generally all the conditions are commoner in males for the lymphoid conditions and about equal between the sexes for the myeloid diseases.

It can be seen that all the conditions are uncommon. Table 2.2 estimates

Table 2.1 Incidence (per 1000 100 per year) of specific haematological malignancies 1984–9 by sex and age band

Disease		Age group		
		15–19	20–24	25–29
Acute myeloid leukaemia	M	0·5	1·0	0·7
	F	0·7	0·6	1·1
Chronic myeloid leukaemia	M	0·2	0·1	0·2
	F	0·2	0·1	0·2
Myelodysplasias	M	0·1	0·1	0·1
	F	0·1	0·1	0·1
Acute lymphoblastic leukaemia	M	1·7	0·7	0·5
	F	0·8	0·3	0·3
Non-Hodgkin's lymphoma[a]	M	1·4	1·7	1·6
	F	0·6	0·7	1·3
Hodgkin's disease	M	2·9	3·8	4·4
	F	2·8	3·9	2·9

[a]Includes hairy cell leukaemia.

the new case numbers seen in the United Kingdom in a year, to give a better idea of the burden of the disease. This table is ordered by how common the condition might be, and it demonstrates that about half the disease burden is due to Hodgkin's disease followed by non-Hodgkin's lymphoma (20%) and the acute leukaemias (10%).

Hodgkin's disease

Descriptive epidemiology

Incidence

Hodgkin's disease reaches a peak of incidence in those aged in their 20s and declines thereafter, and in the United Kingdom has a rate in adolescents between 3 and 4 per 100 000 per year. At its peak the sexes are roughly equal whilst at other ages there is a male predominance. Figure 2.1 shows the overall age specific incidence.

If the commonest subtype of Hodgkin's disease, nodular sclerosing, is

Table 2.2 Estimated annual case expected numbers in England and Wales by age (sexes pooled)

Disease	Age group			
	15–19	20–24	25–29	Percentage
Hodgkin's disease	112	157	136	52
Non-Hodgkin's lymphoma	39	51	53	19
Acute lymphoblastic leukaemia	51	20	16	11
Acute myeloid leukaemia	30	36	20	11
Chronic myeoid leukaemia	7	14	15	5
Myelodysplastic syndrome	5	3	3	1
Totals	244	281	243	

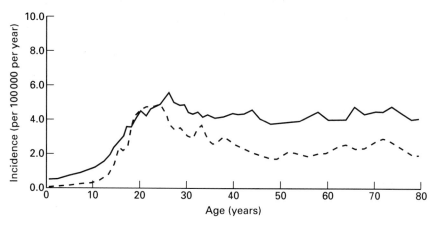

Fig 2.1 Age-specific incidence of Hodgkin's Disease 1984–8 from parts of the United Kingdom. ——, male; – – –, female

isolated from this total, it can be demonstrated that the adolescent peak is due in large part to that subtype alone.[2]

An examination of international comparative data demonstrates other unusual features. Some countries have not an adolescent excess but a childhood peak. This is shown, in summary, in Table 2.3. These conditions tend to be in Asia or developing countries and the overall rates are generally low.[3] This view has been recently challenged when more data have been examined (Grufferman, personal communication). However, in those countries with a clear adolescent peak there is a wide variation in rates (Table 2.4). This cannot be entirely explained by diagnostic difficulties or small case numbers, especially in this age group.

The higher rates are seen in Europe and North America but the highest and most consistent rates come from the United States. The fewer high European rates are inconsistent with a general European rate averaging out at between 3 and 4 per 100 000 for 15–24 year olds, while the rate in the United States is between 4 and 5.[3] The interpretation of registry data for Hodgkin's disease is generally suspect, however.

Table 2.3 Incidence (per 100 000 per year) of Hodgkin's disease in adolescents in those countries which have childhood peaks c 1982–7

Population	Age group	
	15–19	20–24
California (black population)	1·2	1·7
Costa Rica	2·0	1·7
Hong Kong	0·5	0·3
Bangalore	0·7	0·2
Japan	0	0
New Zealand (Maori population)	0	1·2

Table 2.4 Incidence (per 100 000 per year) of Hodgkin's disease in adolescents in countries with adolescent peaks, c 1982–7

Population	Age	
	15–19	20–24
Puerto Rico	1.7	3.4
Canada	3.7	5.8
United States (SEER)	4·4	5·7
Kuwait	0·5	2·7
Belarus	2·7	2·9
Denmark	2·4	3·9
Finland	1·8	2·4
France (Doubs)	1·0	5·8
Germany (East)	3·9	3·9
Republic of Ireland	4·0	4·7
Turin	1·8	3·2
Norway	0·8	3·1
Zaragoza	1·0	4·1
United Kingdom	3·0	3·7
Australia (New South Wales)	1·8	3·7
New Zealand	1·3	2·5

Social class and area variability

Several studies have suggested that Hodgkin's disease is an "upper social class" disease. This is difficult to interpret. However, it may indicate that the area in which the cases live appears also to influence the occurrence of this peak. The condition is much commoner in adolescents in higher socioeconomic status urban areas and least common amongst isolated rural communities. The adolescent peak is confined to those living in upper social class built-up areas.[4]

Clustering

Hodgkin's disease is almost unique in that at this age group the cases display a marked propensity for close case aggregation. Using modern techniques to study spatial clustering, which require spatial boundaries by electoral wards, or non-boundary methods, such as the nearest neighbour technique, show roughly similar results. When examining any geographical area, clustering appears most commonly in the adolescent age group. However, in isolated rural populations where the disease is least frequent in that age group the condition clusters most frequently. This is shown in Table 2.5: in these areas almost 1 in 3 cases can be spatially linked to another case.[5]

Table 2.5 Clusters frequency in relation to residential distance from urban areas

	Inner (urban)	Intermediate	Outer (rural)
Clustered cases	21	44	9
All cases	182	273	31
Percentage clustered	11·5	16	29

25

Seasonality

There is some suggestion also that, in the younger age groups only, an excess of cases occur in the winter months[6] and also in younger married couples.[7] Recently additional data on seasonality has been made available from Scotland and shows very similar results to that reported by Newall (Douglas, personal communication), with an annual cyclical range at presentation.

Secular trends

In the United Kingdom there is no recent evidence for an increase in the incidence rates in this age group, using very good data sets, and there is probably a decline in rate in older Hodgkin's disease cases. In North America, however, there is evidence for a marked increase in Hodgkin's disease in adolescents since the 1970s which is independent of diagnostic accuracy or biopsy rates.[8] This is found in several good quality data sets from the United States and Canada.

A perusal of less good but recent European and Australasian data (Table 2.6) shows a complex picture of increase and no change. Those non-American countries which do show some increase have all shown mixed and inconsistent results compared to North America, and this is partly ascribable to changes in medical diagnostic practice[9] and to the variable quality of registrations in different registries.

Risk factors in Hodgkin's disease

Careful studies of families suggests that Hodgkin's disease has a genetic basis. It is likely the disease occurs more commonly in genetically susceptible individuals. A susceptibility has been associated with a weak risk conferred by certain alleles in the HLA-DP region.[10][11] This association links in with the clues from the descriptive epidemiology of rural isolation, seasonality, and clustering to suggest that, at least as a very late stage event, some infective agent(s) are involved in the pathogenesis of the disease and the HLA area has been shown in other conditions to mediate responses to infectious agents.

Table 2.6 Increase in incidence of Hodgkin's disease in persons age 15–44 between 1973 and 1987 in selected countries

No increase	Some increase	Marked increase
Norway	Hungary	United States
Poland	Yugoslavia	Canada
Sweden	Israel	
Romania	Switzerland	
United Kingdom	Finland	
Germany (East)	Spain	
Denmark	France	
Italy	Germany (West)	
Australia		
New Zealand		

A good deal of effort has been made to identify candidate agents and much attention has fallen on the Epstein–Barr virus (EBV).[12] Initially this was because of some similarities with Burkitt's lymphoma from Africa, an epidemiological association with infectious mononucleosis, and studies from serum banks on risk over a period of many years.[13] There are grounds for supposing this relationship is more complex than was at first supposed, however. When modern techniques to detect the EBV genome directly in affected cells are employed, the situation becomes confused. When a search for the 6·5 kbasepair fragments of the *EBV* gene is made in Hodgkin's disease cases, the virus could readily be found in childhood cases (about 50%) and in those cases aged over 50 years (about 75%) but in those aged 15–34 years only in 16%. This is shown in Table 2.7.

If EBV were to be the causal agent one would expect most of this to be found in those clustered nodular sclerosis cases in adolescents, and this is not so. It may be that EBV transiently infects cells and then disappears before the onset of the disease. This, however, is thought unlikely by virologists and thus leaves the adolescent peak largely unexplained. Research workers have assumed the peak is consequential on other viral involvement. Other candidate viruses include HHV6.[14] However, it is also a possibility that the observed clustering is consequential of any infection and is dominated by those unknown genes which confer susceptibility. If this were to be the case there is no particular reason why the pathogenic process should be triggered by viruses. Other aspects of impaired immunity may thus have a role to play.

As to other causes of Hodgkin's disease, apart from some possible links with skin conditions such as eczema, there are few clues.[15] Inherited conditions which cause immune deficiency also cause Hodgkin's disease.[16] The weak occupational risks apply to older persons, and what was once thought to be a link with tonsillectomy and appendectomy is now

Table 2.7 EBV positivity by age and histological subtype

Selection procedure	Age and histological subtype							
	Paediatric	15–34 years			35–49 years	>50 years		
		HDNS	HDMC	Other[a]		HDNS	HDMC	Other[a]
Non-selected	2/2	2/22	2/4	0/2	2/8	6/7	2/2	—
Selected for age	5/11	—	—	—	—	10/16	7/11	2/2
Selected for age and subtype	—	—	2/8	—	—	—	—	—
Total	7/13	2/22	4/12	0/2	3/8	16/23	9/13	2/2

HDMC, mixed cellularity Hodgkin's disease; HDNS, nodular sclerosing Hodgkin's disease.
[a] "Other" includes cases of lymphocyte predominance and lymphocyte-depleted Hodgkin's disease. Only non-selected cases or those selected on the basis of age were included in the age analysis. The histological subtypes of cases in the young adults and the 35–49 year age brackets are not given because the numbers in these groups were small; positive results were obtained from both HDMC and HDNS cases.

unsupported.[17]

It may be important to note that the description of Hodgkin's disease differs from non-Hodgkin's lymphoma, while the few known risk factors are similar.

Non-Hodgkin's lymphoma, acute lymphoblastic leukaemia, and acute myeloid leukaemia

There are virtually no epidemiological studies which target adolescents. Most reported surveys either ignore this age group or pool it with others to obscure any effects of that small group.

It is probable that the epidemiology of non-Hodgkin's lymphoma in adolescents is in some respects similar to that of Hodgkin's disease, but with greater emphasis on pathogenic pathways other than viral which create immunodepleted individuals. For example, some inheritance syndromes of impaired immune function exist which typically develop a non-Hodgkin's lymphoma in adolescent life.[16] Links between non-Hodgkin's lymphoma and other chronic diseases such as glomerulonephritis also exist, but at an older age.

Unlike Hodgkin's disease, there are few consistent data to suggest that adolescent non-Hodgkin's lymphoma clusters or is increasing in incidence.

Acute lymphoblastic leukaemia (ALL) in adolescents is likely in its epidemiology to be similar in many ways to childhood ALL, excluding the childhood peak cases, i.e. similar in those over 8–9 years of age. Risk factors are largely unknown at this age, and further studies are currently underway to investigate possible aetiology factors in both children and adolescents.

Acute myeloid leukaemia (AML) in adults has a very different spectrum of known risk factors, being largely based on sources of chemicals which alter DNA through adduct formation. AML in childhood is largely a mysterious disease, in some instances associated with possibly random cytogenetic changes and in others with potential ionising irradiation exposure. Little is known of what causes these conditions in adolescents.

Acknowledgements

The work for the UK described in this article was funded by the Leukaemia Research Fund. My colleagues involved with this work include Dr PA McKinney, Dr FE Alexander, and Dr R McNally.

1 Cartwright RA, Alexander FE, McKinney PA, Ricketts TJ. *Leukaemia and lymphoma: An atlas of distribution within areas of England and Wales 1984–1988.* London, Leukaemia Research Fund, 1990.

2 Alexander FE, McKinney PA, Williams J *et al.* Epidemiological evidence for the 'two-disease hypothesis' in Hodgkin's disease. *Int J Epidemiol* 1991; 20: 354–61.

3 Parkin M, Muir CS, Whelan SL. *Cancer incidence in five continents.* Volume 6. Lyon, IARC, 1992.

4 Alexander FE, Ricketts TJ, McKinney PA, Cartwright RA. Community lifestyle characteristics and lymphoid malignancies in young people in the UK. *Eur J Cancer* 1991; **27**: 1486–90.

5 Alexander FE, Ricketts TJ, McKinney PA, Cartwright RA. Community lifestyle characteristics and incidence of Hodgkin's disease in young people. *Int J Cancer* 1991; **48**: 10–14.

6 Newell GR, Lynch HK, Gibeau JM, Spitz MR. Seasonal diagnosis of Hodgkin's disease among young adults. *J Nat Cancer Inst* 1985; **74**: 53–6.

7 Fogel TD, Peschel Re, Papac R. Hodgkin's disease in married couples. *Cancer* 1985; **55**: 2495–7.

8 Glaser SL, Swartz WG. Time trends in Hodgkin's disease incidence: The role of diagnostic accuracy. *Cancer* 1990; **66**: 2196–204.

9 Coleman M, Esteve J. *Trends in cancer incidence.* Lyon, IARC, 1993.

10 Chakravarti A, Halloran SL, Bale SJ, Tucker MA. Etiological heterogeneity in Hodgkin's disease: HLA linked and unlinked determinants of susceptibility independent of histological concordance. *Genet Epidemiol* 1986; **3**: 407–15.

11 Bodmer J, Tonks S, Oza AM *et al.* HLA-DP based resistance to Hodgkin's disease. *Lancet* 1989; **i**: 1455–6.

12 Jarrett RF, Gallagher A, Jones DB *et al.* Detection of Epstein–Barr virus genomes in Hodgkin's disease: relation to age. *J Clin Pathol* 1991; **44**: 844–8.

13 Mueller N. Epidemiologic studies assessing the role of the Epstein–Barr virus in Hodgkin's disease. *Yale J Biol Med* 1987; **60**: 321–7.

14 Clark DA, Alexander FE, McKinney PA *et al.* The seroepidemiology of human herpes virus-6 (HHV-6) from a case-control study of leukaemia and lymphoma. *Int J Cancer* 1990; **45**: 829–33.

15 McKinney PA, Alexander FE, Roberts BE *et al.* Yorkshire case control study of laeukaemias and lymphomas parallel multivariate analyses of seven disease categories. *Leukemia and Lymphoma* 1990; **2**: 67–80.

16 Magrath IT, editor. *The non-Hodgkin's lymphoma.* London: E. Arnold, 1990.

17 Mueller N, Swanson GM, Hsieh C-C, Cole P. Tonsillectomy and Hodgkin's disease: Results from companion, population-based studies. *J Nat Cancer Inst* 1987; **78**: 1–5.

3: Trends in adolescent cancer with time

RICHARD DOLL

Introduction

Concern that the total mortality from cancer, after standardisation for age, has not fallen in this country, and has actually increased in most developed countries over the last 30 years, is widespread and is contrasted unfavourably with the frequent reports of discoveries about the causes of cancer and of improvements in treatment. In fact, this unsatisfactory situation is largely attributable to the delayed effect of smoking in the older section of the population. When the mortality attributable to smoking is removed, the total mortality from cancer due to other causes is found to have diminished.[1] More detailed examination of the incidence and mortality data by cancer site and age group reveals a diversity of trends, with reductions in the incidence and mortality in young adults, whose experience best reflects recent changes in behaviour and the environment, and increases in only a few types, mostly for reasons that are well known.[2] Some cancers are becoming more common for reasons that are unknown and they deserve intensive research, but there is no justification for the fear that the conditions of modern society are causing a grossly increased risk of the disease. What they are doing is causing such a big fall in mortality from many non-malignant conditions that the proportion of deaths attributed to cancer has increased and cancer as a cause of death has, in consequence, become much more prominent.[2]

Despite the general concern, the trends in cancer in adolescents have attracted very little attention, for, I suspect, two reasons: one good and one, probably, bad. The first is the rarity of all cancers in adolescents—the minimum incidence of cancer being at ages 5–14 years with only a very slight increase at ages 15–19 years—so that very large populations have to be studied to obtain stable rates or enough cases for a case-control study. The second is a suspicion that those cancers that do occur are unlikely to be due to environmental or behavioural factors, because many years of exposure to such factors are usually required before they cause much risk, so that they are unlikely to be important causes of disease before middle life. Alternatively, it is thought, they may act on the fetus in utero, but, in this case, they are likely to have exhausted most of their effect in the first decade after the child's birth. Very little has, in consequence, been written about adolescent cancer in the epidemiological literature.

Material

To obtain numbers sufficiently large for the trends not to be grossly affected by random fluctuation, I have examined the data from the national cancer registry for the whole of England and Wales, have interpreted adolescence loosely as extending from 10 to 24 years of age, and have limited the review to 13 types of cancer, of which 9 affect both sexes, 3 only females, and 1 only males, which together account for 86% of all cancers in this age group in both sexes. These 13 types are cancers of bone, soft tissue, and brain, melanoma and non-melanoma of the skin, Hodgkin's disease, non-Hodgkin's lymphoma, and lymphatic and myeloid leukaemias in both sexes; cancer of the testis in males; and cancers of the cervix, ovary, and thyroid in females (the number of thyroid cancers in males being too few for useful analysis). Even with national data the numbers of cases of any one type are too small to provide stable five-year age-group and five-year calendar rates. I have, therefore, examined the incidence rates over the whole age range, standardized for age, in only two periods: 1971–80 (no reliable data being available before 1971) and 1981–7 (no data having been available for later years at the time of the analysis).

Problems in interpreting temporal changes

Interpretation of temporal changes in the incidence of cancer is unfortunately seldom straightforward, as these changes can be made to appear artificially in three ways when the true incidence of cancer is actually constant: namely, by changes in the efficiency of the reporting system and in the efficiency of the medical services in diagnosing cancer, and by changes in medical fashions in diagnosis, similar cases being given one label in one epoch and another label in another epoch.

The first cause of temporal change is unlikely to have had much influence on the recorded incidence at young ages in Britain since the early 1970s, as registration has been thought to have always been over 95% complete throughout[3] and it seems unlikely that improvements in registration could account for an increase of more than 2–3%. The second cause should also have had very little effect on the incidence of the types of cancer under consideration, except perhaps on the incidence of thyroid cancer, which can be seriously affected by the intensity with which people's necks are examined. Small thyroid nodules may be asymptomatic and, although some lesions may appear malignant under the microscope, they may have remained asymptomatic for many years and might even remain asymptomatic permanently if not looked for. The third cause could, however, have substantial effects on the recorded incidence of several cancers. Dividing

31

lines between Hodgkin's disease, non-Hodgkin's lymphoma, and lymphatic leukaemia, and between lymphatic and myeloid leukaemia, are in some instances arbitrary and although distinctions between these diseases are now mostly well established, the dividing lines have changed over time and can certainly have been drawn in different places by different pathologists.

Changes in incidence

The results summarised in Table 3.1 show, first, that there has been an overall increase of 17% in males and 8% in females. This is too large to be an artefact or due to chance, and must reflect a real increase in the incidence of at least some of the types of malignant disease studied. The most substantial increases of more than 20% have occurred in four types, two in both sexes (melanoma and non-melanoma of the skin) one in males (testis) and one in females (thyroid). The increase in both melanoma and non-melanoma skin cancer is striking and has occurred in each of the three five-year age groups under study. In the United States Kaposi's sarcoma associated with AIDS has been a major contributor to the increase in non-melanoma skin cancer in young men,[4] but it can have played little or no part in this age group in the United Kingdom. In the regions covered by the Thames Cancer Registry, where AIDS-related cancers are most likely to have occurred, the 216 skin cancers recorded at ages 10–24 years in 1980–89 included only three Kaposi's sarcomas against none in the 130 cases in the preceding decade (Coleman, personal communication). Occupational causes and the use of immunosuppressive drugs to support transplants cannot have played any material part in this age group, and the

Table 3.1   Comparison of incidence (per 1000 000 per year) of cancer at age 10–24 in England and Wales 1971–80 to 1981–7, standardized for age

Type of cancer	Male		Female	
	Incidence 1981–7	Percentage change since 1971–80	Incidence 1981–7	Percentage change since 1971–80
Bone	12·5	+4	9·3	+4
Soft tissue	6·5	+14	5·6	+10
Skin, melanoma	5·5	+56	9·5	+28
Skin, non-melanoma	4·9	+22	6·1	+29
Cervix uteri	NA	NA	7·4	+10
Ovary	NA	NA	8·4	−7
Testis	25·2	+21	NA	NA
Brain	16·0	+5	12·9	+3
Thyroid	*	*	6·4	+33
Hodgkin's disease	27·7	−5	23·1	+9
Non-Hodgkin's lymphoma	13·8	+12	6·9	+5
Lymphatic leukaemia	14·5	+18	8·8	+13
Myeloid leukaemia	8·2	−11	6·8	−12
13 cancers	134·8	+17	111·2	+8

NA, not applicable; *, not given, because based on too few cases to be reliable.

only other known cause of both conditions is exposure to ultraviolet radiation. But has there really been a sufficient increase in sun exposure and, perhaps, in sunburn of children since the 1960s to account for 56% and 28% increases in males and females in melanomas and 22% and 29% increases in non-melanomatous skin cancers?

One of the other large increases, of 21% in cancer of the testis, is a continuation of the trend that has been going on in this country since the 1930s and in many other developed countries at least since the 1940s. The increase is occurring in each of the three five-year age groups studied, but in the United Kingdom, and also in the United States, it is most marked at 20 years of age and over. In Scandinavia, however, where the rates are double those in the United Kingdom, the recent increase has been most marked at 15–19 years of age (Möller, personal communication). The only factors that are known to have contributed to the increase in testis cancer are an earlier age of sexual maturity and an increased prevalence of undescended testicle at birth; but neither accounts for more than a very small part of the increase—and anyhow, why has there been an increase in undescended testis? The reasons are shrouded in mystery, as is the reason for the maximum increase occurring at a younger age in Scandinavia.

The reason for the fourth large increase, of 33% in thyroid cancer in females, is equally unclear (no data are given for males as the incidence in males is too low for any reliable evidence of trend to be obtained). Could it be an artefact of more intensive case finding? The fatality of the disease is low. Two deaths occurred over the whole age range in the five years 1986–90 although 44 cases a year were diagnosed in the two years 1986–7 and it may be that some or all of the increase is an artefact due to a greater efficiency in the detection of small lumps in the neck which would not have declared themselves as clinical cancers for many years—if indeed they did so ever. Intensive case finding is probably the explanation for much of the large increase in thyroid cancers in children in the districts near Chernobyl since 1990, although some real increase in incidence has probably also occurred in that area, which is not surprising in view of the very large exposure that young children had to radioactive iodine.

Several other types of cancer have shown smaller, but material, increases, most notably lymphatic leukaemia (of 18% in males and 13% in females) and cancers of the soft tissues (of 14% in males and 10% in females). I can see no reason to doubt that the small increase in the incidence of the latter is real. Several studies have suggested that soft tissue sarcomas have increased in incidence at older ages due to exposure to dioxins in the manufacture of chlorophenol herbicides. The evidence for such a causation is, however, extremely weak, and other causes should, I think, be sought. The increase in lymphatic leukaemia may, however, be a nosological artefact, as there has been almost as big a decrease in myeloid leukaemia. The distinction between these two types of leukaemia should now be clear, but it was not always so in the past and much of these changes could be due to changes in classification. The rest could be due to the classification as lymphatic leukaemia of some cases of non-Hodgkin's lymphoma, which has also increased in incidence, although to a smaller extent. Some support for the idea that the changes are artificial is provided by the small peak in leukaemia at around 15–17 years of age which was found 30 years ago in the mortality data for England and Wales, Scotland, Canada and the United States.[5] At that time Lee found it to be concentrated on acute myeloid leukaemia in the British registration data, but it is now most clearly present in the British national data for lymphatic leukaemia. The peak is small, but it is undeniably there and the reason for it has yet to be found.

Two further increases have been small, but I suspect real: namely, one of 10% in cervix cancer, limited to ages 20–24 years and almost certainly due to increased infection with carcinogenic types of human papilloma virus and one of 12% in males and 5% in females in non-Hodgkin's lymphoma. The increase in non-Hodgkin's lymphoma is accompanied by an increase at all other ages and is a continuation of an increase that has been going on at least since 1950 and has occurred in many other countries. In adolescence the increase is not due to AIDS or to immunosuppression for the treatment of transplants. There is some reason to think that it may be due to the spread of a viral infection,[6] or, in adults, to the use of agricultural chemicals,[7 8] but it has been postulated[9]—and given some theoretical reasons in justification—that it may, like the increase in skin cancers, be due to increasing exposure to sunlight.

Only three types of cancer have remained practically unchanged— cancers of the bone and brain, with increases of between 3% and 5% in each sex, and Hodgkin's disease, for which an increase of 9% in girls has been partly compensated for by a decrease of 5% in boys.

Finally, two types of cancer have become less common: myeloid leukaemia, to which I have already referred, and cancer of the ovary, which has shown a decrease of 7%. The numbers of cases of ovarian cancer are not large, just under 50 a year nationally, and much, if not all of the decrease, could be due to random fluctuation. It is, however, limited to females over 15 years of age and it could be due to the use of oral contraceptives: that is, if many of the cases are adenocarcinomas, which are certainly prevented by oral contraceptives at older ages.

Changes in mortality

These changes are, fortunately, not all mirrored in mortality, which has shown a reduction of 15% in males and 20% in females, over a slightly longer period (that is, up to 1981–90) as is shown in Table 3.2.

All but one type shows a decline in mortality averaged over both sexes, or in the one sex in which it occurs, which varies from 3% for lymphatic leukaemia to 60% for testis cancer, despite the incidence of these diseases having increased. The only increase recorded is a small increase of 6% in the mortality from soft tissue sarcomas (both sexes combined), which serves to strengthen the belief that the recorded increase in incidence (12%)

Table 3.2   Comparison of mortality (per 1000 000 per year) of cancer at ages 10–24 years in England and Wales 1971–80 to 1981–90, standardized for age

Type of cancer	Male		Female	
	Mortality 1981–90	Percentage change since 1971–80	Mortality 1981–90	Percentage change since 1971–80
Bone	7·4	− 11	5·7	− 2
Soft tissue	3·1	− 7	2·9	+ 19
Skin, melanoma	1·2	− 12	1·0	− 37
Skin, non-melanoma	0·1	*	0·0	*
Cervix uteri	NA	NA	1·0	− 5
Ovary	NA	NA	1·9	− 44
Testis	3·0	− 60	NA	NA
Brain	8·6	− 5	6·3	− 15
Thyroid	*	*	0·1	*
Hodgkin's disease	4·0	− 30	2·7	− 31
Non-Hodgkin's lymphoma	5·6	− 26	2·5	− 36
Lymphatic leukaemia	12·3	+ 6	5·8	− 12
Myeloid leukaemia	7·1	− 20	5·3	− 27
13 cancers	52·1	− 15	35·0	− 20

NA, not applicable; *, not given, because based on too few cases to be reliable.

is real. With such a marked difference between the trends in incidence and mortality of most of the cancers in adolescence it is evident that treatments must have improved and the fatality rates for many of them (as estimated crudely by relating the mortality in 1986–90 to the incidence in 1986–7) are indeed encouragingly low, now being less than 20% for melanoma, Hodgkin's disease, and cancers of the cervix and testis, in addition to non-melanoma of the skin and thyroid cancer. Two types, however, stand out as having a high fatality rate (as judged crudely in this way) namely lymphatic leukaemia, with a rate of 77%, and myeloid leukaemia, with a rate of 82%. The lymphatic leukaemias at these ages are mostly different in origin to the lymphatic leukaemias under 5 years of age, which respond so well to treatment, so that a difference in response is not surprising. It was not so long ago, however, that lymphatic leukaemia in childhood had a similar high fatality. The best hope for progress in reducing the high fatality rates of these diseases at 10–24 years of age is, I suggest, through collaborative effort and the admission of all young people affected by them to controlled trials, such as those carried out in the United Kingdom under the aegis of the Medical Research Council that have enabled such steady progress to be made in the treatment of childhood leukaemia.

Conclusion

This brief summary of the trends in the incidence and mortality of cancer in adolescents over a 20-year period in England and Wales provides substantial evidence that not all cancers in this age group are due to unalterable biological characteristics and that many of them must be

35

contributed to by environmental and behavioural factors that are potentially capable of control. Extension to other countries could strengthen the evidence by showing that geographical variations in incidence may be even greater. As yet we have clear ideas about the reasons for only a small part of this variation. The rest provides an opportunity for productive research. Cancers in adolescents are uncommon, but particularly tragic when they occur. Their causes are difficult for the epidemiologist to study because of their rarity, but their study is facilitated by the fact that, because of the subject's age, the events that have caused the cancers can have occurred only in the relatively recent past. I hope this book may stimulate research into the nature of these events and how they can be avoided.

1 Peto R, Lopez A, Boreham J et al. Mortality from tobacco in developed countries: indirect estimation from national vital statistics. *Lancet* 1992; **339**: 1268–78.
2 Doll R. Are we winning the war against cancer? A review in memory of Keith Durrant. *Clin Oncol* 1992; **4**: 257–66.
3 Hawkins MM, Swerdlow AJ. Completeness of cancer and death follow-up obtained through the National Health Service Central Register for England & Wales. *Br J Cancer* 1992; **66**: 408–13.
4 Doll R. Progress against cancer: an epidemiological assessment. *Am J Epidemiol* 1991; **134**: 675–8.
5 Lee JA. Acute myeloid leukaemia in adolescents. *Br Med J* 1961; **1**: 988–92.
6 Memon A, Doll R. A search for unknown blood-borne oncogenic viruses. *Int J Cancer* 1994; **58**: 366.
7 Cantor KP, Blair A, Everett G et al. Pesticides and other agricultural risk factors for NHL among men in Iowa and Minnesota. *Cancer Res* 1992; **52**: 2447–55.
8 Saracci R, Kogevinas M, Bertazzi P. Cancer mortality in workers exposed to chlorophenoxy herbicides and chlorophenols. *Lancet* 1991; **338**: 1027–32.
9 Cartwright R, McNally R, Staines A. The increasing incidence of non-Hodgkin's lymphoma (NHL): the possible role of sunlight. *Leukaemia Lymphoma* 1994; **14**: 387.

PART II
Clinical features

4: Epithelial cancer

PETER SELBY, L RIDER, C JOSLIN, and CLIFFORD BAILEY

Introduction

Cancers arising from epithelial surfaces are the commonest cancers in adults. Carcinomas of the breast, lung and gastrointestinal tract account for 50% of new cancers arising in the countries of the European Union.[1] In adolescents the picture is entirely different, with a much smaller proportion of epithelial cancers, a different distribution of primary sites, and a very wide diversity among the primary sites. Adolescents with epithelial cancers are, fortunately, rare, and relatively little attention has been paid to this group compared to the more readily identifiable groups of patients with lymphoma, leukaemia, sarcomas, and germ cell tumours discussed elsewhere in this book.

In this chapter we examine the problem of epithelial cancers arising in adolescents from a number of standpoints. First, we have examined the scale of the problem and its nature as it might present to a major unit dealing with adolescents with cancer serving a population of several million. For this purpose we have used our own population within Yorkshire as recorded within the Yorkshire Cancer Registry. Second, we have looked at the literature available which discusses this topic usually under the heading of the individual primary sites of cancers. This allows us to make some comments about aetiology and pathology of these rare cancers. Finally, we have examined the survival of patients and the clinical pattern of management of patients with epithelial cancer arising in adolescents in order to deduce some common themes about optimal approaches to their management which might be built into the development of adolescent services in the UK and elsewhere.

The medical literature on cancer in adolescents is rather sparse and fragmented, and there is little consensus about methods of presentation or age groups that should be described. We are unaware of any formal reviews of cancer in adolescents which separate the topic from the paediatric age group and which seek to draw general themes from the literature. We have decided, rather arbitrarily, to set a broad definition of adolescents for the purposes of our examination of the literature and our own data. However, we will break this down into narrower age groups to allow those who wish to work with different definitions to draw conclusions from our observations. The definition of adolescents used in this paper is the age group 15–23 years inclusive. The lower limit is relatively high, which may be in part arbitrary but also reflects the pattern of services that have developed in our own region within which the 13–15 age group have been comprehensively cared for within a paediatric unit. The upper limit is deliberately high to allow us to examine epidemiological and clinical patterns at the lower end of the age range for a number of common epithelial cancers which are not found in teenage.

Cancer registration

The Yorkshire Cancer Registry is one of the registries for cancer contributing the mandatory data for the United Kingdom National Cancer Registration Scheme. Established in 1957 and serving a population of approximately 3·6 million, the Yorkshire Cancer Registry currently registers over 20 000 new cancer cases each year. The data in this chapter relate to the population who were in the age group 15–23 years in the period under examination (1975–91).

The Cancer Registry operates a multiple source system of registration which ensures high ascertainment of cases. Data sources include hospitals (NHS and private), general practitioners, pathology laboratories, screening programmes, hospices, death certificates, and specialist tumour registers. Data are collected primarily by peripatetic registration officers, employed and trained by the registry, who visit designated hospitals in the region to abstract clinical information from case notes of cancer patients. All pathology laboratories in the region routinely send copies of histopathology reports to the Cancer Registry which serve to validate the diagnosis.

Follow-up is passive. Copies of all death certificates of cancer patients are routinely received from the Office of Population Censuses and Surveys and these are linked to the computerised cancer registrations. Where a death certificate is the only information received, the case is followed up through the general practitioner and appropriate hospitals. The index data for computing incidence and survival is the date of first active treatment or first hospital visit. Treatment data collected are for the first nine weeks from date of first active treatment.

Patients

The data on all patients between the ages of 15 and 23 years inclusive who presented with cancer in the Yorkshire region between 1975 and 1991 were examined. The distribution of cases according to the type of cancer is shown in Table 4.1. Figure 4.1 shows the number of cases per year.

The numbers in each year are insufficient for us to comment precisely on any secular trends in the incidence of cancer in this age group in our region,

Table 4.1   All cancers in adolescents in the Yorkshire Registry (1975–91)

Type of cancer	Number of cases
Epithelial cancer	249
Carcinoma in situ of the cervix	1450
Carcinoid	35
Bone sarcoma	89
Soft tissue sarcoma	68
Melanoma	68
Testicular cancer	168
Brain tumours	122
Hodgkin's disease	311
Non-Hodgkin's lymphoma	109
Leukaemia	172

and this topic is discussed elsewhere in this book by Sir Richard Doll. Some changes were, however, so prominent that they are apparent even in the small numbers of each individual cancer in adolescents seen in this population. There has been a dramatic increase in the numbers of patients diagnoses with carcinoma in situ of the cervix (Figure 4.2). Part of the increase can be explained by a change in the diagnosis of these cancers, i.e. around 1984 pathologists started to report CIN IIIs to the registry, and this practice was reflecting the national trend. However, there is also evidence to show that there has been a real increase in incidence of these cancers in younger age groups. The numbers of invasive carcinoma of the cervix are too small to draw any conclusions about the implications of the changes of carcinoma in situ in this age group from the data available here (Figure 4.3). The data on thyroid cancer even in the numbers available to us support trends reported elsewhere in this book by Doll (Figure 4.4).

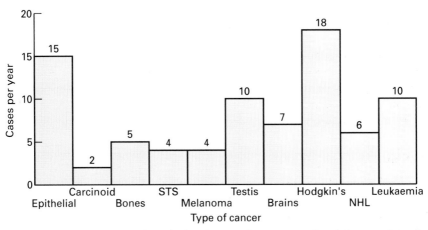

Fig 4.1 Average number of cases of each type of cancer seen in adolescents in each year in the Yorkshire Healthcare Region between 1975 and 1991 (population 3·6 million)

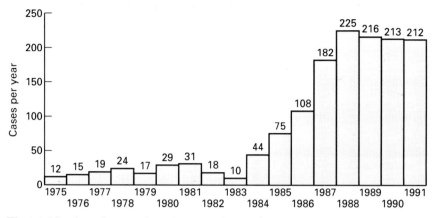

Fig 4.2 Number of cases of carcinoma in situ of the cervix uteri seen in each year in the Yorkshire Healthcare Region between 1975 and 1991

Table 4.2   Sites of epithelial cancers in adolescents

Salivary glands	3	Skin basal cell carcinoma	46
Nasopharynx	14	Squamous cell carinoma	6
Other ENT	3	Breast	14
Thymoma	6	Cervix (invasive)	37
Oesophagus	3	Ovary	22
Stomach	8	Vaginal	2
Colorectal	17	Bladder	9
Hepatic	9	Kidney	5
Pancreas	2	Thyroid	41
Bronchial	2	Adrenal	1
		[Carcinoid]	35
		Total	285

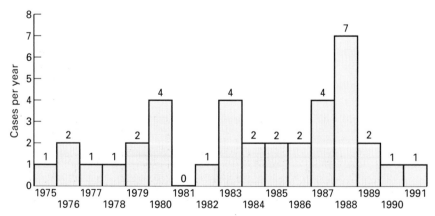

Fig 4.3 Number of cases of invasive carcinoma of the cervix seen in each year in the Yorkshire Healthcare Region between 1975 and 1991

Table 4.3 Age distribution for the commoner epithelial cancers occurring in adolescents

| | Years | | | |
	15–17	18–20	21–23	Total
Nasopharynx	7	6	1	14
Stomach	0	3	5	8
Colorectal	3	8	6	17
Breast	0	0	14	14
Cervix	0	5	31	36
Ovary	3	5	14	22
Kidney	1	2	2	5
Thyroid	8	14	19	41
Total	22	43	92	

Sites of epithelial cancers in adolescents

The sites of the epithelial cancers in this age group are shown in Table 4.2. The very wide range of different sites is immediately obvious. The "commoner" among this collection of rare and varied epithelial cancers are shown in Figure 4.5 with small groups that have some anatomical or medical features in common grouped together. The commonest epithelial cancer in our chosen age range for adolescents is cancer of the thyroid, closely followed by invasive carcinoma of the cervix, adenocarcinomas of the ovary, adenocarcinomas of the colon and rectum, adenocarcinoma of the breast, undifferentiated carcinoma of the nasopharynx, and the carcinomas of the stomach and oesophagus. Hepatomas and renal and bladder cancers are less frequent. If these data are set in the context of the number of cases that might be seen in an adolescent unit serving a population of 3–4 million people, we see that invasive cancer of the cervix and cancer of the thyroid would occur in more than two patients in each year, and colorectal cancer or ovarian cancer in one or two patients in each

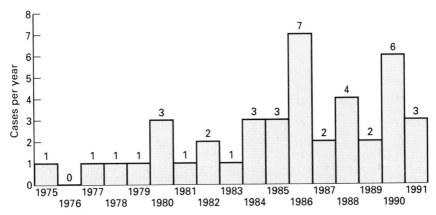

Fig 4.4 Number of cases of carcinoma of the thyroid observed in adolescents in the Yorkshire Healthcare Region between 1975 and 1991

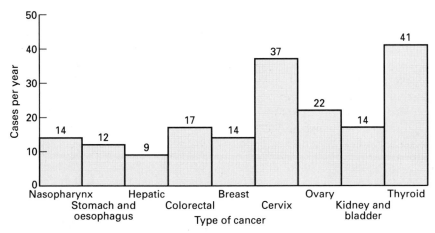

Fig 4.5 Number of cases of the epithelial cancers which are among those more common in adolescents seen in the Yorkshire Health Region between 1975 and 1991 (total cases)

year, but the number of patients with epithelial cancers of the nasopharynx, upper gastrointestinal tract, liver, breast or genitourinary tract would be only one patient every one or two years.

In Table 4.3 the patients have been grouped into the age bands 15–17 years, 18–20 years, and 21–23 years, inclusive in each case. It can be seen that most of the epithelial cancers are, as expected, occurring in the age group 21–23 years. Among these "commoner" epithelial cancers only 22 occur in the age range 15–17 years and 43 in the age range 18–20 years. Particularly it can be seen that breast cancer in our population did not occur under the age of 20 years over an observation period from 1975–1991 and that most cases of epithelial ovarian cancer occurred in the older group. Very few invasive cancers of the cervix were seen, and no cancers of the stomach or oesophagus occurred under 18 years of age. However, colorectal cancers, ovarian cancers, kidney cancers, and thyroid cancers occurred in significant numbers in our two younger age groups. Undifferentiated carcinoma of the nasopharynx occurs particularly in the age group 15–20 years, inclusive, and may be seen as one of the few epithelial cancers to be specific to the teenage years.

Aetiological factors of epithelial cancers in adolescents

Very little laboratory research or epidemiological work has specifically addressed issues relating to aetiological factors in epithelial cancers that occur in the age group 15–23 years.[2] It is however possible to identify a small number of specific associations. Undifferentiated carcinoma of the nasopharynx which is discussed in greater detail below is strongly associated with Epstein–Barr virus (EBV) infection.[2-6] This leads to its high incidence in east Asian countries and larger studies usually relate to populations from that part of the world. Undifferentiated thymoma is less clearly associated with EBV, but some data support this proposal.[7] Specific studies of hepatitis B infection in hepatoma in adolescents are not available, but in those parts of the world where this cancer is common the association is likely. The association of invasive carcinoma of the cervix with human papilloma virus infection is increasingly clear, and seems likely to play a part in this cancer in young adults and in teenagers. Lung cancer is exceedingly rare in adolescents, reflecting the long duration of exposure to cigarette smoke which is necessary before the disease becomes common. Specific studies of dietary associations with carcinomas in adolescents have not been done and would be extremely difficult given the numbers available.

Two clear iatrogenic causes of carcinoma in adolescents have been described. Cyclophosphamide treatment in the paediatric age group is associated with carcinoma of the bladder.[2] Diethylstilboestrol treatment of mothers leads to clear cell carcinoma of the vagina in their daughters.[8] In the gastrointestinal tract, long-standing and extensive inflammatory colitis is clearly associated with carcinoma. However, this becomes apparent in young adults not in adolescents and cannot be identified specifically as a cause of adolescent gastrointestinal cancer.

Patients who develop their cancers as part of distinct familial syndromes tend to be younger than those who develop sporadic carcinomas. This is a relatively consistent observation across a number of cancer sites, and is biologically plausible. However, although young adults in the cancer families are at risk, adolescents in general are not. Breast cancer in the high-risk families, renal cancer in von Hippel–Lindau and related familial syndromes, and colorectal cancer in the polyposis syndromes and non-polyposis familial carcinomas of the colon occur in younger adults but in the main not in adolescents.[2]

This brief survey of aetiological factors in adolescent cancer supports the general statement that virally induced cancers and iatrogenic cancers are a feature of adolescence. Specific genetic risks are associated with younger age of onset but this is rare in adolescents and some environmental causes, prominently cigarette smoke, require lengthy exposures and produce cancers late in life.

Patterns of care for adolescents with cancer

The rarity of epithelial cancers in adolescents means that very few doctors will have experience of many of these patients. Most epithelial cancers are first diagnosed and treated by the same specialist who would treat the cancers in adults. We have examined the specialty of the doctor giving the first treatment to patients with thyroid, gastrointestinal, breast, ovarian, cervical, nasopharyngeal, and thymic cancers within the Yorkshire Registry and find that treatments were given by general surgeons (82 patients), gynaecologists (56 patients), and ear, nose, and throat (ENT) specialists (12 patients). Few patients are seen by oncologists in the first instance. In order to examine the pattern of referral from the district of diagnosis into special centres, we have looked at the patients treated in a hospital not in their own district. Within the Yorkshire Healthcare Region during the period of this study there were the 17 healthcare districts. Two districts within the city of Leeds (population 750 000) each contained teaching hospitals and there was throughout this period a large centralised radiotherapy centre in that city at Cookridge Hospital. In the city of Hull there is a smaller radiotherapy centre.

If we examine the district of origin of all patients we find only a small proportion of patients with most cancers were treated in a hospital not in their own district. This implies only a small proportion of patients were referred to special centres (Table 4.4). Nasopharyngeal cancer and breast cancer are seen to be referred more frequently than the other epithelial cancers reflecting the use of radiotherapy given in only two of the healthcare districts and specialised clinics treating patients with head and neck cancer.

Survival

Minimum follow up is three years for patients with epithelial cancers. Figures 4.6 and 4.7 show the percentage survival for the commoner epithelial sites and Table 4.5 gives precise estimates with 95% confidence limits. Figure 4.6 shows excellent results for patients with carcinomas in skin excluding melanoma, only moderate results comparable to those achieved in adult life for adolescents with colonic and rectal cancer, and disappointing results for nasopharyngeal cancer in this group (see below). Stomach cancer in adolescents, as in adult life, has a gloomy prognosis however it is managed. In Figure 4.7 excellent survival results for carcinoma of the thyroid are seen with the anticipated moderate result for carcinoma of the cervix and ovary. The small number of cases with cancer of the kidney do relatively badly and the poor results for adolescents with

Table 4.4   Cancers in adolescents

Site	Number of cases†	Treated in Leeds‡	Treated at Cookridge (Radiotherapy Centre)§
Nasopharynx	14	1 (7%)	7 (50%)
Stomach	8	1 (13%)	0 (0%)
Colon	14	3 (21%)	2 (14%)
Rectum	3	1 (33%)	1 (33%)
Skin	52	13 (25%)	4 (8%)
Breast	14	2 (14%)	9 (64%)
Cervix	36	9 (25%)	5 (14%)
Ovary	22	5 (23%)	6 (28%)
Kidney	5	0 (0%)	2 (40%)
Thyroid	41	15 (37%)	11 (27%)
Total	209	50 (24%)	47 (22%)

† Number of cases in Yorkshire 1975–91 among people aged 15–23.
‡ Number of these cases treated at a centre in Leeds (excluding Cookridge).
§ Number of these cases treated at Cookridge.

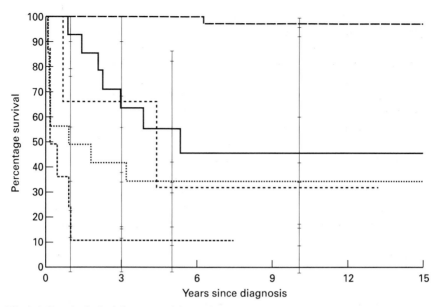

Fig 4.6 Survival of adolescents with carcinoma, ——, nasopharynx (14 cases); ----, stomach (8 cases); ····, colon (14 cases); ----, rectum (3 cases); ———, skin (excluding melanoma) (3 cases)

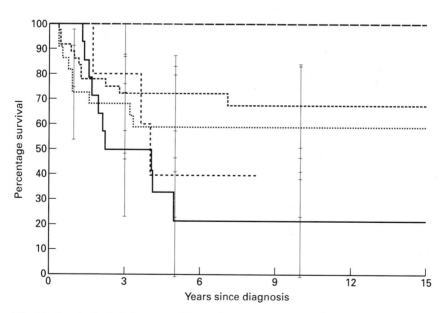

Fig 4.7 Survival of adolescents with carcinoma. —— breast (14 cases); ----, cervix (36 cases); ····, ovary (22 cases); ----, kidney (5 cases); ———,thyroid (41 cases)

47

Table 4.5 Cancer in adolescents 1975–91

Survival rates (%)	1 year		3 years		5 years		10 years		15 years		Number of cases
Nasopharynx	92·9	(100–79)	64·3	(89–39)	56·3	(83–30)	46·9	(75–19)	46·9	(75–19)	14
Stomach	12·5	(35–0)	12·5	(35–0)	12·5	(35–0)	12·5	(35–0)	12·5	(35–0)	8
Colon	50·0	(76–24)	42·9	(69–17)	35·7	(61–11)	35·7	(61–11)	35·7	(61–11)	14
Rectum	66·7	(100–13)	66·7	(100–13)	33·3	(87–0)	33·3	(87–0)	33·3	(87–0)	3
Skin	100		100		100		97·4	(100–92)	97·4	(100–92)	52
Breast	100		50·0	(76–24)	22·2	(47–0)	22·2	(47–0)	22·2	(47–0)	14
Cervix	86·1	(97–75)	72·2	(87–58)	72·2	(87–58)	67·4	(84–51)	67·4	(84–51)	36
Ovary	72·7	(91–54)	68·2	(88–49)	59·1	(80–39)	59·1	(80–39)	59·1	(80–39)	22
Kidney	100		80	(100–45)	40·0	(83–0)	40·0	(83–0)	40·0	(83–0)	5
Thyroid	100		100		100		100		100		41

95% confidence limits in brackets.

breast cancer are very striking, reflecting the aggressive nature of this disease in this age group.

General clinical management issues in epithelial cancers in adolescents

The review of our cases and of the published literature allows a few conclusions about management of adolescents who present with epithelial cancers. Adolescents are almost invariably fully fit and able to tolerate a full complement of anticancer treatments. As discussed thoroughly elsewhere in this book all adolescents will require a full range of psychosocial supportive care which needs to be provided either with or in consultation with specialists in the management of these young people.

For cancers of the gastrointestinal tract, gynaecological cancers, genito-urinary cancers, and thyroid cancers, the results of treatment in our patients and in general in the literature are similar to those in adults and there is no evidence that distinct technical management approaches should be employed in adolescents. Thus, for instance, in colorectal cancer, adequate surgical resection with clear resection margins for primaries in the colon and in the rectum are appropriate. Postoperative radiotherapy has been shown to improve local control. For node-positive patients it would seem appropriate to recommend adjuvant chemotherapy within carefully controlled trials, as would be standard in the adult population. Patterns of care appropriate to the stage of the disease which are established in adults should be pursued for carcinoma of the cervix, ovary, kidney, thyroid, hepatoma, and for the even rarer cancers in adolescents.

The poor outcomes in breast cancer in this age group need careful consideration. Current advances in chemotherapy techniques, particularly with peripheral blood stem cell support, hold out the possibility of better outcomes, particularly when used in carefully selected patients in the adjuvant context. Carefully planned and ultimately controlled research programmes in this age group seem appropriate. In our series the disease has an appalling prognosis, patients are young and fit, and a full range of multimodality approaches to treatment are applicable.

Nasopharyngeal carcinoma

Carcinoma of the nasopharynx in adolescents requires special considera-tion. The disease is rare in industrialised countries but about one third of nasopharyngeal carcinomas of the undifferentiated type are diagnosed in adolescents or young adults. As already mentioned, the disease is much commoner in east Asia. The incidence is approximately one case in 100 000 among the white populations of Europe and North America but may rise as high as 20 to 25 in 100 000 in southeast Asia and Hong Kong. It may be as high as 100 in 100 000 in northern Africa.[29] There is a suggestion that nasopharyngeal cancer may be commoner among black teenagers.[10] There are three histological subtypes which are shown in Table 4.6.[6,11] A staging

Table 4.6   Pathology of nasopharyngeal carcinoma

Type	Pathologic type	Occurrence in childhood	EBV-associated
1	Squamous cell	Rare	No
2	Non-keratinizing	Uncommon	Yes
3	Undifferentiated	Usual	Yes

system in use for nasopharyngeal cancer is shown in Table 4.7. The disease commonly presents with involved cervical lymph nodes and advanced stage primary tumours (stage T3 or T4). Modifications of the staging system have been reported as in Table 4.8.[12]

In general, patients presenting with early stage disease are reported to have a good prognosis when managed by radical radiotherapy alone with more than 75% long-term survival. Unfortunately patients with T3 or T4 tumours have much worse prognosis with less than 30% long-term disease-free survival (Table 4.9).

The poor prognosis of patients presenting with advanced nasopharyngeal

Table 4.7   Tumour, node, metastasis (TNM) classification for tumours of nasopharynx

Primary tumour

TO	No evidence of primary tumour
Tis	Carcinoma in situ
T1	Tumour confined to one site of nashpharynx or no tumour visible (positive biopsy only)
T2	Tumour involving two sites (both posterosuperior and lateral walls)
T3	Extension of tumour into nasal cavity or oropharynx
T4	Tumour invasion of skull, cranial nerve involvement, or both

Nodal involvement

N0	No clinicially positive node
N1	Single clinically positive homolateral node 3 cm or less in diameter
N2	Single clinically positive homolateral node more than 3 cm but not more than 6 cm in diameter, or multiple clinically positive homolateral nodes, none more than 6 cm in diameter, or bilateral or contralateral lymph nodes, none more than 6 cm in greatest dimension
N2a	Single clinically positive homolateral node more than 3 cm but not more than 6 cm in diameter
N2b	Multiple clinically positive homolateral nodes, none more than 6 cm in diameter
N2c	Bilateral or contralateral positive nodes, none more than 6 cm in greatest dimension
N3	Metastasis in a lymph node more than 6 cm in greatest dimensions

Distant metastasis

M0	No evidence of metastasis
M1	Distant metastasis present

Stage grouping, American Joint Committee

Stage I	T1, N0, M0
Stage II	T2, N0, M0
Stage III	T3, N0, M0 or T1 or T2 or T3, N1, M0
Stage IV	T4, N0 or N1, M0 or any T, N2 or N3, M0 or any T, any N, M1

carcinoma in adolescence has led to consideration of combined modality primary treatment with the addition of chemotherapy to radiotherapy. Table 4.8 reviews 10 papers published between 1980 and 1990 in which uncontrolled studies are reported of chemotherapy added to radiotherapy

Table 4.8   Modified TNM classification of nasopharyngeal carcinoma as proposed by Ho[12]

Primary tumour	
T0	No evidence of primary tumour
Tis	Carcinoma in situ
T1	Tumour confiend to nasopharyngeal mucosa or no tumour visible but biopsy positive
T2	Tumour extended to the nasal fossa, oropharynx, or adjacent muscles or nerves below base of the skull
T3	Tumour beyond T2 limits and subclassified as follows:
T3a	Bone involvement below base of the skull
T3b	Involvement of base of skull
T3c	Involvement of cranial nerves
T3d	Involvement of orbit, laryngopharynx, or infratemporal fossa
Nodal involvement	
N0	No clinically positive node
N1	Nodes wholly in the upper cervical level above larynx
N2	Nodes between larynx and supraclavicular area
N3	Nodes palpable in lower third of the neck or supraclavicular area
Distant metastasis	
M	Distant metastasis present

Stage grouping		
Stage I	T1	N0
Stage II	T2	and/or N1
Stage III	T3	and/or N2
Stage IV	T3	(any T)
Stage V	M1	

Table 4.9   Nasopharyngeal cancer in adolescents

Author	Patients	Stages	Treatment	Outcome
Gasparini (1988) Milan[13]	12	T3 T4	VAC + RT	75% DFS at 5 years
Pao (1989) St Judes[14]	29	T3 T4	Varied CT + RT	30%
Berry (1980) Princess Margaret Hospital[15]	25	T3 T4	RT	37%
Ingersol (1990) MD Anderson + Stanford[16]	57	T4	RT	40%
			RT + CT	60%
Kim (1989) Atlanta[17]	7	T3 T4	CT + RT	86%
Jenkin (1981)[18]	12	T3 T4	RT ± CT	30%
Roper (1986)[19]	18	T3 T4	CT + RT	7/9 at > 2 yrs
			RT	0/9 at > 2 yrs
Lobo-Sanahuija (1986)[20]	18	T3 T4	CT + RT	83%
Lombardi (1982)[21]	27	T3 T4	CT ± RT	No benefits from CT
Jereb (1980)[22]	16	T3 T4	RT	No benefits from CT
	2		CT + RT	

CT, chemotherapy; RT, radiotherapy; VAC, vinicristine, actinomycin D, cyclophospha-mide; DFS, disease-free survival

in this disease. The reports are not conclusive. Five papers suggest considerable improvement in outcomes with as much as 75% five year disease-free survival for patients with advanced disease treated with combined modality approaches using chemotherapy and radiotherapy. However, others have concluded that evidence of benefit is absent. In the absence of randomised prospective trials it will always be difficult to draw conclusions from studies of this kind. Nevertheless, the evidence is sufficiently encouraging to suggest that patients should always be considered for combined modality approaches when they present with advanced nasopharyngeal carcinoma. Patients with truly early and localised disease after detailed staging investigation can be managed by radical radiotherapy alone.

Conclusions

Epithelial cancers account for a substantial proportion of cancers in adolescents when the broader age group 15–23 years is considered. However, many of these are occurring in young adults rather than teenagers and therefore present different management problems. Very small numbers of patients present with primary cancers in each epithelial site, and none of these cancers are truly common. Practice in this area will be dominated by gynaecological, gastrointestinal, ENT and breast cancer. Thyroid cancer is the commonest but at present the results are good with current management practices. Particular concern must be expressed about the increasing incidence of some cancers in adolescents (see Doll, this volume).

The majority of patients with epithelial cancer will need medical care similar to that for adults. However, they may need to be managed partly or in consultation with a unit with expertise in the special psychosocial and family problems presented by teenagers. The principal philosophy underpinning the care of adolescents with epithelial cancer has to be close collaboration between the multidisciplinary team with special expertise in each epithelial cancer site and a similar team with special expertise in the problems of these young people. Many doctors from different disciplines will inevitably be involved in their care, and close integration and good communications will be necessary in maintaining high cure rates and good quality of life.

Acknowledgements

Professor Selby would like to acknowledge support from the Imperial Cancer Research Fund and the Yorkshire Cancer Research Campaign, and Dr Clifford Bailey from the Candlelighters Children's Cancer Charity.

1 Muir CS, Boyle P. The burden of cancer in Europe. *Eur J Cancer* 1990; 26: 1111–13.
2 Pratt CB, Douglass EC. Management of the less common cancers of childhood. In: Pizzo PA, Poplack DG, eds. Principles and practice of pediatric oncology, Philadelphia, JP

Linnincott, 1993; 913–38.

3 Klein G, Giovanella BC, Lindahl T *et al.* Direct evidence for the presence of Epstein–Barr virus DNA and nuclear antigen in malignant epithelial cells from patients with poorly differentiated carcinoma of the nasopharynx. *Proc Natl Acad Sci USA,* 1974; **71**: 4747–51.

4 Huang DP, Ho JHC, Henle W *et al.* Presence of EBNA in nasopharyngeal cancer and control patients tissues related to EBV serology. *Int J Cancer* 1978; **22**: 266–74.

5 Henle G, Henle W. Epstein–Barr virus specific IgA serum antibodies as an outstanding feature of nasopharyngeal carcinoma. *Int J CAncer* 1976; **17**: 1–8.

6 Naegele FR, Champion J, Murphy S *et al.* Nasopharyngeal carcinoma in American children: Epstein–Barr virus specific antibody titer and prognosis. *Int J Cancer* 1982; **29**: 209–12.

7 Leyvraz S, Henle W, Chahinian AP *et al.* Association of Epstein–Barr virus with thymic carcinoma. *N Engl J Med* 1985; **312**: 1296–9.

8 Melnick S, Cole P, Anmderson D, Herbst A. Rates and risks of diethylstilbestrol related clear cell carcinoma of the vagina and cervix: An update. *N Engl J Med* 1987; **316**: 514–16.

9 Gastpar H, Wilmes E, Wolf H. Epidemiologic, etiologic and immunologic aspects of nasopharyngeal carcinoma. *J Med* 1981; **12**: 257–84.

10 Easton JM, Levine PH, Hyams VJ. Nasopharyngeal carcinoma in the United States: A pathologic study of 177 US and 30 foreign cases. *Arch Otolaryngol* 1980; **106**: 88–91.

11 Shanmugaratnam K, Sobin L. Histological typing and upper respiratory tract tumours. *World Health Organisation* 1978; **19**: 23–33.

12 Ho JHC. Clinical staging and recommendations. In de The G, Ito Y, eds, *Nasopharyngeal Carcinoma: Etiology and Control.* Lyon: International Agency for Research in Cancer, 1979, 594–5.

13 Gasparini M, Lombardi F, Rottoli L *et al.* Combined radiotherapy and chemotherapy in stage T3 and T4 nasopharyngeal carcinoma in children. *J Clin Oncol* 1988; **6**: 491–4.

14 Pao WJ, Hustu HO, Douglass EC *et al.* Pediatric nasopharyngeal carcinoma in long term follow up of 29 patients. *Int J Radiat Oncol Biol Phys* 1989; **17**: 299–305.

15 Berry MP, Smith CR, Brown TC *et al.* Nasopharyngeal carcinoma in the young. *Int J Radiat Oncol Biol Phys* 1980; **6**: 415–21.

16 Ingersol L, Woo SY, Donaldson S *et al.* Nasopharyngeal carcinoma in the young: A combined MD Anderson and Stanford experience. *Int J Radiat Oncol Biol Phys* 1990; **19**: 881–7.

17 Kim TH, McLaren N, Alvarado CS *et al.* Adjuvant chemotherapy for advanced nasopharyngeal carcinoma in childhood. *Cancer* 1989; **63**: 1922–6.

18 Jenkin RDT, Anderson JR, Jereb B *et al.* Nasopharyngeal carcinoma: A retrospective review of patients less than thirty years of age. *Cancer* 1981; **47**: 360–6.

19 Roper HP, Essex-Cater A, Marsden HB *et al.* Nasopharyngeal carcinoma in children. *Pediatr Hematol Oncol* 1986; **3**: 143–52.

20 Lobo-Sanahuja F, Garcia I, Carranza A, Camacho A. Treatment and outcome of undifferentiated carcinoma of the nasopharynx in childhood: A 13 year experience. *Med Pediatr Oncol* 1986; **14**: 6–11.

21 Lombardi F, Gasparini M, Gianni C *et al.* Nasopharyngeal carcinoma in childhood. *Med Pediatr Oncol* 1982; **10**: 243–50.

22 Jereb B, Huvos AG, Steinherz P, Unal A. Nasopharyngeal carcinoma in children: Review of 16 cases. *Int J Radiat Oncol Biol Phys* 1980; **6**: 487–91.

5: Lymphoma: clinical features, management and results of treatment

JS MALPAS, JE KINGSTON, and TA LISTER

Introduction

It is generally accepted that the management of cancer in adolescent patients has its own special problems, and this is certainly true of the lymphomas. Adolescence has been defined for this account as between 15 and 20 years of age. There are well defined differences between childhood and adult lymphoma, and this chapter explores how far the adolescents reflect the features of either childhood or adult disease, and whether these in turn affect response to treatment or survival.

There are many large series of lymphomas reported: Padmalatha et al[1], Lange et al.[2], Murphy et al.[3] and Kennedy et al.[4] In these studies the age range falls within the period of adolescence as defined above, but unfortunately the features of either Hodgkin's disease or non-Hodgkin's lymphoma (NHL) in the adolescent age group have not been defined, and it is not possible to study such factors as incidence, male/female ratio, histopathology, or distribution of the various stages of disease or outcome from these large studies.

Between 1974 and 1990 a total of 1669 children, adolescents and adults with Hodgkin's disease or NHL were seen at St Bartholomew's Hospital in London. Follow up is virtually complete on all these patients, and a total of 89 adolescents with Hodgkin's disease and 21 adolescents with NHL are available for comparison.

Clinical features in Hodgkin's disease

The main clinical features of adolescents with Hodgkin's disease are given in Table 5.1. It can be seen that the male preponderance seen in childhood has largely disappeared by adolescence. More than half of patients are at an early stage of disease, and there is a high proportion of nodular sclerosing histology.

Table 5.1   Hodgkin's disease in 15–20 year age group, St Bartholomew's Hospital 1974–1990

Number	89	
Median age	18 years	
Male	45	
Female	44	
Male:female ratio 1·01:1		
Stage I	7	(9%)
Stage II	44	(49%)
Stage III	22	(27%)
Stage IV	14	(16%)

Histology
Nodular sclerosing	72 (80%)
Lymphocyte proliferative	8 (9%)
Mixed cellularity	7 (8%)
Lymphocyte depleted	1 (2%)

These clinical features were compared to 69 children and 423 adults with Hodgkin's disease to see if they were significant.

Male:female ratios

In children there were 45 boys and 26 girls, giving a male:female ratio of 1·7:1·0. This male preponderance was also seen in the adult age group (over 20 years): in those aged between 21 and 35, the ratio was 1·9:1·0, and in those aged between 36 and 50, it was 2·4:1·0. In the adolescent group there were 45 boys and 44 girls, illustrating the increasing frequency of Hodgkin's disease in adolescent girls. This difference in gender ratios is statistically significant at $p = 0·02$.

Table 5.2   Stage at presentation in adolescent Hodgkin's disease compared with children and adults, St Bartholomew's Hospital 1974–90

Age (years)	0–15	15–20	>20
Number	69	89	423
Stage I	19 (28%)	7 (8%)	80 (19%)
Stage II	29 (42%)	44 (49%)	137 (32%)
Stage III	15 (22%)	24 (27%)	118 (28%)
Stage IV	6 (9%)	14 (16%)	88 (21%)

Stage of the disease

The Ann Arbor classification[5] has been used throughout, so that the three groups are comparable. Pathological staging in children was not carried out after 1972, whereas it continued in adolescents and adults where radiotherapy was to be used for initial therapy.

It can be seen from Table 5.2 that more children presented at an earlier stage of the disease than adults, and that the presenting stage of adolescents falls somewhere between these two. Thus, 67% of children present with stage I and II disease, compared with 51% of adults, and adolescents are in

Table 5.3   Histology in adolescent Hodgkin's disease compared with children and adults, St Bartholomew's Hospital 1974–90

Age (years)	0–15	15–20	>20
Number	69	89	423*
Nodular sclerosing	44 (64%)	72 (80%)†	255 (60%)
Lymphocyte proliferative	14 (20%)	8 (9%)	56 (13%)
Mixed cellularity	11 (16%)	7 (8%)	89 (21%)
Lymphocyte depleted	0 (0%)	1 (2%)	12 (3%)

* Significant $p = 0.038$.
† 11 unclassified.

between, at 58%. Since both adolescents and adults are pathologically staged they are comparable, and the difference is not statistically significant ($p = 0.04$).

Histology

During the period 1974–90, all histology was reviewed by a single histopathologist, and reported using the criteria of Lukes and Butler.[6] These criteria should therefore be identical across the three groups, and comparable. Histological differences have been previously recognised, such as the lower incidence of lymphocyte-depleted, and higher incidence of lymphocyte-predominant histologies in children, and are again confirmed. The very high proportion of adolescents presenting with nodular sclerosing disease is of interest, with type I predominating (Table 5.3). The frequency in girls and the association with mediastinal masses may have some bearing on the outcome, for it is notable that of the 10 deaths occurring in this series, 9 were of patients with nodular sclerosing histology. Eighty-one per cent of adolescents showed nodular sclerosing histology, compared with 64% of children and 60% of adults. This is statistically significant ($p = 0.04$).

Clinical features of non-Hodgkin's lymphoma

The main features of the 21 adolescents with NHL are given in Table 5.4. Although this number appears small, it nevertheless represents approximately 10% of the NHL cases occurring in the adolescent age range in England and Wales during the period. Sixteen of the 21 are male, showing a marked male preponderance. This is similar to the childhood NHL, where there are 59 boys and 20 girls, giving a male:female ratio of 3:1·0. Over the age of 20, in 988 adults, this ratio falls to 1·3:1·0. The comparison of adult and adolescent gender ratios is highly significant at $p = 0.001$.

Stage of disease

Since 1972, patients at St Bartholomew's Hospital with NHL have not been pathologically staged. Clinical staging has followed very similar lines in children, adolescents, and adults. The early use of lymphography has

Table 5.4   Non-Hodgkin's lymphoma in 15–20 year old patients treated at St Bartholomew's Hospital 1974–90

Number	21	
Median age	17 years	
Male	16	
Female	5	
Male:female ratio 3.0:1		
Stage I	Localised	0
Stage II		9 (42%)
Stage III	Disseminated	2 (10%)
Stage IV		10 (48%)
Histology		
High grade	19	
Low grade diffuse	2	
Follicular	0	

been replaced by computed tomography, and bone marrow examinations have been done on all patients. Staging procedures, therefore, are very comparable between the three age groups considered.

However, when the staging classification has been applied, there have been major differences between children and those over the age of 15. In adolescents and adults, the Ann Arbor staging classification[5] has been applied until recently; now the Cotswold modification[7] is used.

It became evident during the late 1970s that the Ann Arbor classification was insufficiently discriminating for children with NHL, and it was decided to stage all children by the classification proposed by Murphy and colleagues, and introduced at St Jude's Children's Research Hospital.[8] The St Jude classification differs in two important respects from the Ann Arbor system, in that the presence of intrathoracic disease or bulky abdominal disease places the child in a more advanced stage. In the present analysis it was thought wiser to compare the relatively localised categories of stages I and II in both staging classifications, and a disseminated group (stages III and IV in both systems).

When this is done, it can be seen (Table 5.5) that there is relatively little difference in the presentation staging of NHL between the three age

Table 5.5   Stage at presentation in adolescent non-Hodgkin's lymphoma compared with children and adults

Age (years)	0–15†		15–20‡		>20‡	
Number	79		21		988	
Stage						
I (localised)	7 (9%)		0 (0%)		171 (17%)	
II	15 (19%)	} 28%	9 (43%)	} 43%	158 (16%)	} 33%
III (disseminated)	27 (34%)		2 (10%)		120 (12%)	
IV	30 (38%)	} 72%	10 (47%)	} 57%	539 (55%)	} 67%

† St Jude classification.
‡ Ann Arbor classification.

Table 5.6 Histopathology in adolescent non-Hodgkin's lymphoma compared with children and adults

Age	0–15	15–20	>20
Number	79	21	988
High grade	73 (92%)	19 (90%)	450 (45%)
Low grade	3 (4%)	2 (10%)	308 (32%)
Follicular	0 (0%)	0 (0%)	230 (23%)
Not available	3 (4%)	0 (0%)	0 (0%)

groups. Approximately three quarters of both children and adults are in a more advanced stage at presentation, and just under two thirds of the adolescent group. There would therefore appear to be no significant differences between the three groups ($p = 0.4$).

Histology

When histology is compared, the well documented predominance of high grade histology of childhood NHL compared with the high and low grade histologies of adult lymphoma can be clearly seen. Adolescent histology of NHL closely resembles that seen in childhood (Table 5.6), only a small number presenting with other than high grade histology.

Response to therapy: Hodgkin's disease

Management of Hodgkin's disease in the last two decades has not remained static. Initially the importance of pathological staging, so that the extent of disease was clearly defined, was a necessary preliminary to the use of radiotherapy in the early stages of the disease. Chemotherapy, on the other hand, was reserved for more advanced disease. There was general agreement that stage IVA and B disease should be treated with multidrug chemotherapy, mustine, vincristine, procarbazine and prednisolone (MOPP)[9] chemotherapy being most frequently used. Other multidrug chemotherapies such as mustine, vinblastine, prednisolone, procarbazine (MVPP)[10] and chlorambucil, vincristine, prednisolone, and procarbazine (chlorambucil VPP)[11] were introduced with the main aim of reducing toxicity without loss of effectiveness, and this can be said to have been achieved. More recently, anthracycline-containing regimens have been used with equal effectiveness.

In childhood Hodgkin's disease the deleterious effects on growth of standard adult radiotherapy doses soon led to the exploration of lower doses and reduction of field size combined with multidrug chemotherapy. Of the children reported in this series, the majority will have received in-field irradiation together with chlorambucil VPP.

In adolescents, growth considerations have not been so paramount, and therapy has more closely followed that used in adults. Table 5.7 shows that using the same criteria for complete response, good partial response and poor partial response in all groups, excellent results are seen (major

Table 5.7 Response to initial therapy in Hodgkin's disease

Age (years)	0–15		15–20		>20	
Number	69		89		423	
Complete response	60	(89%)	64 (74%)	(86%)	299 (70%)	(81%)
Good partial response	2		11 (12%)		47 (11%)	
Poor partial response			6 (7%)		19 (45%)	
Fail			1 (1%)		6 (1.5%)	
Progress	7 (11%)		7 (8%)		33 (8%)	
Deaths/unknown	0		0		19 (4.5%)	

responses of over 80%). Adolescents show no significant difference in their response to treatment ($p=0.9$), and the very high incidence of nodular sclerosing Hodgkin's disease, which seems to carry a less favourable prognosis, does not seem to affect response to initial treatment.

Survival

When the 15–20 age group staging is reviewed, no difference is seen in the survival of the various stages. At a follow-up of 18 years all stages are doing well (Figure 5.1).

Adolescents treated for Hodgkin's disease in a similar manner to adults would appear to do better (Figure 5.2). Survival at 18 years is 80%, compared to 82% in children and just over 60% in adults. They thus tend to resemble children in terms of both response and outcome.

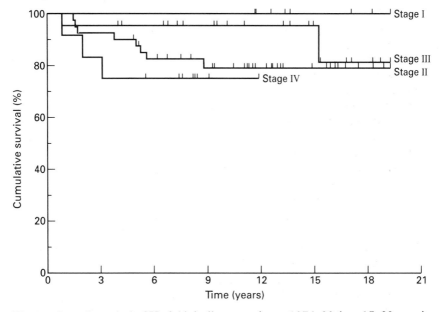

Fig 5.1 Overall survival of Hodgkin's disease patients, 1974–90 (age 15–20 years). Stage I, $n=7$; stage II, $n=41$; stage III, $n=22$; stage IV, $n=12$; $P=0.29$; $\chi^2_3=3.78$

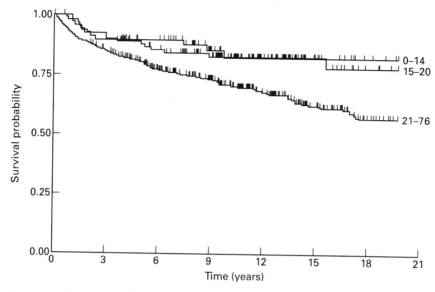

Fig 5.2 Survival of Hodgkin's disease patients by age

Response to therapy: non-Hodgkin's lymphoma

Introduction

Since nearly all NHL in children is of high grade, it is necessary only to compare the results achieved in the high grade pathologies in all three groups. High grade lymphomas have been treated with multidrug chemotherapy regimens since the early 1970s. The major innovation has been the addition of an anthracycline in the so-called CHOP regimen[12] and the realisation of the importance of central nervous system prophylaxis. Although many agents have been added to the original CHOP protocol, and some improvement in response or survival claimed in small selected institutional studies, their efficacy has not been confirmed in large randomised studies (Fisher *et al*[13]). When children, adolescents or adults have been treated with a full course of an anthracycline-containing programme with cranial prophylaxis where appropriate, it is possible to compare these groups. If response is examined using the criteria of CR,

Table 5.8 Response to initial therapy in high-grade non-Hodgkin's lymphoma

Age (years)	0–15	15–20	>20
Number	73	21	450
Complete response	69 (94%)	12 (57%)⎫81%*	166 (36·9%)⎫54.9%
Good partial response	—	5 (24%)⎭	81 (18%)⎭
Poor partial response	—		46 (10%)
Fail	2 (2·5%)	3 (14%)	72 (16%)
Death during induction	2 (2·5%)	1 (1%)	67 (9%)
Not accessible			2 (0·1%)

*Significant, $p = 0.001$.

GPR, and PPR, it is evident that the adolescent group respond much better than the adults (Table 5.8) and slightly less well than the children. This is significant ($p = 0.001$).

Survival

Univariate log rank analysis shows that the 16 adolescents treated in an identical manner to their adult counterparts achieved a survival identical to the children and better than the adults (Figure 5.3).

Steady improvements in outlook have been seen in childhood NHL, and since 1985 survival rates of over 70% have been seen in children.[14] This small group of adolescents therefore falls somewhere between the 20% long term survival seen in the total adult population, and the 62% survival for children.

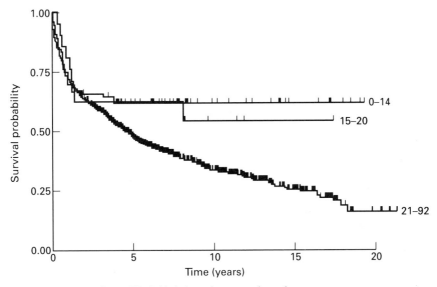

Fig 5.3 Survival of non-Hodgkin's lymphoma patients by age

Management of Hodgkin's disease

In general the results for Hodgkin's disease are so good that attention must now be turned to the reduction of short term and long term toxicity. The comparable outlooks for children and adolescents managed very differently from each other, one group being treated by chemotherapy and radiotherapy without pathological staging, and the other by radiotherapy or chemotherapy alone after pathological staging, are similar to those reported by Donaldson and her colleagues,[15] who compared these two approaches in children. In their study of 171 children there was equal survival in the two groups treated with these different management plans. At the time of the report there was no excess morbidity or mortality as a result of either treatment programme, except that the boys treated with chemotherapy had been rendered infertile. The authors also noted the same deleterious effect on outcome of large mediastinal masses in nodular sclerosing Hodgkin's disease in both groups of children, and recommended that combined modality therapy was preferred in this subgroup.

In a review of 6345 patients with Hodgkin's disease[4] the 10-year survival for 454 patients aged under 17 years was 86%, and in 2024 patients aged 17–34 it was some 10% less. Age was a significant prognostic factor, but unfortunately this study did not single out the adolescent age group for particular attention.

In attempts to use less toxic chemotherapy, a number of regimens have been tried. Anthracycline-containing regimens such as adriamycin, bleomycin, vinblastine, and decarbazine (ABVD)[16] show equivalent efficacy and a much less harmful effect on fertility. More recently, however, concern has been expressed with regard to the long-term cardiotoxicity and pulmonary toxicity of such regimens.

In an attempt to obviate long-term toxic effects, the vincristine, etoposide, epidaunorubicin, and prednisolone (VEEP) regimen was investigated. Early reports[17] suggested that it had activity and was not toxic. However, further experience (JE Kingston, personal communication) suggests that there is an unacceptable early relapse rate, and this particular combination has now been abandoned.

Management of non-Hodgkin's lymphoma

Although adolescents in this series have done better than adults as far as survival is concerned, their long term event-free survival is much less satisfactory than in children, and while long term toxicity is nevertheless a concern, the major problem is to improve response rate to make these durable. In one of the largest series of childhood and adolescent NHL studies, Murphy et al.[3] reviewed 338 consecutive newly diagnosed children and adolescents treated at St Jude Children's Hospital between 1962 and 1986, with a further follow up of between 1·8 and 23 years. The children were aged between 7 and 21 years, so that many fall within the defined range of adolescence of this study. On both univariate and multivariate analysis of event-free survival, age was not a factor. In the St Jude series, adolescents did as well as children, stage for stage. Murphy and her colleagues point out that histological subtypes were not a significant factor; what caused the differences in survival was the use of protocols that successively reduced the duration and intensity of therapy, and eliminated radiotherapy. A major factor for the improved results was the recognition that T-lymphoblastic lymphomas needed treatment similar to that for acute lymphoblastic leukaemia, whilst B-cell lymphomas needed short term therapy including fractionated cyclophosphamide, high dose methotrexate, high dose cytarabine, and intrathecal therapy. This confirmed earlier work in a seminal study by Anderson and colleagues[18] in which a four-drug regimen of cyclophosphamide, vincristine, methotrexate, and prednisone

(COMP) was compared to a modified regimen including cyclophosphamide, vincristine, methotrexate, daunomycin, prednisolone, cytarabine, thioguanine, asparaginase, and carmustine (the so-called modified LSA_2-L_2 programme). The latter regimen was shown to be more successful in disseminated T-lymphoblastic lymphoma, while the four-drug cyclophosphamide regimen was more effective in all other forms of high-grade NHL.

A feature of the present series is that the deaths in children and adolescents were nearly all due to disease (adolescents 80%; children 93%). Robertson et al.[19], reviewing the causes of 479 deaths in 883 children treated between 1974 and 1985 (a similar period to that of the present investigation), also found that 377 (79%) were related to disease, compared with 18% due to treatment. They did not find any increase of treatment-related deaths over the period surveyed.

Long term toxic effects

Morbidity and mortality from the late effects of chemotherapy, radiotherapy, or the two combined, is increasing, and is a consequence of the increased intensity of therapy. Various aspects of these late effects are specifically dealt with in other chapters in this volume. The adolescents in this study have been subject to two ongoing investigations, and the information given should be considered when planning future treatment programmes for younger age groups.

Cardiotoxicity

There is much concern over the toxic damage that may occur to the myocardium following anthracyclines. Among several studies, toxic damage seen on cardiac testing some years after treatment has been noted in over 50% of children.[20] In this context, serial studies of cardiac function in eight children are in this series treated for NHL with varying doses of doxorubicin are of interest. Eight children aged between 3 and 12 were treated with a total cumulative dose of up to 469 mg/m² of doxorubicin. At the conclusion of this therapy, ejection fraction measurements were carried out, and in some cases serial studies were performed (Table 5.9). All children had normal ejection fractions. When they had passed through adolescence (incidentally, without any symptoms referable to the cardiovascular system) they were again studied using nuclear angiography. Again, all ejection fraction measurements were normal, except, interestingly, in the two girls in the series, where the measurements were borderline before and after exercise (solid lines in Figure 5.4). Measurements of ventricular wall thickness, also an important parameter, were borderline in one girl.

It appears that children who have normal ejection fractions on completion of therapy are likely to pass through adolescence without subjective or objective evidence of cardiotoxicity. The only cause for concern was the two girls. Silber et al.[21] have shown that at every age and for

Table 5.9 Cardiotoxicity in adolescents treated as children with doxorubicin for non-Hodgkin's lymphoma

Patient	Date of birth	Diagnosed	Dose of doxorubicin (mg/m²)	Dates of study	Ejection fraction (exercise)	Ventricular wall thickness (mm)	Cardiac symptoms
PB (M)	30.11.59	1974	185	24.11.75	0·56		No
				13.12.90	0·60 (0·60)	—	
DB (M)	23.3.65	1976	212	1.3.76	0·64		
				21.6.76	0·66		
				15.7.76	0·63		
				22.3.77	0·64		
				1978	0·60		
				9.10.80	0·66		
				26.9.91	0·54 (0·69)	10	
GC (M)	27.1.70	1976	469	10.10.79	0·69		
				19.12.91	0·53 (0·64)	10	No
PC (M)	16.6.70	1979	360	2.12.81	0·72		
				3.5.82	0·72		
				13.2.92	0·62 (0·59)	9	No
IH (M)	24.7.76	1979	408	11.8.81	0·70		
				29.1.92	0·63 (0·69)	8	No
CH (M)	5.4.70	1979	390	Sept. 81	"Normal"		
				5.12.91	0·65 (0·78)	8	No
CD (F)	29.6.67	1979	310	5.1.82	0·70		
				11.3.92	0·55 (0·58)	6	No
LS (F)	13.9.67	1976	192	15.3.76	0·63		
				21.7.76	0·66		
				28.4.77	0·68		
				1978	0·66		
				13.12.90	0·56 (0·44)	8	No

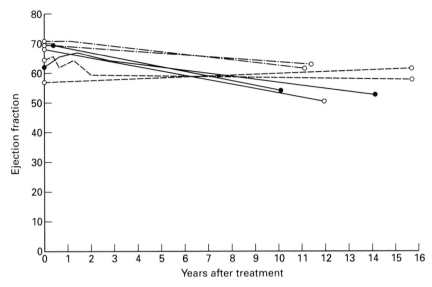

Fig 5.4 Serial cardiac ejection fraction measurements following therapy with doxorubicin

every cumulative dose of doxorubicin, boys are less likely to be affected than girls. The average age of children treated in this present study and followed through adolescence was 8 years, and at this age for a median dose of 400 mg/m^2 of doxorubicin, the expectation of abnormality in boys is 50% and in girls is 78%. It is worth noting that in the adolescents with a mean age of 18 in this analysis, treatment with a total of 400 mg/m^2 of doxorubicin resulted in an expectation of only 33% abnormality in boys and 64% in girls on the criteria outlined.[22] Adolescents therefore seem to be tolerating anthracycline drugs rather better than children.

It is evident that there is no safe dose of anthracycline, and that there is a progression of susceptibility, which is marked in the very young, decreases through adolescence, and is least evident in adults. There is also a gender difference, girls being far more susceptible than boys. The explanation for this is difficult, but it may be a consequence of the differing distribution of anthracycline in the two sexes, based on body fat characteristics.[21]

Fertility in adolescents treated for Hodgkin's disease

Testicular function following treatment for Hodgkin's disease was studied by Shafford et al.[22] Eleven boys who had mostly received chlorambucil VPP formed part of this series, and have undergone series studies during adolescence or early adulthood. Some show disturbing findings. All patients included were over 16 years of age, and had been off treatment for a minimum of 6 years. Basal levels of follicle stimulating hormone (FSH), luteinising hormone (LH) and testosterone levels were measured, and testicular size was measured using a Praeder orchidometer.

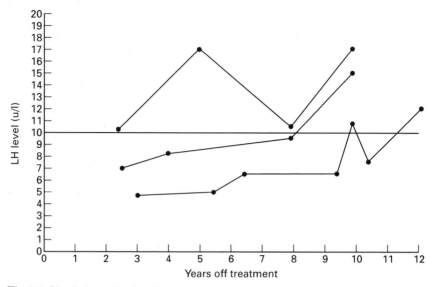

Fig 5.5 Rise in basal levels of luteinising hormone following the end of treatment

All patients were offered the opportunity of seminal analysis.

Germ cell dysfunction was considered to be present if basal FSH levels rose above 8 units/l; confirmatory evidence for this was a testicular volume of less than 15 ml and a low sperm count. Leydig cell function was considered disordered if the LH level rose above 10 units/l with or without a low testosterone (<9 mmol/l).

Of the 11 adolescents in the series, 8 were azoospermic, 1 was oligospermic between 7 and 15 years off therapy, and 2 were not tested. All except one had testicular volumes below 15 ml. Estimation of hormone levels showed that all had normal testosterone levels, but it was disturbing that serial measurements indicated a falling trend. All had elevated FSH levels, and five had elevated levels of LH, which on serial measurements appeared to be rising (Figure 5.5). All the children passed through puberty normally, and had normal Leydig cell function at the time. No boy developed gynaecomastia, but the serial fall in testosterone levels, with a rising LH, may possibly predict Leydig cell failure in the future.

The effect of chemotherapy on the girls in the series, as far as fertility was concerned, was much less severe. Only one girl, who had resistant disease and was eventually treated with high dose melphalan supported by bone marrow transplantation, developed ovarian failure, and is infertile. Of the 14 girls, 4 have conceived, 5 have been investigated and shown to be ovulating, and 4 others, who are awaiting investigation, are menstruating normally. All these girls are passing through adolescence or young adulthood normally, but will need careful follow up. In a study on gonadal status and reproductive function following treatment for Hodgkin's disease, Ortin et al.[23] followed 92 girls and 148 boys. Their finding in boys was identical to that reported by Shafford *et al.*[22] In their study, 87% of the 86 girls had normal menstrual function, but all those who underwent pelvic irradiation without oophorpexy had ovarian failure. Two of those girls developed ovarian failure following further chemotherapy for relapsed Hodgkin's disease. Whether ovarian failure with early menopause will be seen in children treated for Hodgkin's disease remains to be seen, although it has been reported in young adult patients.[24]

Conclusion

This account has attempted to focus specifically on the adolescent period (15–20 years of age), and to address the question of whether there are significant differences between this group of patients and either children or adults. There appear to be differences between adolescents and the other age groups in respect of some of the clinical features of Hodgkin's disease and NHL, in particular the high incidence of nodular sclerosing histology in adolescent girls with Hodgkin's disease, but response to therapy and survival are good, and overall survival is better than that seen in young and middle-aged adults. Complications due to cardiotoxicity have not been a feature in this group of adolescents, but gonadal function has been markedly impaired in adolescent boys.

Acknowledgements

Our thanks are due to Ms Sharon Love, of the ICRF Medical Statistics Laboratory, Lincoln's Inn Fields, London, for the statistical studies contained in this paper, and to Mrs Jo Barton for preparation of the manuscript.

1 Padmalatha C, Ganick DJ, Hafez G-R, Gilbert EF. Hodgkin's disease and non-Hodgkin's lymphoma in children and young adults. *Med Pediatr Oncol* 1982; **10**: 175–84.

2 Lange B, Littman P. Management of Hodgkin's disease in children and adolescents. *Cancer* 1983; **51**: 1371–7.

3 Murphy SB, Fairclough DL, Hutchison RE, Berard CW. Non-Hodgkin's lymphomas of childhood: analysis of the histology, staging and response to treatment of 338 cases at a single institution. *J Clin Oncol* 1989; 7: 186–93.

4 Kennedy BJ, Loeb V, Peterson V *et al.* Survival in Hodgkin's disease by age and stage. *Med Pediatr Oncol* 1992; **20**: 100–4.

5 Carbone PP, Kaplan HS, Musshoff K *et al.* Report of the Committee on Hodgkin's Disease Staging Classification. *Cancer Res* 1971; **31**: 1860–1.

6 Lukes RJ, Butler JJ. The pathology and nomenclature of Hodgkin's disease. *Cancer Res* 1966; **26**: 1063–81.

7 Lister TA, Crowther D. Staging for Hodgkin's disease. *Seminars in Oncol* 1990; **17**: 696–703.

8 Murphy SB. Classification, staging and end results of treatment of childhood non-Hodgkin's lymphomas: dissimilarities from lymphomas in adults. *Seminars in Oncol* 1980; 7: 322–4.

9 DeVita VT, Serpick AA, Carbone PP. Combination chemotherapy in the treatment of advanced Hodgkin's disease. *Ann Intern Med* 1970; **73**: 881–95.

10 Nicholson WM, Beard MEV, Crowther D *et al.* Combination chemotherapy in generalised Hodgkin's disease. *Br Med J* 1970; 3: 7–10.

11 Dady PJ, McElwain TJ, Austin DE *et al.* Five years experience with Chl.VPP—effective low-toxicity combination chemotherapy for Hodgkin's disease. *Br J Cancer* 1982; **45**: 851–9.

12 McKelvey EM, Gottlieb JA, Wilson HE. Hydroxyldaunorubicin (Adriamycin) combination chemotherapy of malignant lymphoma. *Cancer* 1971; **28**: 306–17.

13 Fisher RI, Gaynor F, Dahlberg S *et al.* Comparison of a standard regimen (CHOP) with three intensive chemotherapy regimens for advanced non-Hodgkin's lymphoma. *N Engl J Med* 1993; **328**: 1002–6.

14 Murphy SB, Magrath IT. Workshop on Pediatric Lymphomas: current results and prospects. *Ann Oncol* 1991; **2**: 219–23.

15 Donaldson S, Whitaker SJ, Plowman PN *et al.* Stage I-II pediatric Hodgkin's disease: long-term follow-up demonstrates equivalent survival rates following different management schemes. *J Clin Oncol* 1990; **8**: 1128–37.

16 Santoro A, Bonadonna G, Valagussa P *et al.* Long term results of combined chemotherapy-radiotherapy approach in Hodgkin's disease: superiority of ABVD plus radiotherapy versus MOPP plus radiotherapy. *J Clin Oncol* 1987; **5**: 27–37.

17 O'Brien MER, Pinkerton CR, Kingston JE *et al.* 'VEEP' in children with Hodgkin's disease—a regimen to decrease late sequelae. *Br J Cancer* 1992; **65**: 756–60.

18 Anderson JR, Wilson JF, Jenkin RD *et al.* Childhood non-Hodgkin's lymphoma—the results of a randomised therapeutic trial comparing a 4-drug regimen (COMP) with a 10-drug regimen (LSA2-L2). *N Engl J Med* 1983; **308**: 559–65.

19 Robertson CM, Stiller CA, Kingston JE. Causes of death in children diagnosed with non-Hodgkin's lymphoma between 1974 and 1985. *Arch Dis Child* 1992; **67**: 1378–83.

20 Lipschultz SE, Colan SD, Gelber RD *et al.* Late cardiac effects of doxorubicin therapy for acute lymphoblastic leukaemia in childhood. *N Engl J Med* 1991; **324**: 808–15.

21 Lipshultz SE, Lipsitz R, Mone SM *et al.* Female sex and higher drug dose as risk factors for late cardiotonic effects of doxorubicin therapy for childhood cancer. *J Engl J Med* 1995; **332**: 1738–43.

22 Shafford EA, Kingston JE, Malpas JS. Testicular function following the treatment of Hodgkin's disease in childhood. *Br J Cancer* 1993; **68**: 1199–204.

23 Ortin TT, Shostak CA, Donaldson SS. Gonadal status and reproductive function following treatment for Hodgkin's disease in childhood: the standard experience. *Int J Rad Oncol* 1990; **19**: 873–80.

24 Chapman RM, Sutcliffe SB, Malpas JS. Cytotoxic-induced ovarian failure in women with Hodgkin's disease. *J Am Med Assoc* 1979; **242**: 1877–81.

6: Management of soft tissue sarcomas

CLIVE HARMER

Introduction

Soft tissue sarcomas are rare, with only 1200 new patients being diagnosed each year in the United Kingdom—representing 1 in 50 000 of the population. There does appear to be a real increase in incidence in all age groups. In adolescents there has been an increased incidence of 10% in females and 14% in males during the last decade, compared with the previous decade (Sir Richard Doll, this volume). Furthermore, soft tissue sarcomas are the only tumours to demonstrate an increase in mortality in the adolescent age group, of approximately 6%.

Within the 11–20 year age range there occur two broad categories of soft tissue sarcoma. The first group are those which typically present in children and are exemplified by the rhabdomyosarcoma. The second group are those typically occurring in adults, of which malignant fibrous histiocytoma is now the most common. It is because the histology and natural history of these two groups are so fundamentally different that their management is also quite dissimilar. Furthermore, management of each group is complex and they will therefore be considered separately.

In the four year period from January 1990 to December 1993 456 new patients were referred to the Royal Marsden Hospital with the diagnosis of sarcoma; 3% were aged 10 or less and 89% were aged 21 or over. There were only 16 new patients aged 11–16 and 18 aged 17–20 (each approximately 4% of the total). The majority of patients in the 11–16 age range had sarcomas of "paediatric" type whereas in the 17–20 year age range the majority were of "adult" type. In each age range males predominated, comprising 56% of the total.

Soft tissue sarcomas of paediatric type

Rhabdomyosarcoma (RMS) is the most frequently encountered sarcoma of paediatric type. It forms a model for the other, much rarer varieties which include extraskeletal Ewing's sarcoma and peripheral neuroecto-dermal tumours.

Rhabdomyosarcoma

Rhabdomyosarcoma is a highly malignant tumour that may arise in any part of the body where striated muscle is found but can also occur in those sites where striated muscles are not normally found. It is the most common soft tissue sarcoma in children and adolescents, with 70% of cases occurring before the age of 10.

Histology

Embryonal RMS is the commonest subtype (60% of all RMS), occurring typically in the head and neck or genitourinary region. It has been described as "low grade RMS", but such a designation is misleading because an aggressive therapeutic strategy is mandatory. It is characterised by sheets of primitive round cells and differentiating rhabdomyoblasts. Cross-striations or muscle-specific proteins such as desmin may be identified. Botryoid RMS is a variant of the embryonal type simply occurring in hollow organs, such as the vagina, nasal sinuses, or bladder, said to resemble a bunch of grapes.

Alveolar RMS is characterised by alveolar spaces lined by primitive round cells. It is also designated high grade RMS. It is less common than the embryonal type and typically arises from the extremities, especially the hands or feet, of older adolescents. Mixed embryonal and alveolar types should be designated alveolar, out of respect of their more aggressive natural history. Chromosomal translocation t(2;13) (q37;q14) is characteristic.

The pleomorphic RMS rarely occurs in either children or adolescents. Its natural history is similar to that of the other "adult" sarcomas and it is therefore considered later in this chapter. The primary sites of rhabdomyosarcoma are indicated in Table 6.1.

Presentation and natural history

Like any other soft tissue sarcoma, RMS produces a local swelling. When large enough this will cause discomfort and pain. Tumours arising in the orbit may cause displacement of the globe with diplopia. Nasal blockage or deafness will be caused by a tumour arising in the nasopharynx or middle

Table 6.1   Distribution of primary sites of rhabdomyosarcoma

Site	Relative frequency (%)
Head and neck	40
Orbit	10
Non-parameningeal	10
Parameningeal	20
Genitourinary	25
Bladder–prostrate	10
Paratesticular vagina uterus	15
Limbs	15
Other	20

Adapted from the SIOP 1984–8 study of 289 cases.

ear; epistaxis and cranial nerve palsy may occur. Tumours arising in the bladder or prostrate region can cause dysuria, haematuria, or retention. Vaginal discharge or bleeding occur with those tumours originating in the female genital tract.

Rhabdomyosarcoma grows rapidly and infiltrates along tissue planes. Regional lymph node metastasis may be the presenting symptom and occurs early, especially in the alveolar subtype, with enlarged nodes appearing in the epitrochlear, axillary, popliteal, or inguinofemoral regions. Cervical lymphadenopathy is common with head and neck primary tumours. The principal site of haematogenous spread is to the lungs, present in 10–30% of patients at presentation, but rarely symptomatic. Other sites of metastases include bone and bone marrow; pain and anaemia may result.

Biopsy and other investigations

Open biopsy is mandatory, with fresh tissue being obtained for cell surface markers and chromosome studies. Fine needle aspiration cytology will not yield adequate tissue for special stains and immunocytochemistry to differentiate from lymphoma or other small round-cell tumours. Examination under anaesthesia may be required, especially for the head and neck or genitourinary sites. If there is significant doubt about the histology further biopsy must be achieved prior to treatment.

A plain chest radiograph is likely to be clear and, if so, should be followed by computed tomography (CT) of the thorax. CT of the primary site is of considerable help in delineating both the origin of tumour and its extent. Magnetic resonance imaging (MRI) is often superior but may not be available. Ultrasound may be complementary and has the advantage of easy repetition. Bone marrow aspirate plus trephine should be obtained initially as occult spread may have occurred. Plain radiographs and a bone scan would be appropriate if there were any distant site of pain. A full blood count and biochemistry will also be required.

Staging

Historically a postsurgical staging was used but depended on whether disease had been completely resected or not. With the wider acceptance of preoperative chemotherapy in an attempt to reduce the need for aggressive surgery or even to avoid it altogether, such a staging system is obsolescent. The presurgical staging system has therefore gained acceptance, having been proposed by the International Union against Cancer (UICC) and adopted by the International Society of Paediatric Oncology (SIOP). This allows comparison of results between different institutions and relates to prognosis (see Tables 6.2 and 6.3).

Treatment

Following confirmation of the diagnosis and complete staging, it is crucial for the patient to be seen by a multidisciplinary team devoted to treatment of these rare tumours. Only by such initial agreement can the

Table 6.2   TNM clinical classification of rhabdomyosarcoma

T1	Tumour confined to organ or tissue of origin
T1a	5 cm or less in size
T1b	More than 5 cm in size
T2	Tumour involves contiguous organs or structures
T2a	5 cm or less in size
T2b	More than 5 cm in size
N0	No clinical or radiographic evidence of regional lymph nodes
N1	Clinical or radiographic evidence of regional lymph nodes
M0	No distant metastases (clinical, radiographic or bone marrow)
M1	Evidence of distant metastasis

Modified from *TNM Classification of Malignant Tumours.*[1]

optimum scheduling of chemotherapy, surgery, and radiotherapy be achieved.

Chemotherapy   Rhabdomyosarcoma is a chemosensitive tumour. The most effective drugs are ifosfamide, doxorubicin, vincristine, cyclophosphamide, and actinomycin D. When used as single agents the response rates are 25–43%. In order to increase these figures a variety of combinations has evolved following cooperative national and international study group results. The combination of vincristine and actinomycin D (without radiotherapy) is usually effective in achieving local tumour control in microscopically completely resected non-alveolar RMS. With the addition of local radiotherapy this combination was found to be as effective in maintaining local control as a three-drug regimen with cyclophosphamide added for patients who had microscopic residual disease after surgery.

Cyclophosphamide has generally been replaced by ifosfamide (plus mesna) as this yields a higher response rate.[2] More recently introduced agents comprise carboplatin (which is less neurotoxic and nephrotoxic but more myelosuppressive than platinum) and epirubicin (which may have less cardiotoxicity than doxorubicin).

Although great advances have been made, progress is still urgently needed for patients with locally advanced and metastatic disease. More aggressive treatments are therefore being piloted with the goal of rapidly eliminating as many tumour cells as possible and preventing the development of drug resistance. Increased toxicity can be predicted but the achievement of complete remission is of critical importance.[3] Further improvements are likely to be achieved both by incorporation of as many active agents as possible to try and overcome drug resistance and by the use

Table 6.3   Clinical stage grouping of rhabdomyosarcoma

Stage	Primary	Nodes	Metastases
I	T1	N0	M0
II	T2	N0	M0
III	T1 or T2	N1	M0
IV	T1 or T2	N0 or N1	M1

Modified from *TNM Classification of Malignant Tumours.*[1]

of regimens of higher dose intensity to achieve a higher rate of complete remission.

Initial treatment with chemotherapy has gained general acceptance, with the aim of using less aggressive methods of local treatment. In all European studies, primary intensive chemotherapy is given, unless complete non-mutilating excision of the primary tumour is feasible.

In the SIOP MMT-89 study, primary chemotherapy alone is continued as long as tumour response can be documented before considering local treatment with either surgery or radiotherapy. The intensity and duration of chemotherapy are stratified according to site and tumour extent.[4]

Second line chemotherapy combinations together with radical surgery if feasible, and/or radical dose radiotherapy, are considered for patients with progressive disease. The optimal duration of drug treatment after complete remission remains unknown but the present tendency is to shorten overall treatment time to perhaps as little as 6 months. High dose chemotherapy followed by autologous bone marrow transplant or peripheral blood stem cell rescue may be an attractive strategy for selected high risk patients, although the results of treating established metastatic disease remain disappointing. Newer drugs under investigation include etoposide and high dose melphalan.

Surgery It is rarely possible to undertake complete excision with safe

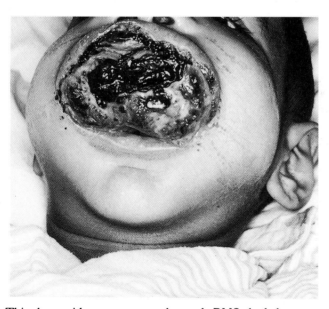

Fig 6.1 This boy with recurrent embryonal RMS had been treated with chemotherapy but the primary tumour in the hard palate had not been resected following complete remission. He was barely able to breathe or swallow. Radiotherapy delivered a dose of 60 Gy in six weeks, which he tolerated easily and which resulted in complete regression

73

margins at presentation without causing functional or cosmetic impairment; thus initial treatment with chemotherapy is almost universal. Surgery should not be considered until tumour reduction has been achieved by drugs and, in patients who achieve a reliable complete remission, may be avoided altogether. Every patient must therefore be assessed as an individual in combined consultation. For younger adolescents whose bones and soft tissues must continue to grow, surgery is usually preferred to radiotherapy. However, in older adolescents where growth is complete, radiotherapy has the advantage of being a more comprehensive regional treatment. Lymph node block dissection may occasionally be necessary but again should be a secondary excision rather than initial treatment.

The goal of surgical exploration after chemotherapy is to achieve local control whilst avoiding radiotherapy. Irradiation can be avoided when no trace of tumour is found or when all residual tumour has been removed. However, in patients who do achieve complete remission, surgical exploration after drug treatment should be undertaken only when it will result in a good outcome both from the point of view of function and cosmesis; otherwise it should be omitted and radiotherapy given instead. Sarcomas unresectable after initial chemotherapy can often be removed following second line drug treatment or irradiation.

Radiotherapy RMS is markedly radioresponsive, but the role of radiotherapy has diminished over the last two decades as more effective drug combinations have become established and the disadvantages of late radiation damage have become recognised, especially in the younger adolescent. An identical scenario has been enacted in the management of Ewing's sarcoma of bone.

The Intergroup Rhabdomyosarcoma Study (IRS) first set of trials ran between 1972 and 1978. For patients with localised disease which had been completely resected, the role of radiotherapy was assessed in patients treated with adjuvant chemotherapy. The addition of radiotherapy did not affect local recurrence or survival such that it is no longer offered for this category of patients.

For gross residual disease, doses of 50–60 Gy over 5–6 weeks are required. For microscopic disease doses of less than 50 Gy are associated with high control rates. Local control is less probable for tumours more than 5 cm in size. A wide margin must be allowed around the tumour volume and a shrinking field technique should be employed. Careful planning is mandatory with the addition of lead shielding to as much of the adjacent normal tissue as is possible, especially the growing end of a long bone.

Interstitial radiotherapy using iridium-192 implanted into the tumour bed or an intracavitary mould is effective at specific sites where small volume radiotherapy is adequate.[5] The trunk or vagina are examples where these techniques can deliver a high continuous dose with the inverse square law ensuring a rapid fall off in dose to adjacent critical structures.

Recent analysis has demonstrated that, even for patients with completely resected localised disease, those with unfavourable histology (alveolar) and/ or extremity tumours, treatment without radiotherapy showed an unexpectedly high relapse rate. It is therefore now accepted that irradiation is always used in these two subsets of patients.

In an attempt to improve the therapeutic ratio, a number of studies are looking at the use of two (or more) fractions of radiotherapy per 24 hours. To permit recovery of normal tissue, the interval between fractions should be at least six hours. When smaller than normal sized fractions are used, this technique is known as hyperfractionation, typically given over a long overall treatment period.

Accelerated radiotherapy also utilises more than one fraction each day but with the overall treatment period being shortened. This is theoretically attractive for rapidly dividing tumours but is limited by acute toxicity. Definitive results are awaited.

It is not normal practice to irradiate the entire muscle compartment as in the treatment of adult-type sarcomas. A margin of 2–5 cm around the original tumour dimension (before chemotherapy) is usually regarded as adequate, with the phase II volume introduced after 40 Gy being confined to the size of the original tumour.

Prophylactic irradiation of regional lymph nodes is not recommended, as it is to be hoped that prior drug treatment would have eliminated any microscopic node involvement. However, particularly for head and neck sites, inclusion of the immediately adjacent lymph node area can often be accomplished with minimal additional morbidity. Unresectable chemoresistant lymph node disease would of course demand radical dose irradiation.

Treatment options are summarised in Table 6.4.

Orbital tumours

Orbital tumours rarely metastasise and have an excellent prognosis. Exenteration is unnecessary and initial chemotherapy should be given. Subsequent radiotherapy is often avoided in children because of impaired growth of periorbital bone but this restraint does not apply to older adolescents for whom the entire orbit can easily be treated to 50 Gy (with protection of the lacrimal fossa and lens).

Parameningeal tumours

Invasion into the central nervous system remains a frequent cause of treatment failure. Radiotherapy to the skull base plus any intracranial extension is therefore always advised following initial drug treatment up to a dose of 55 Gy, but whole brain irradiation is rarely necessary. Surgery is limited to biopsy.

Bladder/prostate and vagina/uterus

At these sites the radical surgical approach has now been largely replaced by more aggressive initial chemotherapy. Thus organ-conserving surgery is usually possible, for example by undertaking only partial cystectomy with preservation of the trigone; a histologically proven complete response would permit avoidance of irradiation. Limited field radiotherapy or brachytherapy (which might be either interstitial or intracavitary) is

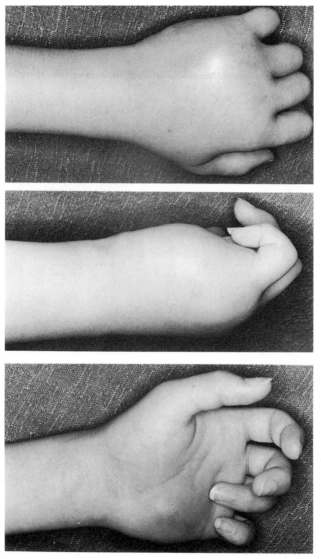

Fig 6.2 A 17 year old trainee beautician presented with a 7 cm mass. Biopsy showed alveolar RMS and simultaneous biopsy of an enlarged epitrochlear node was positive. She was treated with multiple drug chemotherapy and, following complete remission, high dose melphalan with peripheral blood stem cell rescue. The primary tumour recurred and resection was thought to be incomplete such that radical dose radiotherapy followed. She now has axillary node enlargement, 20 months after her original presentation

Table 6.4 Treatment strategy for rhabdomyosarcoma

Disease extent	Treatment options
Localised	
Complete resection	Vincristine + actinomycin (VA) × 4 (9 weeks)
Incomplete resection	VA + ifosfamide (IVA) × 4
Regional	IVA + doxorubicin (VAIA) × 6
	Surgery if functional and cosmetic operation possible
	Radiotherapy if incomplete resection, inoperable, or para-meningeal
Metastatic	Multidrug intensive—add platinum/carboplatin/etoposide
	Megachemotherapy—marrow or stem cell rescue

Adapted from Pinkerton et al.[6]

indicated for microscopic or macroscopic residual tumour.[7] Either second line drug treatment or radiotherapy can be employed in patients demonstrating an initial poor response before mutilative surgery is contemplated.

Paratesticular tumours

These easily accessible tumours have a favourable prognosis and require initial retrograde inguinal orchidectomy, followed by drug treatment. For postpubertal adolescents adjuvant radiotherapy to retroperitoneal nodes may be indicated.[8] For patients presenting with nodal involvement the CT scan will need to be repeated after initial chemotherapy; radiotherapy or node dissection will be required.

Extremity lesions and alveolar subtype

Primary tumours of the extremities have a poorer prognosis and a higher incidence of alveolar type with a high recurrence rate. Following drug treatment, both wide surgical excision and radiotherapy are recommended.

Prognostic factors and results (Table 6.5)

Relapse is rare after five years. The five year survival for completely resected local disease is just over 80%, falling to 70% when there is microscopic residue. For patients with gross residual disease the figure falls to 50–60%. Long-term survival for those presenting with metastatic disease

Table 6.5 Prognostic factors for rhabdomyosarcoma

Favourable factors	Unfavourable factors
Tumour limited organ of origin	Adjacent tissues invaded
5 cm or less in greatest dimension	More than 5 cm
No regional lymph nodes	Node involvement
Orbit paratesticular gynaecological	Extremity/parameningeal
Embryonal histology	Alveolar histology
Rapid response to chemotherapy	Incomplete response
Complete resection	Macroscopic residue
Microscopic residue	Distant metastases

Table 6.6   Four year survival of T1 tumours according to site[9]

Site	Patients surviving (%)
Orbit	90
Head and neck	
Non-parameningeal	79
Parameningeal	62
Genitourinary	
Bladder prostate	80
Paratesticular vagina uterus	96
Limbs	63
Other	53

remains at less than 25%. See Table 6.6 for four year survival data.

The major cause of treatment failure is local or regional relapse, although this is often salvageable with the use of second-line chemotherapy, additional surgery, or irradiation. Less than half of all failures are due to distant metastases (which may be associated with locoregional recurrence).

The future

To achieve maximum tumour control with minimum morbidity demands the closest cooperation of the histopathologist, paediatrician, medical oncologist, surgeon, and radiotherapist. There has been considerable progress over the past few decades, and further improvements will continue to rely on the trials presently being conducted in Europe and the United States. For good prognosis patients the intensity and length of drug treatment is likely to be reduced, together with elimination of alkylating agents and avoidance of radiotherapy. For those patients with poor prognosis more intensive multidrug chemotherapy, possibly with bone marrow transplant or the use of peripheral stem cells, complemented by adequate surgery and radiotherapy, should yield improved survival.

Peripheral neuroectodermal tumours and extraosseous Ewing's sarcoma

Peripheral neuroectodermal tumours (PNET) are extracranial extraspinal small round-cell malignant tumours supposedly of neuroectodermal origin. When arising within the thoracic cavity they are referred to as Askin's tumours. Their natural history and thus treatment are similar to extraosseous Ewing's sarcoma, being comparable to Ewing's sarcoma arising in bone. They occur in adolescents and young adults but are less common in children. They are highly aggressive and rapidly growing, producing an extensive primary mass soon associated with regional lymphadenopathy and metastases to the lung (and skeleton).

Optimal management comprises initial intensive combination chemotherapy using ifosfamide, vincristine, and doxorubicin (IVAD).

In the adolescent male this should be preceded by sperm banking. Initial investigations should include both bone marrow and bone scan. Surgical resection of the primary site should always be considered with the addition of radical dose radiotherapy as necessary. Combination drug treatment would then continue for at least six months.[10]

For patients with initially localised tumours the three year disease-free survival from diagnosis is 50%. The median relapse-free period is about two years with the latest relapses occurring as late as four years. Patients with metastatic disease demonstrate less than 20% survival at three years, despite initial good response.

Sarcomas of adult type

In the Royal Marsden Hospital series the majority of sarcomas diagnosed in the 17–20 year age range were of adult type but there was also a significant incidence in the 11–16 year age range.

Histology

There are more than 15 types of adult soft tissue sarcoma which can be classified into three categories. The most familiar are those whose line of differentiation is clear such as fibrosarcoma, angiosarcoma, malignant peripheral nerve sheath tumour, liposarcoma, and leiomyosarcoma; about half of all adult sarcomas fall into this category. The second large category comprises malignant fibrous histiocytoma (MFH) and sarcomas not otherwise specified, where the line of differentiation is not clear. MFH is now the most common adult soft tissue sarcoma diagnosis, demonstrating a pleomorphic picture, often with a storiform pattern. The third and smallest category comprises those of easily recognisable pattern but of no normal tissue equivalent. These include synovial sarcoma, alveolar soft part sarcoma, epithelioid sarcoma, and clear cell sarcoma (thought to be the soft tissue equivalent of malignant melanoma).

Immunocytochemistry has become invaluable in distinguishing these varieties, with electron microscopy being complementary. More recently, cytogenetics and molecular genetics have been found to give invaluable additional information.[11]

Grade

Despite the fascinating array of different histological types of sarcoma occurring in adults, the majority tend to behave in a similar fashion such that treatment is tailored to other features. The most important of these is the histological grade which is the single prognostic factor most closely related to behaviour and prognosis (and thus treatment). A three-point grading system is usually adopted comprising good, intermediate, and poor differentiation. The accepted grading criteria include cellularity, cellular pleomorphism, mitotic activity, and necrosis. So important is grade that it forms the basis of the staging system in both Europe and the United States.

Table 6.7   TNM stage grouping of adult sarcomas

Stage	Grade	T	N	M
IA	G1	T1	N0	M0
IB	G1	T2	N0	M0
IIA	G2	T1	N0	M0
IIB	G2	T2	N0	M0
IIIA	G3	T1	N0	M0
IIIB	G3	T2	N0	M0
IVA	Any	Any	N1	M0
IVB	Any	Any	Any	M1

Modified from *TNM Classification of Malignant Tumours.*[1]

Staging

Grade 1 tumours are designated stage I; grades 2 and 3 become stages II and III respectively (see Table 6.7). The TNM clinical classification[1] denotes a tumour measuring 5 cm or less in its greatest dimension as T1; greater than 5 cm indicates T2. Unlike the paediatric sarcomas, adult sarcomas rarely involve regional lymph nodes (the rare exceptions being clear cell sarcoma and epithelioid sarcoma). Regional node involvement should always be confirmed (at least by fine needle aspiration cytology) as it demands the designation of stage IVA disease and is a very strong adverse prognostic factor, frequently accompanied by or soon followed by distant metastatic disease which carries the designation of stage IVB.

Natural history and presentation

As with sarcomas of paediatric type, those of adult type present as a swelling arising in the soft tissues. Pain will follow if the tumour becomes large enough or invades adjacent bone or nerves. Regional lymph node enlargement is characteristically absent and, although pulmonary metastases are likely to develop in half of all large high grade tumours, they rarely cause symptoms at the time of diagnosis. Other sites of metastasis are much less common and usually appear only subsequent to pulmonary involvement. The primary tumour can present at any site in the body although the majority arise in the limbs and limb girdles. Very large tumours can evolve in sites such as the buttock and retroperitoneum without being noticed.

Biopsy and investigations

For small superficially placed sarcomas, complete excision biopsy is appropriate; indeed this is often done in ignorance of the diagnosis. For deep tumours an incision biopsy is required but its site must be correctly placed so as to be readily encompassed by the subsequent resection.[12] The less traumatic alternative is insertion of a trocar and cannula via a 1 cm skin incision with multiple fragments of tumour being removed with biting forceps. Tru-Cut biopsy or fine needle aspiration cytology may not permit accurate grading but may be useful for preliminary outpatient assessment.

Once the definite diagnosis of sarcoma has been confirmed, together with the histological type and grade, routine haematology, biochemistry, and a chest radiograph will be required. If the latter is negative, computed tomography (CT) of the thorax will exclude occult metastases. Detailed imaging of the primary site is essential to assess operability and can be undertaken using either CT or MRI. There has developed a consensus that MRI is superior, although CT is usually adequate.

Treatment of the primary tumour

For sarcomas of adult type, surgery is the definitive and potentially curative treatment. Postoperative radiotherapy will often be required; preoperative radiotherapy may render an otherwise inoperable tumour removable. Adjuvant or neoadjuvant chemotherapy is not of proven benefit such that the major role for drug therapy is treatment of symptomatic metastases.

Surgery

When surgery is used as sole treatment, the recurrence rate following local excision is greater than 90%; with wide excision approximately 40% of patients will recur, and for radical limb-sparing compartmental resection the local relapse rate is 25%. Even amputation fails occasionally, especially for proximally situated sarcomas. Amputation should not be contemplated as preferred treatment but rather thought of as an admission of failure. A significant proportion of patients referred to the Royal Marsden Hospital Sarcoma Unit request a second opinion as amputation has been recommended elsewhere; a limb-sparing operation can usually be undertaken, the only worthwhile exception being when fracture has occurred and the limb is already useless as well as painful.

The surgeon's goal is a wide excision in all three dimensions, including the deep aspect, whilst preserving as much function as possible (and preferably being cosmetically acceptable). A considerable degree of surgical expertise and experience is mandatory, with the corollary that such patients benefit by being referred to a specialist unit. The change in emphasis over the last decade has been away from total compartmental resection towards a functional wide resection,[13] complemented by radical dose radiotherapy whenever the resection margins are narrow or the tumour of intermediate or high grade. Many patients are referred with local recurrence when the same principles apply.

Advances in reconstructive surgery, especially the development of the myocutaneous flap, have extended the possibilities of limb salvage. Major arteries are seldom invaded by sarcoma but occasionally resection is required for adequate clearance and continuity can be restored by standard vascular techniques. The disability following sacrifice of major peripheral nerves may still be less than that of amputation and requires individual consideration.[9] No artificial limb can replace the function of the hand even after sacrifice of the radial or ulnar nerve; resection of the sciatic nerve when involved by a tumour of the buttock or hamstrings is followed by surprisingly little dysfunction, although often the tumour can be stripped off with the perineurium, leaving the nerve intact. Frank invasion of a long bone is uncommon and would be an indication for preoperative radiotherapy. Stripping of the periosteum can then be achieved with resection of a sliver of cortex when necessary.

Tumours arising in the head and neck have an overall five year survival of only 50%,[14] with local disease being the cause of death in the majority. Radical resection is rarely possible and irradiation should always be added. Retroperitoneal sarcomas have the worst prognosis of any site, largely due to late presentation and difficulty in complete removal.

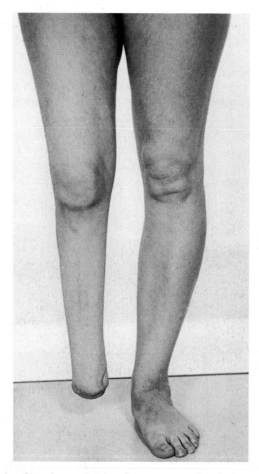

Fig 6.3 Following Syme's amputation four years previously for a clear cell sarcoma arising on the dorsum of the foot this girl was referred with biopsy positive inguinal lymphadenopathy and pulmonary metastases. This type of tumour is one of the few adult-type sarcomas which does metastasise to regional lymph nodes. The preferred initial treatment would have been wide local excision with radiotherapy as the mutilating surgery had not prevented subsequent dissemination

Radiotherapy

Wide local excision, usually complemented by radical dose radiotherapy, has become established as the treatment of choice for adult soft tissue sarcomas. The patient should be seen preoperatively in combined consultation. It is Royal Marsden Hospital policy for all patients with grade 2 or 3 tumours to receive wide field irradiation, irrespective of the margins of surgical clearance, as these tumours have a greater propensity for locoregional recurrence (as well as metastasis). However, there is no need for radiotherapy in grade 1 tumours when the margins of excision are confirmed as adequate on histology. Thus the majority of patients will receive both modalities of treatment but there is a significant number who do not require the addition of irradiation. This fact forms the basis of our preference of giving radiotherapy only after histological examination of the resected tumour and is in contrast to those centres which recommend preoperative radiotherapy in every case, thereby giving unnecessary irradiation to some patients.

Adult sarcomas are less radiosensitive than paediatric sarcomas so high dose treatment is mandatory. A dose–response relationship has been

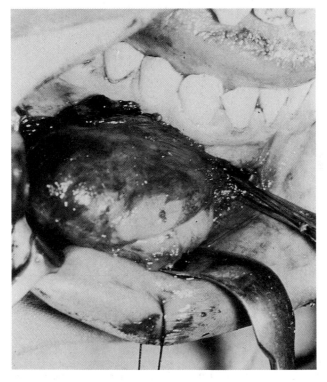

Fig 6.4 This 15 year old boy presented with a synovial sarcoma adjacent to the mandible. It was completely resected, including stripping of the periosteum. Radiotherapy delivered 63 Gy in 30 fractions over 6 weeks through oblique wedged portals. He remains asymptomatic in complete remission 14 years later

documented.[15] A dose of 60 Gy delivered in 30 daily fractions over a period of six weeks is standard. Wide field external beam treatment is necessary as these tumours tend to spread along fascial planes. The phase I volume is therefore large but, using a shrinking field technique, a considerably reduced phase II volume will encompass only the tumour bed after the first 50 Gy have been delivered. When macroscopic (or microscopic) residual disease is present, the dose can sometimes be escalated to 66–70 Gy over seven weeks, but doses in excess of this will lead to unacceptable late normal tissue damage. The preferred alternative is to undertake a wider re-excision prior to irradiation.

A CT scan, performed in the treatment position, is normally employed in order to optimise the portal arrangement which is typically a pair of

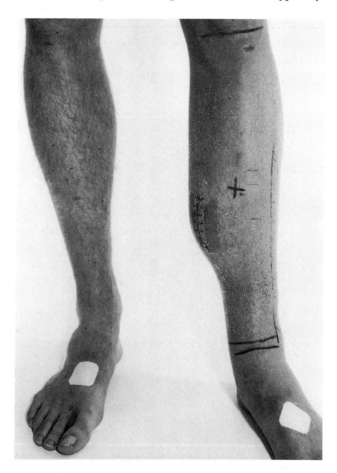

Fig 6.5 This liposarcoma was fixed to the tibia and unresectable short of amputation, which had been recommended and prompted referral for a second opinion. Preoperative radiotherapy was advised and surgery undertaken after 40 Gy when the resected specimen revealed no evidence of residual tumour. He remains in complete remission and enjoys dancing 17 years later

opposing fields, angled so as to ensure sparing of a corridor of normal tissue along the whole length of the field to avoid an encircling fibrosis which can result in lymphoedema. With limb tumours the other major consideration in planning is to avoid as much of the adjacent joint as possible, in order to minimise subsequent painful ankylosis. Throughout treatment the patient should continue with physiotherapy commenced in the immediate post-operative period.

Conformal planning, or at least the careful insertion of lead into the portals to protect as much of the adjacent normal tissue as possible, will also minimise late morbidity.[15] Considerable care must therefore be taken with patient immobilisation, and a shell or similar method of restraint will normally be advantageous. A linear accelerator producing photons at 4–10 MV is preferable to telecobalt. The use of electrons for a superficial tumour should be confined to the booster dose. For sarcomas arising on the trunk, in the head and neck region, or in the retroperitoneum, surgical margins are invariably narrow and radiotherapy will always be required; with the close proximity of sensitive normal organs meticulous planning is mandatory.

At selected sites, a radioactive implant or intraoperative radiotherapy is occasionally possible and can deliver a high target dose with minimal dose to the surrounding normal tissues. Split course radiotherapy has no advantage. Large fraction treatment (hypofractionated radiotherapy), although radiobiologically attractive, did not result in increased local control.[16] Another Royal Marsden Hospital trial compared neutrons with photons but likewise did not demonstrate any improvement.[17] Our experience of delivering simultaneous radiotherapy and chemotherapy is that the increased local reaction prevents the target dose being achieved and is therefore not recommended. Our present pilot study uses hyper-fractionated irradiation with 1·2 Gy fractions being given twice daily to a total of 72 Gy in 60 fractions over a period of six weeks; theoretically this higher dose should reduce local recurrence.

Preoperative radiotherapy is advised only when initial surgery is unlikely to be able to completely resect tumour.[18] The patient is seen in combined consultation after 50 Gy and ideally the operation performed between two and six weeks thereafter. Phase II can then be delivered postoperatively so as to take the final dose up to 60 or 66 Gy, once wound healing is secure. The use of radiotherapy alone is not normally recommended but is occasionally used when a tumour remains inoperable or the patient is not fit enough for radical surgery.[19] Approximately one in three of such patients will demonstrate prolonged local control.

Recurrent tumours should always be considered for further wide surgical excision; radiotherapy will usually be required in addition. Occasionally reirradiation is possible.[20]

The other major role for radiotherapy is in palliation, for example in the treatment of bone metastases or fungating tumours. At least 35 Gy delivered over a period of three weeks will be necessary to relieve

Table 6.8 Five-year actuarial results in 317 patients treated by conservative surgery plus radiation according to stage

Stage	Number of patients	Local control (%)	Overall survival (%)
IA	20	100	100
IIB	35	91	93
IIA	51	85	95
IIB	86	86	68
IIIA	37	90	87
IIIB	85	81	48

Adapted from Willett and Suit.[21]

mediastinal or spinal cord compression and higher doses may achieve prolonged benefit.

Chemotherapy

Drug treatment has an established role for symptomatic metastases and may be of value when recurrent primary tumour becomes inoperable following full dose irradiation. Pulmonary metastases are the cause of the majority of deaths from sarcoma, and the lack of an effective drug in this common situation remains disappointing. The use of thoracic bath irradiation may temporarily ameliorate symptoms but does not prolong survival. Resection of pulmonary metastases (metastasectomy) is of great value in selected patients, similar to its use in osteosarcoma. A long disease-free interval and a limited number of metastases are favourable features; prolongation of survival has been documented.

The most effective agents are doxorubicin and ifosfamide (plus mesna) both of which yield a response rate of 20–25% in non-pretreated patients. Unfortunately these responses are usually only partial and typically short lasting. Toxicity is significant but the occasional complete response does translate into prolonged survival. For regimens comprising standard drug dosage, single agent doxorubicin is as effective as combination chemotherapy and is less toxic.[22] Recent studies have demonstrated the importance of a good initial performance score, regardless of the chemotherapy given.

The present European Organisation on Treatment and Research of Cancer (EORTC) study compares ifosfamide ($5 g/m^2$) and doxorubicin ($50 mg/m^2$) with ifosfamide and doxorubicin ($75 mg/m^2$) plus granulocyte macrophage colony stimulating factor (GM-CSF). The latter reduces myelosuppression and subsequent infection, although the other side effects of hair loss, renal impairment, and cardiomyopathy persist. Dose intensification may be the key to achieving a higher response rate in metastatic disease. However, toxicity will be increased and may be unacceptable.

Adjuvant chemotherapy at the time of initial treatment is aimed at reducing the metastatic rate, which for large high grade sarcomas is 50%. Unfortunately, despite several trials indicating an advantage, there remains no clinically proven value for chemotherapy of sarcomas in the adjuvant setting. Therefore such treatment is not to be recommended, outside of well-constructed research protocols.[18] However, an intriguing outcome from adjuvant studies has been the suggestion of reduction in local recurrence rates (unassociated with reduction in metastases or prolonged survival). The EORTC proposes randomising high risk patients after surgery to intensive chemotherapy or no drug treatment, prior to standard irradiation.

Neoadjuvant chemotherapy is delivered before definitive surgery (or irradiation). The presence of evaluable tumour permits determination of chemoresponse both clinically and histologically on the resected specimen. The primary tumour may also be downstaged such that some initially operable tumours are rendered surgically removable. It has been suggested in the paediatric literature[23] that non-RMS tumours be treated with initial chemotherapy as for RMS. This approach may be illogical in view of their different chemoresponsiveness. Of the 100 patients analysed, the histology was unclassifiable in 25 and some of these were round cell tumours. Furthermore in a review of 62 non-RMS cases treated at St Jude Children's Research Hospital the conclusion was that chemotherapy did not produce any demonstrable gain in survival.[24] However, when confronted by a locally advanced tumour, especially in a younger adolescent where both surgery and radiotherapy would result in severe morbidity, initial chemotherapy may have a role in an attempt to reduce the bulk of disease prior to definitive treatment.

Regional intra-arterial chemotherapy has not been shown to be superior to drugs given intravenously but requires further evaluation. Finally, the potential benefit of immunotherapy and biological response modifiers are being tested in a variety of trials.

Prognostic factors derived from multivariate analysis

Multivariate analysis has been performed on a consecutive series of 421 patients whose initial treatment was at the Royal Marsden Hospital from 1970 to 1990. Tables 6.9 and 6.10 describe the prognostic factors derived from these data.

Table 6.9 Results of multivariate analysis for local recurrence in 421 patients whose initial treatment was at the RMH

Factor	Hazard for	Relative to	Hazard ratio	p-value
Age	Age ≤ 40	Age > 40	0·62	0·03
Site	Lower Limb	Retroperitoneum	0·27	0·0001
Grade	High	Low	2·12	0·003
	Intermediate	Low	2·26	0·026
Clearance	Adequate	Inadequate	0·36	0·0004
Radiotherapy	Used	Not used	0·52	0·006

Adapted from Robinson.[15]

Table 6.10 Results of multivariate analysis for metastasis in 421 patients whose initial treatment was at the RMH

Factor	Hazard for	Relative to	Hazard ratio	p value
Size	≦5 cm	>5 cm	0·46	0·0001
Histology	Unspecified	Others	1·57	0·01
Grade	High	Low	2·43	<0·0001
Time-dependent factors				
Recurrence	Local	None	2·68	<0·0001
Nodes	Nodes	None	1·88	0·04

Adapted from Robinson.[15]

The future

For adolescents presenting with tumours of adult-type histology, definitive treatment will remain wide excision usually followed by radical dose irradiation. The future emphasis will be on adjuvant or neoadjuvant chemotherapy to reduce the number of patients dying of metastatic disease, although the only major advance will occur when a more effective drug becomes available.

Whatever the histological diagnosis, all patients will benefit from initial assessment in a multidisciplinary clinic such that treatment can be individualised to achieve the optimum balance of the available therapeutic modalities. Randomised clinical trials will continue to give the most valuable information regarding improvements in detail of these overall strategies.

Acknowledgements

I warmly acknowledge my colleagues in the Sarcoma Unit: Dr Ross Pinkerton (paediatric oncologist), Dr Ian Judson (medical oncologist), Mr Meirion Thomas (surgeon), Dr Eleanor Moskovic (radiologist), and Dr Cyril Fisher (histopathologist). This manuscript has been prepared by Ms Louise Workman. I am also most grateful to Dr Roger Greenwood for having provided the analysis of Royal Marsden Hospital referrals and to the Photographic Department for the illustrations.

1 Hermanek P, Sobin LH. *TNM classification of malignant tumours.* Fourth edition, 2nd revision. London: Springer-Verlag, 1992.

2 Crist WM, Garnsey L, Beltangady MS *et al.* Prognosis in children with rhabdomyosarcoma: A report of the Intergroup Rhabdomyosarcoma Studies I and II. *J Clin Oncol* 1990; **8:** 443–52.

3 Carli M, Guglielmi M, Sotti G *et al.* Soft tissue sarcomas. In Plowman PN, Pinkerton CR, eds, *Paediatric Oncology: Clinical practice and controversies,* London: Chapman & Hall Medical, 1991, 295–307.

4 Verweij J, Pinedo HM, Suit HD. *Multidisciplinary treatment of soft tissue sarcomas.* London: Kluwer, 1993.

5 Flamant F, Voute PA, Sommelet D. Rhabdomyosarcoma. In: Voute PA, Barrett A, Lemerle J, eds, *Cancer in children: clinical management,* London: Springer-Verlag, 1992.

6 Pinkerton CR, Cushing P, Sepion B. *Childhood cancer management.* London: Chapman & Hall Medical, 1994.

7 O'Connell MEA, Hoskin PJ, Mayles WPM, McElwain TJ, Barrett A. Intravaginal iridium-192 in the management of embryonal rhabdomyosarcoma. *Clinical Oncology* 1991; **3**: 236–9.

8 Horwich A. Rhabdomyosarcoma. In: Horwich A, ed., *Combined radiotherapy and chemotherapy in clinical oncology.* London: Edward Arnold, 1992.

9 Rodary C, Gehan E, Flamant F *et al.* Prognostic factors in 951 nonmetastatic rhabdomyosarcoma in children: A report from the International Rhabdomyosarcoma Workshop. *Med Pediatr Oncol* 1991; **19**: 89–95.

10 D'Angio GJ, Sinniah D, Meadows AT *et al. Practical pediatric oncology.* London: Edward Arnold, 1992.

11 Fisher C. Soft tissue sarcomas: current concepts in pathology. *Clin Oncol* 1992; **4**: 322–6.

12 Westbury G. Surgery in the management of soft tissue sarcoma. *Clin Oncol* 1989; **1**: 101–5.

13 Pitcher ME, Thomas JM. Functional compartmental resection for soft tissue sarcomas. *Eur J Surg Oncol* 1994; **20**: 441–5.

14 Eeles RA, Fisher C, A'Hern RP *et al.* Head and neck sarcomas: prognostic factors and implications for treatment. *Br J Cancer* 1993; **68**: 201–7.

15 Robinson MH. Soft tissue sarcoma. MD thesis, Cambridge University, 1992.

16 Ashby MA, Ago CT, Harmer CL. Hypofractionated radiotherapy for sarcomas. *Int J Radiat Oncol* 1986; **12**: 13–17.

17 Glaholm J, Harmer C. Soft tissue sarcoma: neutrons versus photons for post-operative irradiation. *Brit J Radiol* 1988; **61**: 829–34.

18 Robinson MH, Ball ABS, Schofield J *et al.* Preoperative radiotherapy for initially inoperable extremity soft tissue sarcomas. *Clin Oncol* 1992; **4**: 36–43.

19 Harmer C, Frampton M, Wiltshaw E. Role of radiotherapy and chemotherapy in management of soft tissue sarcomas. In Bloom HJG, ed., *Head and neck oncology.* New York: Raven Press, 1986.

20 Graham JD, Robinson MH, Harmer CL. Re-irradiation of soft-tissue sarcoma. *Brit J Radiol* 1992; **65**: 157–61.

21 Willett CG, Suit HD. Soft tissue sarcomas. In Horwich A, ed., *Combined radiotherapy and chemotherapy in clinical oncology.* London: Edward Arnold, 1992.

22 Verweij J, Pinedo HM. Changing concepts in the systemic treatment of locally advanced or metastatic soft tissue sarcomas. In Verweij J, Pinedo HM, Suit HD, eds, *Multidisciplinary treatment of soft tissue sarcomas.* London: Kluwer, 1993.

23 Sommelet D, Flamant F, Rodary C. A series of 100 soft tissue sarcomas (STS) in childhood excluding embryonal rhabdomyosarcomas (RMS) and schwannomas. *Med Pediatr Oncol* 1991; **19**: 390.

24 Horowitz ME, Pratt CB, Webber BL *et al.* Therapy for childhood soft tissue sarcomas other than rhabdomyosarcoma: a review of 62 cases treated at a single institution. *J Clin Oncol* 1986; **4**: 559–64.

7: Medical management of bone tumours

IAN J LEWIS

Introduction

Bone tumours are among the more common tumours occurring in adolescents. Examination of data produced by the Yorkshire Regional Tumour Registry for the years 1984 to 1988[1] demonstrated an incidence of bone tumours between 6·2 and 7·2 per 100 000 population for those between the ages of 10 and 24. The peak incidence is in those between the ages of 15 and 20 with an overall male preponderance of approximately 3:2. These incidence figures imply that between 120 and 150 new patients with bone tumours will be seen in the United Kingdom in this age group each year. Osteosarcoma and Ewing's sarcoma account for more than 95% of malignant bone tumours in adolescents, with osteosarcoma being about twice as common as Ewing's sarcoma.

Although most bone tumours appear to arise without an obvious predisposing cause, there are a number of recognised associations that can be implicated in the development of osteosarcoma in children and young adults. Osteosarcoma occurs with greatly increased frequency in patients who have hereditary retinoblastoma.[2] This was originally thought to relate to radiotherapy given as treatment for retinoblastoma, but it is now apparent that the increased incidence relates to a predisposition caused by mutation in the *RB* gene on chromosome 13q14.[3] Abnormalities of the *RB* gene have been found in tumours from patients with sporadic osteosarcoma and there is evidence that this occurs predominantly in the paternal gene.[4] However, many osteosarcomas have no detectable abnormality of the *RB* gene.

Osteosarcoma is one of the tumours recognised to occur in patients with the Li–Fraumeni familial cancer syndrome.[5] Many of these families have abnormalities of the p53 gene on chromosome 17p13, and abnormalities of structure, function, or control of p53 also occur in sporadic osteosarcoma.[6 7]

Prior treatment for other tumours with radiation and/or alkylating agents is implicated in about 3% of patients with osteosarcoma.[8] Radiation induced osteosarcoma can occur after many years (median 12–16 years) but this interval may be shortened following alkylating agents or anthracyclines.[9] Osteosarcoma is a recognised second malignancy after treatment for Ewing's sarcoma.[10]

In contrast, Ewing's sarcoma has only been very rarely reported as occurring with specific congenital anomalies or other potential etiological factors. It does not appear to be one of the cancers implicated in familial cancer syndromes, but it is recognised that Ewing's sarcoma is more common in some races. Publications from a number of tumour registries report that the vast majority of patients are white with only a very low incidence in black Afro-Caribbeans.[11]

Clinical presentations

There are many similarities but some differences in the symptoms and signs of osteosarcoma and Ewing's sarcoma. Typically, both types of tumour present with a history of pain and swelling in the involved bone. These tumours, however, occur at different sites. Osteosarcoma most commonly occurs in the metaphyseal regions of the distal femur, proximal tibia, and proximal humerus, whereas Ewing's sarcoma arises throughout the skeleton including the flat bones of the axial skeleton and the diaphyseal regions of the long bones (Figure 7.1). Probably as a result of this site distribution, most patients with osteosarcoma present within 6–10 weeks of onset of symptoms while it is not uncommon for patients with Ewing's sarcoma to have symptoms over many months, particularly when the primary tumour is in the axial skeleton. Systemic symptoms of fever, fatigue, and weight loss occur more frequently in patients with Ewing's than with osteosarcoma, as do metastases at presentation. Between 10% and 20% of patients with osteosarcoma have visible metastases during initial radiological evaluation, most in the lungs with a minority having secondary involvement of other bones. In the current United Kingdom Children's Cancer Study Group (UKCCSG) experience approximately 25% of patients with Ewing's sarcoma have metastases at diagnosis with common sites being lung, other bones, and bone marrow. Lymphatic spread is reported in less than 10% of these, and although central nervous system (CNS) involvement occurs in advanced disease at relapse, it is extremely rare at presentation.

There are a number of uncommon patterns of presentation. Osteosarcoma can occur in less usual sites, for example in the mandible, vertebrae, or sacrum where symptoms will be produced by nerve involvement. More rarely, osteosarcoma can present with multifocal synchronous skeletal tumours suggesting multicentric origin. Primary Ewing's tumours of rib in association with pleural effusion and respiratory symptoms are now more generally referred to as Askin's tumours of the peripheral primitive neuroectodermal tumour (pPNET) family. Ewing's sarcoma of vertebrae commonly produce neurological symptoms of nerve root compression.

Investigations

The diagnosis of bone tumours depends on biopsy. The biopsy should be undertaken by clinicians with appropriate expertise, particularly when subsequent limb-sparing surgery or radical excision is sought. Nowadays,

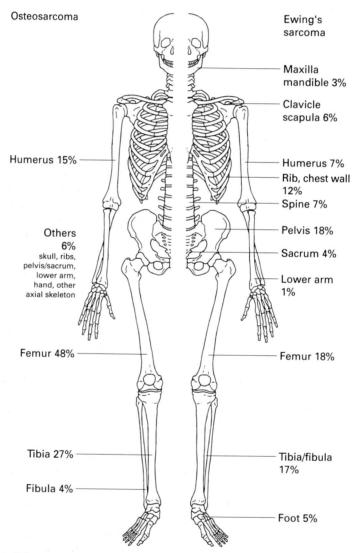

Osteosarcoma

Ewing's sarcoma

Maxilla mandible 3%

Clavicle scapula 6%

Humerus 15%

Humerus 7%

Rib, chest wall 12%

Spine 7%

Others 6%
skull, ribs, pelvis/sacrum, lower arm, hand, other axial skeleton

Pelvis 18%

Sacrum 4%

Lower arm 1%

Femur 48%

Femur 18%

Tibia 27%

Tibia/fibula 17%

Fibula 4%

Foot 5%

Fig 7.1 Primary tumour sites for osteosarcoma and Ewing's sarcoma. Osteosarcoma data from 295 patients in European Osteosarcoma Intergroup Study 80831: Ewing's sarcoma data from 251 patients in UKCCSG ET-1, ET-2

pathological evaluation of these tumours demands not only routine histopathology but immunocytochemistry, cytogenetics and, increasingly, newer methods of molecular diagnosis.

Radiological investigation is an essential part of the evaluation of bone tumours. Plain radiographs of the involved area can offer diagnostic guidance and be helpful in determining the presence of fractures. Ewing's sarcoma typically has a motheaten appearance without new bone formation, but in osteosarcoma new bone formation is common. Both tumours can cause a periosteal reaction and although Ewing's sarcoma is said to cause an "onion skin" appearance and osteosarcoma to cause spiculation, none of these appearances can be relied upon and biopsy remains mandatory. Local tumour evaluation should include computed tomography and/or magnetic resonance imaging, which is thought to be particularly helpful in delineating intramedullary extension.[12]

Investigation for metastatic disease should include plain chest radiograph, computed tomography of the chest, and radionuclide bone scan. Bone marrow aspiration and biopsy should be performed when Ewing's sarcoma is suspected. The current recommendations of the UKCCSG/MRC are to perform two bone marrow aspirates and two bone marrow trephines at sites away from the primary tumour. Other laboratory investigations that can be helpful include full blood count and erythrocyte sedimentation rate or plasma viscosity, serum lactate dehydrogenase, and alkaline phosphatase, the latter tests because of their possible prognostic significance.[13 14] Baseline tests of renal and cardiac function are performed because of specific toxicities associated with the most commonly used chemotherapy agents.

Pathology

Osteosarcoma is a malignant tumour originating in bone, and histological diagnosis is usually made by the presence of a sarcomatous spindle cell stroma producing osteoid (new bone) in combination with the expected radiological appearance. There are several distinct pathological variants of osteosarcoma.[8 15] The most common group are conventional osteosarcomas which can be subdivided into osteoblastic osteosarcoma (50%), chondroblastic osteosarcoma (25%), or fibroblastic osteosarcoma (25%), depending on the apparent predominant differentiation. There is no clear prognostic difference between these subtypes. Osteosarcoma arising from periosteal tissue at the surface of the bone[8] or primary osteosarcoma of the jaw in older patients[16] tend to be associated with a slower disease course and local recurrence rather than distant metastases. One rare variant that can cause some diagnostic confusion with Ewing's sarcoma and other small-cell tumours is the small-cell osteosarcoma[17] occurring in less than 4% of osteosarcoma. Although osteoid production can be found, this may be difficult and diagnosis depends on careful microscopic, immunocytochemical, and ultrastructural studies.

Ewing's sarcoma is one of the small round blue cell tumours of childhood which include neuroblastoma, rhabdomyosarcoma, and lymphoma but to which should be added the other primitive peripheral neuroectodermal tumours (pNETs), small cell osteosarcoma, and chondrosarcomas. These tumours often lack specific morphological features that would allow a precise diagnosis and have therefore been the subject of enormous study and discussion by pathologists. Establishing a pathological diagnosis demands expert advice and modern technology. Light microscopy, electron microscopy, immunocytochemistry, cytogenetics, fluorescent in situ hybridisation and newer molecular techniques of DNA, RNA, and protein detection are all important.[18] Ewing's sarcoma used to be largely a diagnosis of exclusion, but recent developments in tumour classification, cytogenetics, and molecular biology have changed this situation. It is now becoming generally accepted that Ewing's sarcoma is at the undifferentiated end of a spectrum of tumours that include atypical Ewing's sarcoma and pPNETs. These tumours seem to share a specific chromosomal translocation, t(11:12) (q24q12) in more than 80% of cases,[19 20] expression of a specific antigen of unknown function known as MIC 2,[21] and specific chimeric RNA transcripts of fusion proteins associated with the specific translocation and determined by reverse transcriptase polymerase chain reaction (RTPCR).[22]

Treatment of osteosarcoma

It is now established that osteosarcoma is optimally treated with multimodal therapy, requiring both surgery and chemotherapy for the best chance of long term survival. The only exceptions to this statement are low grade periosteal tumours without medullary involvement where local complete excision has been thought to be the treatment of choice.[8 23]

Treatment development of osteosarcoma has been through a number of historical phases. Initially, treatment relied on local tumour therapy, with amputation being the most common option although there was a vogue for using radiotherapy to the primary tumour.[24] Historically, this resulted in published overall survival figures of less than 20% with the vast majority of patients developing metastases within two years.[25]

During the late 1960s and early 1970s, there were a number of studies examining the use of single agent therapy. Doxorubicin[26] and high dose methotrexate[27] were reported to result in shrinkage of metastatic tumours and subsequently, cisplatin[28 29] and ifosfamide[30] were also shown to have activity. Other agents such as carboplatin[31] and etoposide have not been demonstrated to have independent activity in osteosarcoma although studies are continuing. The combination of bleomycin, cyclophosphamide, and actinomycin D (BCD) is also said to have activity[32] although this is disputed.[33]

Early studies of adjuvant chemotherapy using some or all of these agents were reported to result in improved survival rates[34-36] when compared with historical controls. However, some methodological difficulties were subsequently identified and this, together with a series of papers from the Mayo Clinic that reported improved survival with an aggressive surgical policy but no adjuvant chemotherapy, led to these results being challenged.[25 37 38] It was proposed that improvements in prognosis for non-metastatic osteosarcoma may have occurred because of a change in the natural history of the tumour.

The controversy resulted in two prospective randomised trials being undertaken that compared adjuvant chemotherapy with surgery alone in this group of patients. These studies, from the Multi-Institutional Osteosarcoma Study (MIOS)[39] and from UCLA,[40] both demonstrated a clear advantage in relapse-free survival for the patients receiving adjuvant chemotherapy and suggested that the natural history of osteosarcoma was unchanged. The results of these trials were very similar. The MIOS trial employed a multidrug regime based on a regimen known as the T-10 protocol described by Rosen consisting of BCD/high dose methotrexate, doxorubicin, and cisplatin. Recent follow up has demonstrated an eight year event-free survival of 61% for the immediate chemotherapy arm compared with 11% for the control group. The projected overall survival at eight years is 71% for the immediate chemotherapy arm and 51% for patients treated initially with surgery but salvaged after relapse with thoracotomy and chemotherapy.[41] The UCLA study[40] using a similar chemotherapy schedule but without cisplatin, reported 55% disease-free survival at two years in the chemotherapy arm compared with 20% in the surgery alone group.

The chemotherapy schedules used in these trials were based on a series of studies undertaken at Memorial Sloan-Kettering (MSK) Hospital by Rosen et al[42–44] that have had a pivotal role in osteosarcoma therapy. The MSK group developed a number of novel approaches to treatment based around the introduction of prosthetic, limb-sparing surgery instead of amputation. They pioneered the concept of neoadjuvant chemotherapy in an effort both to control local and metastatic disease and to provide time to construct limb prostheses. They utilised multiagent chemotherapy in an effort to prevent drug resistance and introduced the idea that prognosis may be influenced by histologically determined response of the primary tumour to neoadjuvant therapy.[45] They also suggested that patients having a poor histological response to initial therapy could be rescued by switching to schedules containing different chemotherapy agents.[43]

The best known of the Memorial Sloan-Kettering protocols was the T-10 schedule, which when first published reported an actuarial disease-free survival of 93% at 20 months.[43] This protocol used a 16 week initial therapy based on repeated courses of high dose methotrexate, BCD, and doxorubicin. Patients who had a good histological response, defined as tumour necrosis greater than 50%, continued with similar therapy for a further 30 weeks whereas those having a poor histological response were switched to a cisplatin-containing regimen for a similar length of time. The

95

initial report suggested that this switch could indeed salvage patients successfully and the results were so startling that they formed the basis of numerous subsequent studies carried out by multi-institutional cooperative groups and individual institutions throughout the world. Many of these studies have recently been updated in a single volume[46] (Table 7.1).

The use of neoadjuvant therapy as a prerequisite for prosthetic replacement has become standard although it is not clear that this approach offers any survival benefit over initial amputation. Indeed there have been suggestions[41 47] of adverse results in patients having prosthetic replacement and it could be argued that early amputation of resistant osteosarcoma is highly desirable. Nevertheless, the often perceived psychological benefits of limb-sparing surgery have been instrumental in maintaining this approach, even though published studies suggest no long term psychological advantage.[48 49]

Histopathological assessment of the response of the primary tumour to neoadjuvant chemotherapy has been accepted as of valuable prognostic significance following a number of studies,[46] with necrosis of greater than 90% of tumour indicating favourable outcome. The encouraging early suggestion that patients with poor histological response could be rescued by changing chemotherapy has not been borne out by subsequent experience. Studies from the American CCG,[50] the German COSS-82 trial,[51] Istituto Rizzoli,[52] and an update from MSK[13] have all demonstrated good histological responses associated with disease-free survival of greater than 75% but that poor histological responders have a significantly worse prognosis despite tailoring chemotherapy.

MRC/EORTC Studies: The European Osteosarcoma Intergroup

Studies by the MRC and by the European Organisation on Research and Treatment of Cancer have mimicked those elsewhere. Independently, both groups undertook studies during the mid to late 1970s of adjuvant chemotherapy in osteosarcoma but, in both groups, the chemotherapy schedules were of low intensity when compared to those in current use and demonstrated little advantage in disease-free survival over historical reports of amputation alone.[45 54]

The MRC and EORTC together with UKCCSG and SIOP formed the European Osteosarcoma Intergroup (EOI) and initiated a series of studies from 1983 onwards. The first study (80831) started as a pilot study but rapidly grew to a full phase III randomised trial in which a two-drug regimen of doxorubicin/cisplatin, based upon a previously published study by Ettinger et al[55] was compared with a three-drug schedule that incorporated high dose methotrexate in addition to doxorubicin and cisplatin (Figure 7.2). The results showed that in patients with non-metastatic limb primaries, the schedule containing two drugs had a significantly superior disease-free survival (Figure 7.3).[56] This was a slightly surprising result until it was realised that the schedules varied not only in the number of drugs, but also in both the total doses of doxorubicin/

Table 7.1. Results for osteosarcoma of extremities: therapy incorporating chemotherapy

Study group	Number of patients	Chemotherapy regimen	Disease-free survival (%)	Length of follow up	Reference
Memoral Sloan–Kettering (T-10)	79	HDMTX, VCR, DOX, BCD ± CDDP	93 76	2 years 5 years	43 13
German COSS-80	116	DOX, HDMTX + BCD or CDDP	68	4 years	51
German COSS-82	125	HDMTX, DOX, CDDP, IFOS	58	4 years	51
Multi-Institutional Osteosarcoma Study	201	HDMTX, BCD, DOX, CDDP vs no adjuvant therapy	61 11	8 years	39, 41
University of California Los Angeles	59	HDMTX, BCD, VCR, DOX vs no adjuvant therapy IACDDP, DOX ± BCD	55 20 58	2 years (HDMTX)	40
Istituto Rizzoli	127	HDMTX or IDMTX HDMTX, VCR, DOX, BCD ± CDDP	42	5 years (IDMTX)	52
Childrens Cancer Group	192	CDDP, DOX	61	2 years	50
European Osteosarcoma Intergroup	198	CDDP, DOX, HDMTX	41	4 years	56

BCD, bleomycin, cyclophosphamide, actinomycin-D; CDDP, cisplatin; DOX, doxorubicin; HDMTX, high dose methotrexate; IACDDP, intra-arterial; IDMTX, intermediate dose methotrexate; IFOS, ifosfamide; VCR, vincristine.

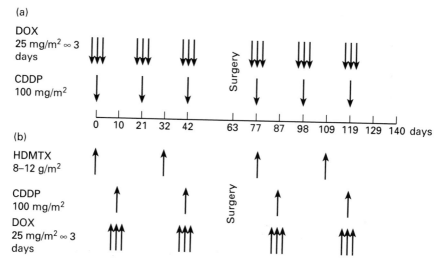

Fig 7.2 Chemotherapy regimens used in European Osteosarcoma Intergroup Study 80831: (a) two-drug regimen (b) three-drug regimen. CDDP, cisplatin; DOX doxorubicin; HDMTX, high dose methotrexate

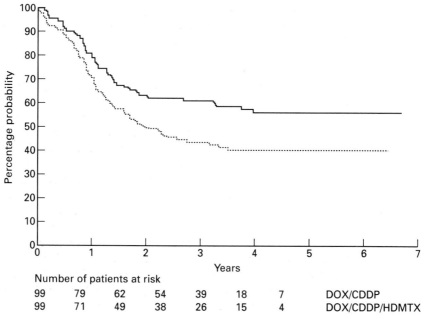

Fig 7.3 Disease-free survival of patients with non-metastatic limb osteosarcoma, from European Osteosarcoma Intergroup Study 80831. Abbreviations as in Figure 7.2. ——, DOX/CDDP; ·········, DOX/DDP/HDMTX. $p = 0.02$, logrank test

cisplatin and the dose intensity with which these two drugs were delivered, suggesting an important role for these variables. The results of this study

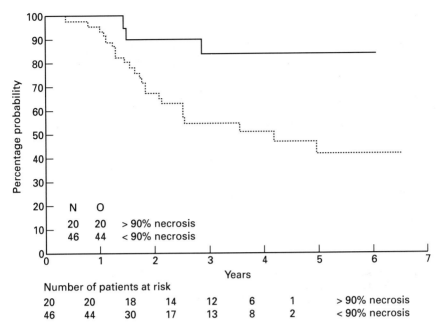

Fig 7.4 Survival of patients with non-metastatic limb osteosarcoma based on histological response following neoadjuvant chemotherapy, from European Osteosarcoma Intergroup Study 80831. ——, >90% necrosis; ········ <90% necrosis. $p=0.008$, logrank test

also supported the contention that histological response was a significant prognostic variable (Figure 7.4).

The two-drug arm doxorubicin/cisplatin was carried through into the second EOI trial (80861). This randomised trial compared this regime with a schedule based upon the Rosen T-10 protocol, termed the "multidrug" arm (Figure 7.5). This schedule differed from the original Rosen protocol in two main respects. Firstly, doxorubicin was included in the preoperative phase of therapy and secondly, all patients were switched to a cisplatin containing regime at 20 weeks because it was not logistically possible to have all postchemotherapy histological specimens systematically assessed for tumour necrosis within the required time in the context of a multinational study of this size. More than 400 eligible patients with primary non-metastatic limb osteosarcoma were entered into this study between 1986 and 1993. Preliminary results suggest no advantage for the 47 week multidrug arm compared to the 18 week doxorubicin/cisplatin arm.

During the latter part of the EOI study 80861, there was extensive debate about subsequent studies. A pilot study of cisplatin, ifosfamide, and doxorubicin (PIA) for patients with axial primaries or metastatic osteosarcoma at diagnosis did not appear to offer any clear advantage over the protocols already in use. The question was raised of the possibility of undertaking a prospective study of the role of total dose or dose intensity, particularly in view of the observations made during study 80831. These suggested that the two-drug arm was superior to the three-drug arm because of one or other of these variables. Because the two-drug arm had been in use from 1983, it became possible to undertake a retrospective analysis of dose and dose intensity in the 290 patients with non-metastatic limb osteosarcoma that had received this schedule. The protocols had contained recommendations for both dose reduction and delay in the event

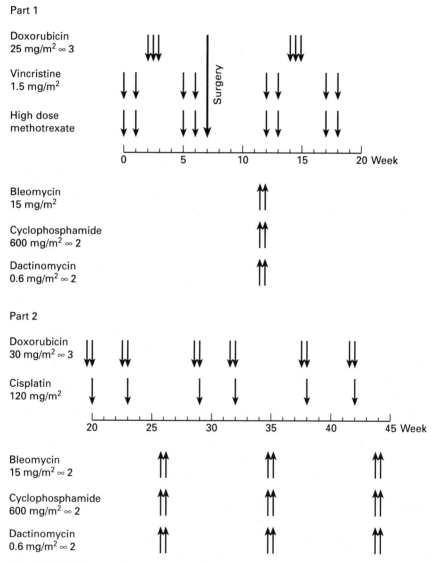

Fig 7.5 Multidrug regimen used in European Osteosarcoma Intergroup Study 80861

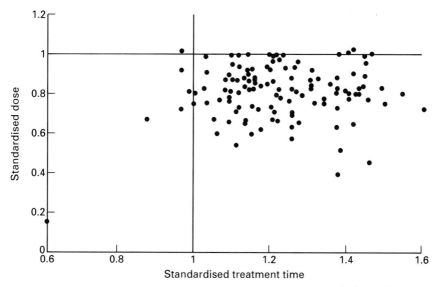

Fig 7.6 Scatter plot of received intensity of doxorubicin and cisplatin for patients on European Osteosarcoma Intergroup Studies 80831 and 80861. Treatment time standardised to 1 if patients' chemotherapy on time. Results greater than 1·0 imply treatment delay; results below 1·0 are for patients who did not receive six planned courses. Dose standardised to 1 for expected dose with no dose reductions, based on planned dose of doxorubicin 75 mg/m^2 × 6 courses. Results below 1·0 imply dose reduction

of particular toxicities and consequently there was a wide scatter of both received dose and time to complete therapy (Figure 7.6). Unpublished analysis of this data (IJ Lewis and D Machin, personal communication) revealed an effect of either dose or dose intensity on survival, although in the context of a retrospective analysis it has not been possible to distinguish between these two variables. It appeared that for patients who received 50% or less dose intensity of cisplatin/doxorubicin, survival was less than 50% at three years compared with greater than 70% survival for those who received a higher dose intensity. A decision was therefore made to design a dose-intensive schedule to try and compare directly with the original doxorubicin/cisplatin arm.

A pilot study was designed in which doxorubicin/cisplatin was given at two-weekly intervals but with granulocyte-colony stimulating factor (GCSF) being given between drug courses in order to lessen neutropenia (Figure 7.7). The pilot data[57] demonstrated that although toxic, this regimen was feasible provided it was given in a clinical setting used to delivering high dose chemotherapy and providing appropriate supportive care. The current EOI study (80931) is therefore a direct randomised comparison of this dose-intensive arm with a conventional doxorubicin/cisplatin arm. The study opened in late 1993 and is currently accruing patients at the same rate as previous trials.

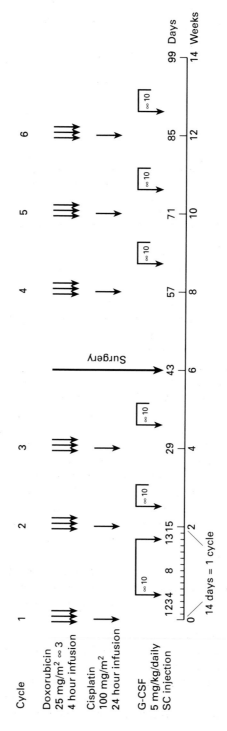

Fig 7.7 Dose-intensive arm of European Osteosarcoma Intergroup Study 80931

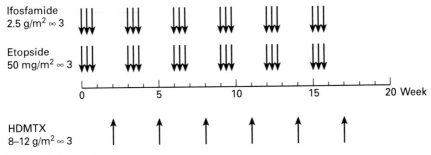

Fig 7.8 Salvage therapy for relapsed osteosarcoma in patients treated initially with doxorubicin/cisplatin. For neoadjuvant use, disease response monitored after two and four courses. Pulmonary metastatectomy performed when feasible. Disease response monitored after two and four courses if there is assessable disease. If no assessable disease, then six courses given. Dose and timing of courses adjusted according to myelosuppression. HDMTX, high dose methotrexate

Treatment of metastatic disease

Patients presenting with metastatic disease at diagnosis have a much poorer outlook than those with primary tumour alone. Those patients that have bone metastases, either at diagnosis or at relapse, have a uniformly fatal outcome despite therapy, but it has become accepted that patients with relatively small numbers of lung metastases at diagnosis may be treated successfully by using an aggressive surgical approach. In the EOI study 80831 five year survival for this group was approximately 25% (V Bramwell, personal communication) after treatment with chemotherapy, primary tumour surgery, and in many cases pulmonary metastatectomy.

Patients who develop metastases following therapy have a poor prognosis although complete surgical resection of pulmonary metastatic disease has been associated with long term survival.[58-60] Factors associated with prolonged survival include complete resection, a small number of metastases, or a longer time from completion of primary therapy to development of metastases and unilateral disease.[61-63] Further chemotherapy in this situation is not of proven benefit but is commonly used and a number of active regimens have been reported in relapsed disease[63 64] including ifosfamide and etoposide in combination.[65] The management of patients with metastatic disease is complex and demands a multidisciplinary approach in deciding whether to use chemotherapy before thoracotomy in order to assess response or whether to use surgery first. For those patients who received initial therapy with doxorubicin/cisplatin, my own approach has been to use a schedule of ifosfamide, etoposide and high dose methotrexate as salvage therapy (Figure 7.8).

The role of radiotherapy is controversial, as osteosarcoma is considered to be largely radioresistant. Radiotherapy may have a role in the palliative treatment of recurrent primary tumours and there is evidence that prophylactic lung irradiation is of benefit in preventing the development of pulmonary metastases.[54] Radiotherapy is commonly used as palliative therapy for unresectable axial skeleton primary tumours and for bony metastases.

Current controversies and future directions

Despite the major advances in osteosarcoma therapy, only just over 50% of patients are long term survivors; this provides an impetus for future developments. There are a number of controversial areas relating to chemotherapy. The debate over the use of presurgical chemotherapy has already been addressed in this chapter. However, its use within Europe appears to have been established. In the United States, the Paediatric Oncology Group have undertaken a randomised trial in which neoadjuvant chemotherapy followed by surgery and adjuvant chemotherapy is being directly compared with initial surgery and adjuvant chemotherapy in patients with non-metastatic extremity osteosarcoma. It is hoped that this trial will be reported during the mid 1990s and will help to resolve this debate.

The role of high dose methotrexate as first line treatment remains somewhat controversial. There is no doubt that single agent high dose methotrexate produced responses in osteosarcoma[27] and that subsequently it has been used as part of many multiagent neoadjuvant and adjuvant chemotherapy regimes (Table 7.1), apparently contributing to improvements in prognosis over the past 20 years. Some initial studies suggested that high dose methotrexate could not be shown to have an independently beneficial effect on outcome,[66] and more recent studies including EOI 80831[56] have been cited as supporting this lack of effect. However, much of the evidence against high dose methotrexate has been in trials where it has been given at lower doses and greater intervals than recommended by Rosen in his T-10 protocol[44] and therefore the overall contribution of this agent remains unresolved.[67]

There are recent studies which suggest that the peak level of methotrexate achieved influences outcome[68] with levels above 1000 μmol/l being associated with improved survival. This influence decreases with the use of cisplatin containing regimes.[69]

There has been a vogue, initially proposed by Jaffe,[70] for using intra-arterial chemotherapy, usually cisplatin, for primary tumour therapy based on the rationale that use of this route would achieve very high local concentrations within a tumour and thereby overcome some theoretical problems such as variable vascularity and drug resistance. This hypothesis was tested within the COSS-86 study in which intra-arterial cisplatin was compared with intravenous cisplatin within the context of a multiagent regime. No benefit of intra-arterial cisplatin on response was shown in this study[71] or others such as those at Istituto Rizzoli[52] and there seems little to justify pursuing this approach.

Is it possible to improve survival rates in osteosarcoma? Future studies will attempt to do this but without increasing the not inconsiderable late effects associated with agents such as cisplatin and doxorubicin. It is important to find out if there is a role for specific agents such as ifosfamide in improving the outcome in osteosarcoma. This is currently being addressed by the Children's Cancer Group. There might be a role for analogues of currently used agents as a means of reducing late effects, for example carboplatin replacing cisplatin. The numbers of patients required for such trials are large and would demand commitment from multinational groups.

Formal studies of dose intensity such as are being addressed in EOI 80931 will hopefully provide a basis for future studies, and technologies such as growth factors and the use of peripheral blood progenitor cells may be used to support these approaches. These approaches would gain extra validity if it were possible to better delineate up-front prognostic groups. Although histological response to initial chemotherapy is a powerful indicator of outcome, methods defining good risk, standard risk, and high risk groups at diagnosis are relatively crude and depend on assessments of tumour size or simple tumour markers such as LDH or alkaline phosphatase.[14] It is to be hoped that better biological markers of prognosis will be identified and studies should be developed to address these points.

Treatment of Ewing's sarcoma

The earliest descriptions of Ewing's sarcoma include the observation that these tumours are radiosensitive.[72] As a result of these reports, radiotherapy was widely used as the main or only form of primary tumour treatment. However, despite this apparently locally effective treatment, more than 90% of patients developed and succumbed to disseminated metastatic disease, demonstrating the aggressive systemic nature of this tumour.[73 74]

Improvements in the prognosis for Ewing's sarcoma only started to occur following the introduction of effective systemic chemotherapy during the late 1960s and 1970s.[74] It is now clear that successful treatment of Ewing's sarcoma demands an integrated team approach to the use of radiotherapy, surgery, and chemotherapy in order to offer the best prospects for both primary tumour and systemic disease control.

Systemic therapy

There are a number of single therapeutic agents that have been shown to have an effect on Ewing's sarcoma. The earliest tumour responses were seen with cyclophosphamide,[75] vincristine,[76] actinomycin D,[77] and doxorubicin.[78] Other agents such as melphalan[79] and more recently ifosfamide[80 81] have been shown to be effective single agents and there is evidence that etoposide enhances the effect of ifosfamide when used in combination.[65]

The use of these agents in combination led to changes in the previously observed history of this tumour and concomitant improvements in survival. Early studies used various combinations of vincristine, cyclophosphamide, actinomycin D, and doxorubicin as adjuvant therapy to radiotherapy[74] and showed survival approaching 50%. Subsequent studies in both single institutional and multi-institutional settings using similar agents and methods of primary tumour control have produced comparable results indicating disease free survival in the region of 50–70% (Table 7.2).

Some of the most important observations have been those from the Intergroup Ewing's Sarcoma Studies (IESS). IESS 1 showed a marked advantage in both survival and local control of a four-drug regime—vincristine, actinomycin D, cyclophosphamide, and doxorubicin—over the same regime without doxorubicin.[82] IESS 2 demonstrated the superiority of this four-drug schedule being delivered in a higher dose intermittent schedule when compared with a moderate dose continuous schedule using the same agents.[83 91]

One of the main changes in therapy during the 1980s was the introduction of ifosfamide into combination chemotherapy schedules either in place of, or in addition to, cyclophosphamide. The German CESS group replaced cyclophosphamide with ifosfamide in their high risk group and showed an apparent survival advantage for this group in CESS 86 when compared to a historically comparable cohort from CESS 81[87–89] although there were other changes in primary tumour therapy that may have contributed.

Primary tumour control

Changing the previously dire outcome of Ewing's sarcoma has focused attention on to the importance of primary tumour control and the relative merits of radiotherapy and surgery.

Traditionally, attempts at primary tumour control have been achieved using radiotherapy. Most of the initial studies of chemotherapy continue to use radiotherapy as the main method of primary tumour treatment, but it soon became obvious that there were problems of both local primary tumour relapse following therapy and late radiation effects on both growth and second malignancy in survivors, leading to a re-evaluation of the role of surgery in primary tumour therapy.[85 93–95]

A review of published studies demonstrated overall local relapse rates of 10–45% (Table 7.2) following radiation to the primary site, with increased local recurrence in central sites of pelvis and upper humerus when compared to distal primary sites of forearm and tibia and fibula. There is a strong body of opinion led by the CESS group[87] that relapse rates relate more to primary tumour volume than to site, and tumours in central areas tend to be larger than distal ones. The CESS group now stratify patients by tumour volume with tumour < 100 ml on clinicoradiological assessment falling into a better prognostic group.

Only if a tumour can be completely surgically removed with clearly demonstrated histological clearance is it feasible to consider eliminating radiotherapy from the management plan. Despite advances in tumour surgery and prosthetics, many Ewing's tumours occur in sites where these requirements are impossible and therefore radiotherapy remains a crucial treatment modality. Surgery is definitely indicted for lesions in expendable or distal bones where complete resection with clear margins can be achieved. The question of debulking large tumours within the axial skeleton remains controversial and, although this has been recommended by the CESS group together with radiotherapy to residual tumour, this approach remains unresolved. More detailed discussion of surgical techniques and prosthetics are beyond the scope of this chapter.

Careful radiotherapy planning by experienced radiation oncologists is crucial to providing both optimum disease control and reduction of associated late effects. Even in patients who received primary chemotherapy, successful radiotherapy planning must be based on the original tumour volume, and the IESS originally emphasised the importance of including whole bone and a 5 cm margin, although they also suggested that it was feasible to elect to exclude one epiphyseal centre at the furthermost point from the primary tumour.[96] This latter approach has become acceptable practice in children and teenagers who have not completed growth. For pelvic and central axis tumours, particular attention must be paid to soft tissue tumour extension and protecting against radiation effects on normal tissue and organs such as lung, heart, bladder, and bowels. Use of surgically implantable spacing devices or moving intra-abdominal organs, for example ovary, may decrease bystander radiation effects. Care with planning radiotherapy in conjunction with ifosfamide or cyclophosphamide should reduce the likelihood of haemorrhagic cystitis.

There has been no clear evidence of a radiation dose–response relationship above 40 Gy. The change in emphasis over recent years towards primary chemotherapy and surgery, where feasible, has meant that radiotherapy is often used for tumours at difficult sites, of large volume, or both, particularly pelvic lesions. Analysis of pelvic tumours in IESS 1 did not demonstrate any dose–response relationship above 40 Gy[97] although there was a suggestion in a study from Istituto Rizzoli of slightly higher local relapse rates of 41% with doses of 40–55 Gy compared with 30% of doses with 56–60 Gy.[84] Because of greater impairment of function and a possible increased risk of secondary malignancies, most studies now limit radiation dose to 55 Gy in conventional fractionation of 180–200 cGy when given as a part of multimodeal treatment with current chemotherapy schedules.

UKCCSG studies

Treatment for Ewing's sarcoma in the United Kingdom has mirrored developments elsewhere in the world. The first national study (ET-1) from 1979 to 1985 recommended vincristine, doxorubicin, and cyclophosphamide to be given for one or two courses of induction therapy followed by the maximally tolerable dose of radiotherapy to the affected bone. Vincristine, doxorubicin, and cyclophosphamide were then alternated with vincristine, actinomycin, and cyclophosphamide for one year and followed by a second year of vincristine, actinomycin, and cyclophosphamide at three week intervals. Surgery was not particularly recommended but was used for distal lesions and expendable bones in less than 25% of patients. Event-free

Table 7.2   Studies of Ewing's sarcoma therapy

Study (years)	Number of patients and disease status	Local treatment	Local control	Chemotherapy	Disease-free survival (%)	Length of follow up	Reference
IESS-1 (72–78)	331 Localised	Radiation (45–65 Gy)	85% (overall) 73% (pelvic)	VAD + Ad	59		
				VAC + Pulmon irrad. VAC	42 24	5 years	82
IESS-2 (78–82)	214 Localised	Radiation (50–55 Gy) Surgery (43%)	91% (overall)	VAC Ad (high) VAC Ad (moderate)	73 56	5 years	83,91
Istituto Rizzoli (72–82)	144 Localised	Radiation (40–60 Gy)	64% (overall) 50% (pelvic)	VAC Ad	41	9 years	84
M Sloan Kettering (72–78)	67 Localised	Radiation (45–70 Gy) Surgery	90% (overall)	T2, T6, T9 VAC Ad + MTX/Bleo	79	2 years	85
SFOP (78–84)	67 Localised	Radiation (45–60 Gy)	88% (overall)	VAC Ad	52	4 years	86
CESS 81 (81–85)	93 Localised	Radiation (46–60 Gy) Surgery (64%)	74% (overall) 64% (central)	VAC Ad	55	6 years	87
							88

CESS 86 (89–91)	140 Localised	Radiation (44–60 Gy) conventional vs. hyperfractionated surgery (75%)	92% (overall) 90% (central)	VAC Ad (standard) VAI Ad (high risk)	71	3 years	89
UKCCSG ET-1 (79–85)	142 All patients (15% metastatic)	Radiation (45–60 Gy) Surgery (25%)	57% (overall)	VAC Ad (low intensity) Localised Metastatic	41 10	10 years	90
UKCCSG (86–92)	226 All patients (40% metastatic)	Surgery Radiation (30–55 Gy)		IVAd/IVA	65	4 years	90

Ad, adriamycin (doxorubicin); Bleo, bleomycin; I, ifosfamide; MTX, methotrexate; VAC, vincristine, actinomycin D, cyclophosphamide.

survival at six years for the whole group of 142 was 35% with event-free survival of 41% for patients with non-metastatic disease and 10% for those with metastases. Patients with axial primary tumours had a worse outcome than those with proximal or distal primary tumours with both increased local and distant relapse.

It became clear that these results were not as good as those being seen elsewhere and on reflection this was most probably due to a relatively poor dose intensity, particularly of cyclophosphamide which was given at a dose of 600 mg/m² three weekly.

The second UKCCSG study (ET-2) tried to address some of these problems and take account of advances elsewhere. Several major empirical changes were made. Firstly, high dose ifosfamide (3 g daily for three days given three-weekly) replaced low/moderate dose cyclophosphamide based on the very encouraging early response data reported from the United States and Europe.[65 88] Secondly, it was decided to change recommendations for local disease control in order to try and reduce both local recurrence rates and late effects. It was recommended that following four courses of intensive IVAd (ifosfamide, vincristine, doxorubicin) all patients would be evaluated for primary tumour excision and where feasible this would be carried out. Patients having complete excision with clear histological margins need not receive radiotherapy but would proceed to further chemotherapy. Patients having an incomplete resection or having unresectable tumour would have radiotherapy concurrently with vincristine and cyclophosphamide prior to further IVAd. Patients with bulk residual disease receive 55 Gy in 30 fractions and those with microscopical residual disease received 45 Gy in 25 fractions. Treatment continued for a total of 16 courses (one year) with actinomycin D being used to replace doxorubicin when reaching threshold dose of 420 mg/m².

Between 1986 and 1992, 226 patients were entered into this study and it is apparent that survival has been much improved over ET-1 with an event-free survival at six years of 57%[90] (Figure 7.9). This change in prognosis is reflected in overall national survival figures studying three-year cohorts within the UKCCSG (Figure 7.10). Further analysis is greatly complicated by the observation that 25% of patients in ET-2 had metastatic disease at diagnosis compared with 15% in ET-1. Almost certainly this occurred as a result of intensified staging recommendations and improved technology that makes further historical comparison difficult. Greater detail about the impact of primary tumour policy changes require further analysis but the data demonstrates that many more patients are having surgical tumour resections than previously.

Many of the problems in interpreting data from ET-1 and ET-2 arise because they are single-arm studies dependent on historical comparison. The number of patients with Ewing's sarcoma in the United Kingdom is really insufficient to try and answer questions in a randomised trial, and in order to address new questions without the potential criticism of always using historical controls, the UKCCSG has come together with the MRC

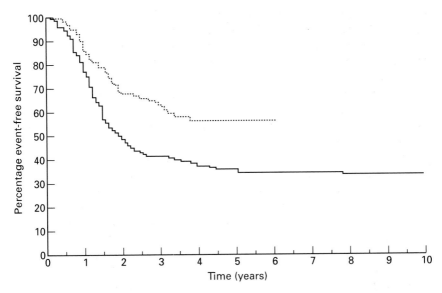

Fig 7.9 Event-free survival for all patients in UKCCSG ET-1 (1979–85) and ET-2 (1986–92). ——, ET-1; ·········, ET-2. $p = 0.002$, logrank test

and the (predominantly German) CESS group to form the European Intergroup Co-operative Ewing's Sarcoma Study (EICESS). The EICESS 92 study is now under way, addressing a number of questions. Firstly, patients are allocated to standard risk (non-metastatic disease, tumour

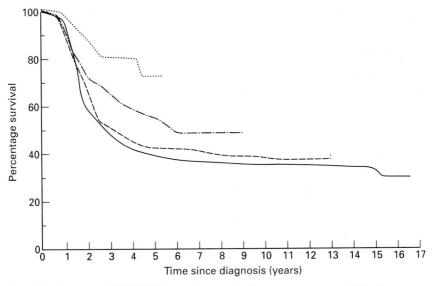

Fig 7.10 Survival of UKCCSG patients with Ewing's sarcoma, 1977–92. ——, diagnosed 1977–80 (63 patients); ——–——, diagnosed 1981–4 (87 patients); —·—·—, diagnosed 1985–8 (86 patients); ·········, diagnosed 1989–92 (84 patients)

volume <100 ml) or high risk (tumour volume >100 ml) groups. The main chemotherapy question for standard risk patients is whether morbidity can be reduced without compromising survival by substituting cyclophosphamide for ifosfamide after an initial ifosfamide based induction and local tumour therapy. The main chemotherapy question for high risk patients is whether the addition of etoposide as a fifth drug to an ifosfamide based regime can improve survival (Figure 7.11). Recommendations for primary tumour therapy are very similar to those in ET-2 except that there is an option to randomise hyperfractionated radiotherapy versus conventional radiotherapy in patients who do not have complete tumour resection

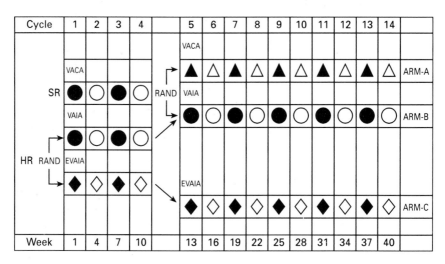

Fig 7.11 EICESS-92 chemotherapy schema. SR, standard risk (<100 ml, favourable response); HR, high risk (>100 ml). Local therapy, surgery or radiotherapy at 12 weeks

with clear histological margins. This is based on evidence that local control may be improved following hyperfractionated radiotherapy.[98]

Other areas to be studied are those of histological response to treatment, ifosfamide nephropathy, and late musculoskeletal effects of treatment. It is expected that this study will accrue at a rate of 150 patients per year and will need to be open for four to five years in order to answer the questions.

Metastatic disease

Historically, it has become evident that virtually all patients with Ewing's sarcoma have micrometastatic disease at presentation. As staging methodologies have improved, increasing numbers of patients are having metastatic disease recognised prior to initiation of therapy and this creates difficulties in trying to evaluate the impact of changes in therapy within a historical context. Nevertheless, it is clear that survival for patients with metastatic disease is greatly reduced when compared to concurrent patients treated on identical schedules.[90] There is evidence that small numbers of patients with pulmonary metastases can be treated successfully, but the outcome of patients with bony metastases is dismal. Historically, pulmonary radiation has been given when lung metastases have been identified, with relapse-free survival of 30% at three years[99] and the current EICESS trial recommends 15–18 Gy bilateral pulmonary irradiation.

This very poor outcome for patients with metastatic disease has led to the development of a number of more intensive treatment approaches using high dose chemotherapy or whole body irradiation with autologous or allogeneic marrow rescue. No firm consensus about the value of these approaches has emerged.[79 100–102]

The outcome for patients who relapse with Ewing's sarcoma is very poor. The current limited number of effective and active agents in Ewing's sarcoma means there is unlikely to be long term value in constructing complex regimes of unproven agents. Treatment for these patients should either be predominantly palliative or else patients could be considered for participation in new agents studies. There is little evidence that further surgery or radiotherapy is more than palliative although this may be of enormous individual benefit. There is an urgent need for planned studies or trials in relapsed patients.

Future directions

It is clear that Ewing's sarcoma and peripheral primitive neuroectodermal tumours (pPNET) are part of a spectrum of disease now called the Ewing's family of tumours.[103] These tumours are now largely defined by specific chimeric transcripts[22] representing balanced translocation between the *EWS* gene on chromosome 22 and either the *FLI1* gene on chromosome 11 or a similar gene for an Ets transcription factor family member on chromosome 21 called *ERG*.[104–106] These exciting discoveries allow for several future developments in both diagnostic evaluation and treatment of this family of tumours.

Firstly, current molecular biological techniques or RTPCR for these transcripts should allow for improved diagnosis of small round blue cell tumours, particularly if they can be combined with similar methodologies identifying small round cell tumours such as tyrosine hydroxylase in neuroblastoma.[107] These techniques also offer potentially sensitive methodologies for detection of occult metastatic disease. Secondly, the identification of different transcript sizes produced by apparently identical translocations raises the issue of whether different transcripts may reflect different biological activity and behaviour. There is no evidence to support this currently,[22 108] but further studies are needed.

The question arises[109] as to whether all pPNET tumours should be treated in the same way despite different phenotypes. My own view is that it would be sensible to treat these tumours in a similar fashion in order to try and truly identify prognostic factors within this family grouping.

Although it is to be expected that these recent exciting discoveries may help in diagnosis and grouping of patients, and may also help our understanding of mechanisms of malignancy, it is not yet clear how this may be translated into eventual therapies. Gene therapy remains a distant hope. More prosaically, advances in the outcome of Ewing's sarcoma in the short term are likely to continue to depend on careful multidisciplinary evaluation and improved supportive care. The availability of haematological growth factors and new harvesting technologies allow for the possibility of developing dose intensive schedules using peripheral blood progenitor cells as rescue and support and it is likely that these approaches will dominate the next few years of studies in high risk Ewing's sarcoma. For standard risk patients the focus will be on trying to improve long term outcome while at the same time trying to reduce late effects of renal and cardiac toxicity[110] or second malignancy. There is a need to identify new active agents in Ewing's sarcoma; it has recently been suggested that paclitaxel may have activity in this tumour.[111] Patients with relapsed or resistant disease should be considered for such studies.

1 Yorkshire Cancer Registry. *Report for the year 1991, including cancer statistics for 1984–1988.* Eds. Joslin C, Rider L, Round C. Leeds: Yorkshire Regional Cancer Organisation, 1991.
2 Draper GJ, Sanders BM, Kingston JE. Secondary primary tumours in patients with retinoblastoma. *Br J Cancer* 1986; 53: 661–71.
3 Friend S, Bernards R, Rogelji S *et al.* A human DNA segment with properties of the gene that predisposes to retinoblastoma and osteosarcoma. *Nature* 1986; 323: 643–6.
4 Teguchide J, Ishisaki K, Sesaki MS *et al.* Preferential mutation of paternally derived *RB* gene as the initial event in sporadic osteosarcoma. *Nature* 1989; 338: 156–8.
5 Birch JM, Hartley AL, Tricker KJ *et al.* Prevalence and diversity of constitutional mutations in the p53 gene among 21 Li–Fraumeni families. *Cancer Res* 1994; 54: 1298–304.
6 Miller CW, Aslo A, Tsay C *et al.* Frequency and structure of p53 rearrangements in human osteosarcoma. *Cancer Res* 1990; 50: 7950–4.
7 Diller L, Kassel J, Nelson CE *et al.* p53 functions as a cell cycle control protein in osteosarcomas. *Mol Cell Biol* 1990; 10: 5722–81.
8 Dahlin D, Unni K. Osteosarcoma of bone and its important recognizable varieties. *Am J Surg Pathol* 1977; 1: 61–72.

9 Newton WA, Meadow AT, Shuada H *et al.* Bone sarcomas as second malignant neoplasms following childhood cancer. *Cancer* 1991; **67**: 193–201.

10 Chan RC, Sutow WW, Lindberg RD *et al.* Management and results of localised Ewing's sarcoma. *Cancer* 1979; **43**: 1001–6.

11 Parkin DM, Stiller CA, Draper GJ, Bieber CA. The international incidence of childhood cancer. *Int J Cancer* 1988; **42**: 511–520.

12 Murphy LA Jr. Imaging bone tumours in the 1990s. *Cancer* 1991; **67**: 1169–76.

13 Meyers PA, Heller G, Healey J *et al.* Chemotherapy for non-metastatic osteogenic sarcoma: The Memorial Sloan-Kettering experience. *J Clin Oncol* 1992; **10**: 5–15.

14 Thorpe W, Reilly J, Rosenberg S. Prognostic significance of alkaline phosphatase measurements in patients with osteogenic sarcoma receiving chemotherapy. *Cancer* 1979; **43**: 2178–81.

15 Huvos AG. *Bone tumours: diagnosis, treatment and prognosis*, 2nd edition. Philadelphia: WB Saunders, 1991.

16 Clark J, Unni K, Dahlin D, Devine K. Osteosarcoma of the jaw. *Cancer* 1983 **51**: 2311–16.

17 Ayala AG, Ro JY, Papadopoules NK *et al.* Small cell osteosarcoma. *Cancer Treatment Res* 1993; **62**: 139–49.

18 Triche TJ. Pathology of pediatrics malignancies. In: Pizzo PA, Poplack DG, editors, *Principles and practice of paediatric oncology.* 2nd edition Philadelphi: JB Lippincott, 1993, 115–52.

19 Aurias A, Rimbaut C, Buffe D *et al.* Chromosomal translocations in Ewing's sarcoma. *N Engl J Med* 1983; **309**: 496–7.

20 Turc-Carel C, Philip I, Berger MP *et al.* Chromosomal translocations in Ewing's sarcoma. *N Engl J Med* 1983; **309**: 497–8.

21 Ambros IM, Ambros PF, Strehl S *et al. MIC2* is a specific marker for Ewing's sarcoma and peripheral primitive neuroectodermal tumours. *Cancer* 1991; **67**: 1886–93.

22 Delattre O, Zucman J, Melot *et al.* The Ewing's family of tumours—a subgroup of small-round-cell tumours defined by specific chimeric transcripts. *N Engl J Med* 1994; **331**: 294–9.

23 Ahuja S, Villacin A, Smith J *et al.* Juxtacortical (paraosteal) osteogenic osteosarcoma. *J Bone Joint Surg [AM]* 1977; **58**: 632–47.

24 Lee S, MacKenzie D. Osteosarcoma: A study of the value of preoperative megavoltage radiotherapy. *Br J Surg* 1964; **51**: 252–74.

25 Carter SK. The dilemma of adjuvant chemotherapy for osteogenic sarcoma. *Cancer Clin Trials* 1980; **3**: 29–36.

26 Carter EP, Holland JF, Wang JJ, Sinks LF. Doxorubicin in disseminated osteosarcoma. *JAMA* 1972; **221**: 1132–8.

27 Jaffe N, Farber S *et al.* Favourable response of metastatic osteogenic sarcoma to pulse high dose methotrexate with citrovorum rescue and radiation therapy. *Cancer* 1973; **31**: 1367–73.

28 Nitschke R, Starling KA, Vats J, Bryan H. *Cis*-diamine-dichloroplatinum (NSC-119875) in childhood malignancies. A Southwest Oncology Group Study. *Med Paediatr Oncol* 1978; **4**: 127–32.

29 Gasparini M, Rouesse J, van Oosteran A *et al.* Phase II study of cisplatin in advanced osteogenic sarcoma. *Cancer Treat Rep* 1985; **69**: 211–3.

30 Marti C, Kroner T, Remagen W *et al.* High dose ifosfamide in adjuvant osteosarcoma. *Cancer Treat Rep* 1985; **69**: 115–7.

31 Lewis IJ, Stevens MCG, Pearson A *et al.* Phase II study of carboplatin in children's tumours. *Proc Asco* 1993; **12**: 412 (abs. 1413).

32 Moseide C, Gutierrez M, Caparros B, Rosen G. Combination chemotherapy with bleomycin, cyclophosphamide and dactinomycin for the treatment of osteosarcoma. *Cancer* 1977; **40**: 2779–86.

33 Pratt CB, Epelman S, Jaffe N. Bleomycin, cyclophosphamide and dactinomycin in metastatic osteosarcoma; lack of tumour regression in previously treated patients. *Cancer Treat Rep* 1987; **71**: 421–3.

34 Cortes EP, Holland JF, Glidewell O. Amputation and adriamycin in primary osteo-sarcoma: A 5 year report. *Cancer Treat Rep* 1978; **62**: 201–7.

35 Jaffe N, Frei N, Traggis D, Bishop Y. Adjuvant methotrexate and citrovorum factor treatment of osteogenic sarcoma. *N Engl J Med* 1974; **291**: 994–7.

36 Sutow WW, Sullivan MP, Fernbach DJ *et al.* Adjuvant chemotherapy in primary

115

treatment of osteogenic sarcoma. A Southwest Oncology Group Study. *Cancer* 1975; **36**: 1598–602.

37 Taylor WF, Ivins JV, Dahlin DC *et al.* Trends and variability in survival from osteosarcoma. *Mayo Clinic Proc* 1978; **53**: 695–700.

38 Lange B, Levine A. Is it ethical not to conduct a prospectively controlled trial of adjuvant chemotherapy in osteosarcoma? *Cancer Treat Rep* 1982; **66**: 1699–704.

39 Link MP, Goorin AM, Miser AW *et al.* The effect of adjuvant chemotherapy on relapse free survival in patients with osteosarcoma of the extremity. *N Engl J Med* 1986; **314**: 1600–6.

40 Eilber F, Giuliano A, Eckard J *et al.* Adjuvant chemotherapy for osteosarcoma: A randomised prospective trial. *J Clin Oncol* 1987; **5**: 21–6.

41 Link MP. The multi-institutional osteosarcoma study—an update. *Cancer Treatment Res* 1993; **62**: 261–7.

42 Rosen G, Marcove RC, Caparros B *et al.* Primary osteogenic sarcoma. The rationale for pre-operative chemotherapy and delayed surgery. *Cancer* 1979; **43**: 2163–77.

43 Rosen G, Caparros B, Huvos AG *et al.* Pre-operative chemotherapy for osteogenic sarcoma: a selection of post-operative adjuvant chemotherapy based on the response of the primary tumour to pre-operative chemotherapy. *Cancer* 1982; **49**: 1221–30.

44 Rosen G. Pre-operative (neo-adjuvant) chemotherapy for osteogenic sarcoma: a ten year experience. *Orthopaedics* 1985; **8**: 659–64.

45 Huvos A, Rosen G, Marcove RC. Primary osteogenic sarcoma. Pathologic aspects in 20 patients after treatment with chemotherapy, en block resection and prosthetic bone replacement. *Arch Pathol Lab Med* 1977; **101**: 14–18.

46 Humphrey GB, Schraffordt Koops H, Molenaar, Postma A (eds). Osteosarcoma in adolescents and young adults: New developments and controversies. *Cancer Treat Res* 1993; **62**: 1–407.

47 Nachman JB. Controversies in the treatment of osteosarcoma. *Med J Austral* 1988; **148**: 105–10.

48 Sugarbaker PH, Berofsky I, Rosenberg SA *et al.* Quality of life assessment on patients in extremity sarcoma trials. *Surgery* 1982; **91**: 17–23.

49 Tebbi CK. Psychological effects of amputation in osteosarcoma. *Cancer Treatment Res* 1993; **62**: 39–44.

50 Provisor A, Nachman J, Krailo M *et al.* Treatment of non-metastatic osteogenic sarcoma of the extremities with pre and post-operative chemotherapy. *Proc Am Soc Clin Oncol* 1987; **6**: 217.

51 Winkler K, Beron G, Delling G *et al.* Neoadjuvant chemotherapy of osteosarcoma: Results of a randomised co-operative trial (COSS 82) with salvage chemotherapy based on histological tumour response. *J Clin Oncol* 1988; **6**: 329–77.

52 Bacci G, Picci P, Ruggieri P *et al.* Primary chemotherapy and delayed surgery (neoadjuvant chemotherapy) for osteosarcoma of the extremities. The Istituto Rizzoli experience in 127 patients treated pre-operatively with intravenous methotrexate (high versus moderate doses) and intra-arterial cisplatin. *Cancer* 1990; **65**: 2539–53.

53 Medical Research Council (MRC). A trial of chemotherapy in patients with osteo-sarcoma (a report to the Medical Research Council by their Working Party on Bone Sarcomas). *Br J Cancer* 1986; **53**: 513–8.

54 Burgers JMV, Van Glabbeke M, Busson A *et al.* Osteosarcoma of the limbs: report of the EORTC-SIOP 03 trial 20781 investigating the value of adjuvant treatment with chemotherapy and/or prophylactic lung irradiation. *Cancer* 1988; **5**: 1024–31.

55 Ettinger LJ, Douglass HO, Higby DJ *et al.* Adjuvant adriamycin and cis-diamine dichlorplatinum (cis-platinum) in primary osteosarcoma. *Cancer* 1981; **47**: 248–54.

56 Bramwell VHC, Burgers M, Sneath R *et al.* A comparison of two short intensive adjuvant chemotherapy regimens in operable osteosarcoma of limbs in children and young adults: The first study of the European Osteosarcoma Intergroup. *J Clin Oncol* 1992; **10**: 1579–91.

57 Ornadel D, Souhami RL, Whelan J *et al.* Doxorubicin and cisplatin with granulocyte colony-stimulating factor as adjuvant chemotherapy for osteosarcoma: Phase II trial of the European Osteosarcoma Intergroup. *J Clin Oncol* 1994; **12**: 1842–8.

58 Perez C, Herson J, Kimball JC *et al.* Prognosis after metastasis in osteosarcoma. *Cancer Clin Trials* 1978; **1**(4): 315–20.

59 Spanos PK, Payne WS, Ivino JC *et al.* Pulmonary resection for metastatic osteogenic sarcoma: *J Bone Joint Surg* 1976; **58A**: 624–8.

60 Han MT, Telander RL, Pairolero PC *et al.* Aggressive thoracotomy for pulmonary metastatic osteogenic sarcoma in children and young adolescents. *J Pediatr Surg* 1981; **16**: 928–33.
61 Putnam JB Jr, Roth JA, Wesley MN, Johnston MR, Rosenberg SA. Survival following aggressive resection of pulmonary metastases from osteogenic sarcoma. Analysis of prognostic factors. *Ann Thorac Surg* 1983; **36**: 516–23.
62 Meyer WH, Schell MJ, Mahesh Kumar AP *et al.* Thoracotomy for pulmonary metastatic osteosarcoma. An analysis of prognostic indicators of survival. *Cancer* 1987; **59**: 374–9.
63 Ward WG, Mikaelian K, Dorcy F *et al.* Pulmonary metastases of stage IIB extremity osteosarcoma and subsequent pulmonary metastases. *J Clin Oncol* 1994; **12**: 1949–58.
64 Morgan E, Baum E, Bleyer WA. Treatment of patients with metastatic osteogenic sarcoma. A report from the Children's Cancer Study Group. *Cancer Treat Rep* 1984; **68**: 661–4.
65 Miser JS, Kinsella TJ, Triche TJ *et al.* Ifosfamide with mesna uroprotection and etoposide: an effective regimen in the treatment of recurrent sarcomas and other tumours of children and young adults. *J Clin Oncol* 1987; **5**: 1191–8.
66 Edmonson JH, Green SJ, Ivins JC *et al.* A controlled pilot study of high-dose methotrexate as post-surgical adjuvant treatment for primary osteosarcoma. *J Clin Oncol* 1984; **2**: 152–6.
67 Gren JL, King SA, Wittes RE, Leyland-Jones B. The role of methotrexate in osteosarcoma. *J Natl Cancer Inst* 1988; **80**: 626–56.
68 Delepine N, Delepine G, Jasmin C *et al.* Importance of age and methotrexate dosage: Prognosis in children and young adults with high grade osteosarcoma. *Biomed Pharmacother* 1988; **42**: 257–62.
69 Graf N, Winkler K, Betlomovic M, Fuchs N, Bode U. Methotrexate pharmacokinetics and prognosis in osteosarcoma. *J Clin Oncol* 1994; **12**: 1443–51.
70 Jaffe N, Knapp J, Chuang VP *et al.* Osteosarcoma, intra-arterial treatment of the primary tumour with cis-diaminnedichloroplatinum-II (CDP). Angiographic, pathologic and pharmacologic studies. *Cancer* 1983; **51**: 402–7.
71 Winkler K, Bielack S, Delling G *et al.* Effect of intra-arterial versus intravenous cisplatin in addition to systemic doxorubicin, high-dose methotrexate and ifosfamide on histologic tumour response in osteosarcoma (Study COSS-86). *Cancer* 1990; **66**: 1703–10.
72 Ewing J. Diffuse endotheloma of bone. *Proc NY Pathol Soc* 1921; **21**: 17–24.
73 Wang CC, Schultz MD. Ewing's sarcoma. *N Engl J Med* 1953; **248**: 571–6.
74 Chan RC, Sutow WW, Lindberg RD *et al.* Management and results of localized Ewing's sarcoma. *Cancer* 1979; **43**: 1001–6.
75 Samuels ML, Howe CD. Cyclophosphamide in the management of Ewing's sarcoma. *Cancer* 1967; **20**: 961–6.
76 Sutow WW, Vietti TJ, Fernbach DL *et al.* Evaluation of chemotherapy in children with metastatic Ewing's sarcoma and osteogenic sarcoma. *Cancer Chemother Rep* 1971; **55**: 67–78.
77 Senyszyn JJ, Johnson RE, Curren RE. Treatment of metastatic Ewing's sarcoma with actinomycin D (NSC-3053). *Cancer Chemother Rep* 1970; **54**: 103.
78 Oldham RK, Pomeroy TC. Treatment of Ewing's sarcoma with Adriamycin (NSC-123127). *Cancer Chemother Rep* 1972; **56**: 635–9.
79 Cornbleet MA, Corringham RET, Prentice HG *et al.* Treatment of Ewing's sarcoma with high dose Melphalan and autologous bone marrow transplantation *Cancer Treat Rep* 1981; **65**: 241–4.
80 De Kraker J, Voute PA. Ifosfamide and vincristine in paediatric tumours. A Phase I study. *Eur Paediatr Haematol Oncol* 1984; **1**: 47–50.
81 Magrath IT, Sandlund J, Raynor A *et al.* A Phase II study of ifosfamide in the treatment of recurrent sarcomas in young people. *Cancer Chemother Pharmacol* 1986; **18**(suppl): 525–8.
82 Nesbit ME, Gehan EA, Burgert EO *et al.* Multimodal therapy of primary non-metastatic Ewing's sarcoma of bone: a long term follow up of the first Intergroup study. *J Clin Oncol* 1990; **8**: 1664–74.
83 Burgert EO, Nesbit ME, Garnsley LA *et al.* Multimodal therapy for the management of non-pelvic localised Ewing's sarcoma of bone: Intergroup Study IESS-11. *J Clin Oncol* 1990; **8**: 1514–24.
84 Bacci G, Toni A, Avella M *et al.* Long term results in 144 localised Ewing's sarcoma patients treated with combined therapy. *Cancer* 1981; **63**: 1477–86.

117

85 Rosen G, Caparros B, Nirenberg A *et al*. Ewing's sarcoma. Ten year experience with adjuvant chemotherapy. *Cancer* 1981; 47: 2204–13.

86 Oberlin O, Patte C, Demeocq F *et al*. The repsonse to initial chemotherapy as a prognostic factor in localised Ewing's sarcoma. *Eur J Cancer Clin Oncol* 1985; 21: 463–7.

87 Jurgens H, Exner U, Gadner H *et al*. Multidisciplinary treatment of Ewing's sarcoma of bone. A 6 year experience of a European cooperative trial. *Cancer* 1988; 61: 23–32.

88 Jurgens H, Bier V, Dunst J *et al*. Die GPO Cooperativen Ewing-Sarkom Studien CESS81/86: Bericht nach $6\frac{1}{2}$ Jahren. *Klin Padiatr* 1988; 200: 243–52.

89 Jurgens H, Donaldson SS, Gobel U. Ewing's sarcoma. In: Voute PA, Barrett A, Lemerle J, eds, *Cancer in children*, UICC 3rd ed., New York: Springer-Verlag, 1992, 295–313.

90 Craft AW, Cotterill S, Imeson J. Improvement in survival for Ewing's sarcoma by substitution of ifosfamide for cyclophosphamide. *AM J Pediatr Hematol Oncol* 1993; 15(suppl A): 531–35.

91 Evans RG, Nesbit ME, Gehan EA *et al*. Multimodal therapy for the management of localised Ewing's sarcoma of pelvis and sacral bones: A report from the second intergroup study. *J Clin Oncol* 1991; 9: 1173–80.

92 Dunst J, Saver R, Burgers JMV *et al*. Radiation therapy as local treatment in Ewing's sarcoma. Results of the co-operative Ewing's sarcoma studies CESS 81 and CESS 82. *Cancer* 1991; 67: 2818–25.

93 Pritchard DJ. Surgical experience in the management of Ewing's sarcoma of bone. *Natl Cancer Inst Monogr* 1981; 56: 169–71.

94 Kinsella TJ, Lichter AS, Miser J *et al*. Local treatment of Ewing's sarcoma; radiation therapy versus surgery. *Cancer Treat Rep* 1984; 68: 695–701.

95 Horowitz ME, Neff JR, Kun LE. Ewing's sarcoma; radiotherapy versus surgery for local control. In: Horowitz ME, Pizzo P (eds), *Pediatr Clin N Amer—Solid Tumours in Children*. 1991; 38: 365.

96 Razek A, Perez CA, Tefft M. Intergroup Ewing's sarcoma study. Local control related to radiation dose, volume and site of primary lesion in Ewing's sarcoma. *Cancer* 1980; 46: 516–21.

97 Evans RG, Nesbit ME, Askin F *et al*. Local recurrence, rate and sites of metastases and time to relapse as a function of treatment regimen, size of primary and surgical history in 62 patients presenting with non-metastatic Ewing's sarcoma of the pelvic bone. *Int J Radiat Oncol Biol Phys* 1985; 11: 129.

98 Marcus RB Jr, Cantor A, Heare TC *et al*. Local control and function after twice-a-day radiation therapy for Ewing's sarcoma. *Int J Radiat Oncol Biol Phys* 1991; 21: 1509–15.

99 Vietti TJ, Gehan EA, Nesbit ME *et al*. Multimodal therapy in metastatic Ewing's sarcoma. An Intergroup study. *Natl Cancer Inst Monogr* 1981; 56: 279–84.

100 Pinkerton R, Philip T, Bouffet F *et al*. Autologous bone marrow transplantation in paediatric solid tumours. *Clin Hematol* 1986; 15: 187–203.

101 Marcus RB, Graham-Pole JR, Springfield DS *et al*. High risk Ewing's sarcoma: End intensification using autologous bone marrow transplantation. *Int J Radiat Oncol Biol Phys* 1988; 15: 53–9.

102 Burdach S, Jurgens H, Peters C *et al*. Myeloablative radiochemotherapy and haematopoietic stem cell rescue in poor prognosis Ewing's sarcoma. *J Clin Oncol* 1993; 11: 1482–8.

103 Horowitz ME, Malawer MM, Delaney TF, Tsokos MG. Ewing's sarcoma family of tumours: Ewing's sarcoma of bone and soft tissue and the peripheral primitive neuroectodermal tumours: p795-821 In: Pizzo PA, Poplack DG, eds, *Principles and practice of pediatric oncology*, 2nd edn, Philadelphia: JB Lippincott, 1993, 795–821.

104 Delattre O, Zucman J, Plougastel B *et al*. Gene fusion with an ETS DNA-landing domain caused by chromosome translocation in human tumours. *Nature* 1992; 359: 162–5.

105 Zucman J, Melot T, Desmaze C *et al*. Combinational generation of variable fusion proteins in the Ewing family of tumours. *EMBO J* 1993; 12: 4481–7.

106 Zucman J, Delattre O, Desmaze C *et al*. Cloning and characterisation of the Ewing's sarcoma and peripheral neuroepithelioma t(11:22) translocation breakpoints. *Genes Chromosom Cancer* 1992; 5: 271–7.

107 Burchill SA, Bradbury FM, Smith B, Lewis IJ, Selby P. Neuroblastoma cell detection by reverse transcriptase-polymerase chain reaction (RT-PCR) for tyrosine hydroxylase mRNA. *Int J Canc* 1994; 57: 671–5.

108 Downing JR, Head DR, Parham DM *et al*. Detection of the (11:22) (q24:q12)

translation of Ewing's sarcoma and peripheral neuroectodermal tumour by reverse transcriptase polymerase chain reaction. *Am J Pathol* 1993; **143**: 1294–300.

109 Kretschmar CS. Ewing's sarcoma and the "peanut" tumours. *N Eng J Med* 1994; **331**: 325–7.

110 Hale JP, Lewis IJ. Anthracyclines: cardiotoxicity and its prevention. *Arch Dis Child* 1994; **71**: 457–62.

111 Hurwitz CA, Relling MV, Weightman SD *et al*. Phase I trial of Paclitaxel in children with refractory solid tumours; A Paediatric Oncology Group Study. *J Clin Oncol* 1993; **11**: 2324–29.

8: Costs and benefits of limb salvage surgery for osteosarcoma

ROBERT J GRIMER

Introduction

Osteosarcoma is a rare primary sarcoma of bone. Approximately 120 cases occur every year in the United Kingdom, the majority being in adolescents with the most common age being 14 years. Boys are slightly more commonly affected than girls. The tumour is presumed to have a peak incidence in adolescents because of the growth spurt which naturally arises at this stage and the potential for disordered growth.[1]

Osteosarcoma used to be considered to be a highly malignant disease, with over 80% mortality despite immediate amputation. The advent of chemotherapy treatment for this condition in the 1970s[2,3] dramatically changed the prognosis of the condition so that now around 60% of cases will be "cured".[4] In the United Kingdom a number of consecutive trials have been carried out under the auspices of the Medical Research Council (MRC) to assess different chemotherapy regimes and the presently favoured regime is one comprising six cycles of cisplatin and doxorubicin at intervals of three weeks.[5]

Coupled with these advances in chemotherapy have come changes in the surgical management of osteosarcoma. Limb salvage surgery is now routinely considered for most cases of osteosarcoma. This type of surgery is complex and expensive, and recognition of this fact has led the UK Department of Health to provide supraregional funding to two centres where this type of surgery is carried out (one in London and the other in Birmingham).

Limb salvage surgery has now been an option for well over 15 years and longer term results are becoming available. It is now possible to stand back and consider whether this type of procedure is cost effective.

Principles of surgical resection

- The tumour must be resectable with a "wide" surgical margin
- Any reconstruction must be effective, durable and relatively free of complications
- Amputation should be considered if the above criteria cannot be satisfied.

Surgical options

The most common site for osteosarcoma to arise is around the knee joint, with 35% of tumours being in the distal femur, 25% in the proximal tibia, and 12% in the proximal humerus. Other sites in order of decreasing frequency are pelvis, fibula, proximal femur, forearm bones, distal tibia, and ribs.

Oncological control is the most important aspect of the surgeon's role. Enneking[6] clearly showed that local control of the tumour was related to adequacy of surgical excision, and this in turn has been shown to be related to response to chemotherapy. It is now standard practice for all patients with osteosarcoma to be offered preoperative chemotherapy with surgery normally taking place after some seven to nine weeks of chemotherapy. In the majority of cases there will be evidence of some necrosis of the tumour with a decrease in peritumoural oedema and clear definition of the margins of the tumour. Despite this it is essential for the surgery to be performed by an experienced orthopaedic oncologist who has carried out careful staging of the tumour and is fully aware of the extent of the tumour in bone and soft tissue. Local recurrence of the tumour implies failure of local control by the surgeon. It is very frequently associated with systemic relapse implying failure of chemotherapy. The aim of the surgical procedure is, however, to achieve sufficient margins to prevent local recurrence no matter what the response to chemotherapy.

Amputation should offer a safer oncological margin than limb salvage, but regrettably this is not always the case. For a proximal tibial tumour an amputation at the site of election in mid thigh will almost always give a satisfactory oncological and functional result, but for the distal femoral tumour very careful assessment of the extent of the tumour needs to be carried out to choose the appropriate level of amputation. This has been clearly shown in a large study by Simon *et al.* who compared the results of limb salvage surgery with amputation for osteosarcoma of the distal femur (Table 8.1)[7]. They showed that, whilst there is an increased risk of local recurrence for patients with limb salvage, this was almost matched by the rate of local recurrence for patients with above-knee amputation. The only way to avoid this complication was to carry out a disarticulation of the hip—a procedure with even greater loss of function than an above-knee amputation. Interestingly the overall rate of metastases and the overall survival rate was not statistically different between all three groups, suggesting that there was possibly no increased risk to life of local

Table 8.1 Rates of local recurrence, metastases and death following surgery for osteosarcoma of the distal femur (from Simon *et al*)[7]

	Limb salvage	Above-knee amputation	Disarticulation at hip
Number	73	115	39
Local recurrence (%)	11	8	0
Metastases (%)	59	57	54
Dead (%)	45	42	46

recurrence. We have found that local recurrence of a tumour following limb salvage surgery is far more likely to arise in patients who have responded poorly to preoperative chemotherapy than in those who have responded well. The effect of chemotherapy is far more significant than the effect of surgical margins at predicting the risk of local recurrence, a finding confirmed in work from Campannacci's unit in Bologna.[8]

Weighing up what is best for any individual patient is a difficult task and has to be done with the fully informed patient. In an adolescent the conflict between preservation of body image and possible consideration of more vigorous function from an amputation needs to be openly discussed. Seeing other patients who have had the proposed surgical treatment is also helpful.

Following resection of the tumour, reconstruction is only required if a non-expendable bone is involved. Unfortunately most osteosarcomas involve structural bones that require replacement. Tumours of the fibula, scapula, and ribs simply require excision with no reconstruction but most other sites will need some form of reconstruction to restore function.

Advantages of amputation as a primary treatment for osteosarcoma

- Once and for all operation (apart from minor refashioning of stump)
- Good functional results of below-knee amputee
- Contact sports possible
- Exoprostheses are expendable

Disadvantages of amputation as a primary treatment for osteosarcoma

- Loss of body image
- Phantom pain
- Problems with limb fitting very common
- Functional results worse the more proximal the amputation
- Many patients never wear an artificial limb
- Stump problems not infrequent
- Continued attendance at limb fitting centre necessary

Methods of reconstruction

- Arthrodesis
- Rotationplasty
- Allograft
- Endoprosthesis

The original methods involved arthrodesis,[9] but the functional results were poor and there was a high complication rate and a long time to full recovery. Rotationplasty has proved popular in Europe for tumours of the distal femur.[10] It involves resection of the whole of the distal half of the thigh apart from the sciatic nerve which is "filleted" out of the back of the leg. The upper tibia is then fixed to the femur and the vessels anastamosed. The leg, however, is rotated 180° in the process so that the foot now points backwards and the ankle is positioned at the level of the knee. The ankle now works like a knee and the patient can be fitted with the equivalent of a below-knee prosthesis, maintaining active extension. The results of this reconstruction are impressive functionally but are often not acceptable cosmetically.

Allografts are popular in North America and have "biological" appeal.[11] Unfortunately there are significant problems with their use, particularly in high grade sarcomas where patients require chemotherapy. There is a very high early complication rate with infection and non-union occurring regularly and 50% of patients will require reoperation within the first year. In the lower limb protected weightbearing must be maintained until union has occurred, often well beyond six months. It was hoped that the long term results of this technique would be good, but unfortunately late complications continue to arise.[12 13]

The preferred method of limb salvage in our centre is with endoprosthetic replacements. This work was first reported by Jackson Burrows in 1975 and increasing experience has been gained over the years.[14–16]

Advantages of endoprosthetic replacement

- Preservation of the limb with distal function
- No disturbance of body image
- Reliable and predictable reconstruction
- Customised to individual patient
- Rapid postoperative recovery
- Socially more acceptable
- Possibility to revert to amputation if it fails
- Improvements in biomechanical engineering result in better endoprosthetic designs and hopefully better results
- Surgery needs to be carried out in specialist centres (hence likelihood of better oncological and functional result)
- Cost effective

> ## Disadvantages of endoprosthetic replacement
>
> - Failure of the implant and further surgery eventually inevitable (except in upper limb or the elderly)
> - Patient needs to protect the implant from trauma and infection
> - Contact sports are not recommended
> - Surgery needs to be carried out in specialist centres (problems with travel and follow-up)

It is now possible to replace all or part of the femur or humerus and to replace portions of the tibia, ulna, radius, and pelvis. In children it is possible to insert customised implants which can be extended during the period of growth to allow the operated limb to maintain an equal length with the normal side. The sites of the various endoprostheses inserted at Birmingham over the past 20 years are indicated in Table 8.2.

The great variety of implants described in Table 8.2 demonstrates the versatility of endoprosthetic replacements. Subject always to the requirement that the tumour must be resected, as much bone and soft tissue will normally be salvaged as possible in order to preserve function of the operated limb. Preservation of joints whenever possible is desirable and even short segment fixation of implants is recommended. We have secured all of our endoprostheses to bone with methylmethacrylate cement and intramedullary fixation.

Replacing any bone with an artificial implant is potentially fraught with problems. This was first discovered with total hip replacement in young adults where failure rates of the implant as high as 57% at five years have been reported.[17] In Dorr's recent paper looking at cemented total hip replacements in otherwise fit people under the age of 30, he found that 42% of the hips had been revised at an average of 9·5 years and 56% of the remaining hips had impending failure.[18] Results for knee replacements in a

Table 8.2 The sites and numbers of endoprostheses inserted at the Royal Orthopaedic Hospital Oncology service up to 1993

Site	Number	Extendable
Distal femur	279	63
Proximal tibia	149	36
Proximal femur	143	6
Proximal humerus	65	4
Pelvis	28	
Total femur	23	2
Total humerus	18	6
Mid femur	15	
Distal humerus	7	
Mid tibia	3	
Distal tibia	3	
Distal radius	2	
Proximal ulna	2	
Mid humerus	1	

young population are not readily available—it would be expected that such a high failure rate would result that total knee replacement is vary rarely indicated in a young person and arthrodesis would normally be preferred. In tumour cases, however, the only alternative to limb salvage is usually amputation and, provided patients are fully informed about the possible outcome of this surgery, the vast majority will opt for limb salvage with an endoprosthetic replacement. The more proximal the site of the tumour the more compelling is the case for limb preservation, the more distal in the lower limb the easier it is to justify amputation.

Functional results

One of the principal indications for limb salvage surgery is the ability to produce a better functional result than would be achieved by amputation. Unfortunately, information about the overall level of achievement of young amputees is not readily available. The well-publicised results of amputees who participate widely and compete in the Paralympics is matched by an equal number who suffer from persistent phantom limb pain and have continuing problems with their prostheses, often to the extent that the artificial limb is left in the cupboard apart from the annual visit to the limb fitting centre.

In general, the more distal the level of amputation the better the functional result that is likely to be achieved. Unfortunately, most bone tumours arise proximally in the limbs and hence high levels of amputation are required. A below-knee amputation produces an extremely successful result in most cases, but is only suitable for the 1% of osteosarcoma patients with tumours of the distal tibia. For tumours of the proximal tibia an above-knee amputation at the site of election 13 cm above the knee can be achieved, and these patients often do well. For distal femoral tumours, as has been shown already, above-knee amputation risks local recurrence and often only a short stump will be left. Alternatively a disarticulation of the hip is required and this produces a poor result with an artificial limb, many young people preferring not to use their prosthesis. Tumours of the proximal femur or proximal humerus require disarticulation of the hip or shoulder respectively and in some circumstances may need hindquarter or forequarter amputation. Hindquarter amputation was described by Sir Gordon Gordon-Taylor in 1935 as "the greatest immolument ever performed on the human skeleton".[19] In the upper limb artificial limbs for proximal amputations are cumbersome and are often used simply for cosmesis.

It is important to assess the functional result of any limb salvage procedure. In 1987 Enneking established what has become the international scale of assessment for functional results in limb salvage.[20] This standard can be used for any joint in the body. Seven different factors are assessed: motion, pain, stability, deformity, strength, functional activity, and emotional acceptance. Each factor is scored either excellent (5), good

Table 8.3 Functional outcome following endoprosthetic replacement at various body sites

	Number	Excellent (%)	Good (%)	Fair (%)	Poor (%)
Proximal humerus	26	4	88	4	4
Proximal femur	31	6	68	26	0
Distal femur	71	39	52	6	3
Proximal tibia	32	16	45	36	3
Total	160	23	59	15	3

(3), fair (1), or poor (0). The maximum overall score is thus 35 points, which implies completely normal functioning. The overall results for a group of patients can then be classified as excellent, good, fair, or poor. This system allows a comparison to be made between patients with different types of limb salvage surgery. Although not perfect it is a useful but not infallible tool.

The results of limb salvage surgery will vary from centre to centre and with the type of reconstruction used. We have recently surveyed a large group of survivors of limb salvage surgery at our centre and assessed their functional outcome (Table 8.3).

Overall 82% of patients had a good or excellent result, implying near normality with some restrictions. All patients are advised to limit themselves to non-contact sports and to avoid running or high impact activities. This advice is often not well received, with many adolescent patients being keen sports players who resent having this activity taken away from them.

The fair results in this group come from patients with replacements of the proximal tibia and proximal femur. In both circumstances it is the lack of muscle control that causes the lower scores. At the hip, the abductors are of prime importance in producing a Trendelenburg negative gait. Following limb salvage surgery these muscles are necessarily detached from the femur and require reinsertion to another muscle group, usually the fascia lata. In older patients in particular the abductors never regain their full power and the patient is left with a limp, although this can be abolished by the use of a stick. This combination will give a fair result. At the proximal tibia, resection will involve detachment of the patella tendon and this will cause problems with knee extension despite a variety of ingenious methods being used to reinsert this. Most patients will still walk with a limp and have difficulty with stairs; they often have to back-knee into slight hyper-extension to lock the knee so they can walk well.

The poor results are due to failure of the prosthesis. The most common and serious cause of failure is infection. The overall incidence of this complication is about 6%, with the vast majority being due to bloodborne infection remote from the time of surgery. It may be due to neutropaenia and sepsis secondary to chemotherapy, but it can also originate from infected central lines and later on from such simple things as an infected

126

ingrowing toenail or a urinary tract infection. All patients with a metal implant are warned of this hazard and are advised to commence antibiotics at the least sign of potential infection. Infection results in pain, swelling, and stiffness and frequently produces a discharging sinus. It can be cured by a two-stage revision, but this is costly and time consuming for the patient. Prevention is very much better than cure.

Failure of endoprostheses

The other causes of failure are implant failure and mechanical loosening. Failure of the implants we currently use is rare, with stem breakage being less than 1%. Wear of the polyethylene bushes surrounding the axle is not uncommon and requires a small operation to replace these—a sort of 30 000 mile service. Frank loosening of the prosthesis also tends to occur with the passage of time and this is not unexpected. Major failure will result in decreasing mobility and increasing symptomatology, resulting in a lower functional score and eventually the patient will require a revision of the implant. This is to be expected in the vast majority of long term survivors. The loose component is removed and replaced with a new one. It will involve a further hospital stay and further time off work but fortunately the functional results following revision usually return to a similar level as the initial implant. The younger the patient at the time of the initial surgery the greater risk of subsequent revision being necessary (Figure 8.1).

In children with growth remaining in the skeleton, allowance has to be made for use of an extensible prosthesis. These can be periodically extended throughout the time of the child's treatment to maintain the limb length of

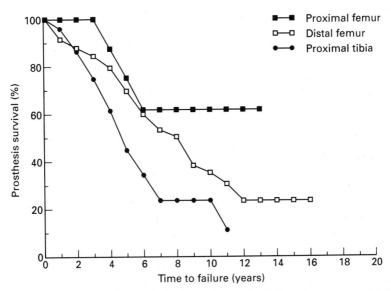

Fig 8.1 Graph showing the survival of an endoprosthesis from insertion until failure (either revision or amputation) in adolescents (<20 years)

the operated limb with that of the opposite limit. One of the problems of operating on the immature skeleton, however, is that the bone which has the intramedullary stem inserted into it will continue to increase in diameter as well as length and this will inevitably lead to loosening of the implant at an early age. For any child or adolescent with a lower limb implant at least one major revision of the implant will be necessary within a few years of completion of growth. The data available to date does not indicate whether these revisions will last as long as implants inserted de novo into adults of a similar age.

One problem for children with extensible prostheses is the repeated hospitalisation necessary for the lengthening procedures. Some children undergo 12 lengthenings over a period of years, and each of these procedures requires a general anaesthetic. The majority of children seem to adapt very well to these repeated spells of hospitalisation. Although the hospital stay is only 48 hours, some time will also be lost from school. The effects of this have not been quantified, nor have the psychological aspects been investigated. It is hoped that a non-invasive lengthening device will be developed in the future, possibly powered by an external electromagnetic field, and this would of course be a much better solution. In contrast, children with amputations will require new sockets or prostheses just as often as they would normally need a new pair of shoes. During the growth spurt an artificial limb may become obsolete almost as soon as it has been manufactured, and this entails frequent time-consuming visits to the limb fitting centres.

Finally, the long term effects of a large metallic implant (largely titanium but some cobalt–chrome) in the body have yet to be evaluated. There is often local staining of tissues, and analysis of this confirms large amounts of metal ions. Whether these are transported further round the body, or whether they have any immunological or teratogenic effect, is still unknown.

Quality of life

Health has been defined by the World Health Organization as "a state of complete physical, psychological and social well being". Any adolescent who has gone through the rigours of being diagnosed and treated for a childhood malignancy will be scarred in some way, but the aim of limb salvage surgery is to minimise this as far as possible. Quality of life studies have been used to assess this.

This chapter makes no attempt to cover the broad and contentious issue of quality of life studies. Many different methods of assessment can be used, all with different advantages and disadvantages. Some have been shown to give reproducible results and others not. Many quality of life studies are limited in their application, being aimed specifically at assessing particular diseases, and hence these studies cannot be used for other conditions.

Furthermore, most studies have been exclusively of adults and hence neither the results nor the technique can be reliably used in adolescents.

The EORTC (European Organization for Research and Treatment of Cancer) has made extensive use of a quality of life questionnaire (the EORTC QLQ-C30) which is a well tested tool specific for patients in cancer trials. It has been widely used and has shown excellent levels of reliability and cross-cultural validity.[21][22] It takes only 10 minutes to complete, and has a high level of patient acceptance. A slightly extended version of this form is currently being piloted in a quality of life study of patients greater than 16 years of age with osteosarcoma in four centres in Europe.

The information that is currently available from quality of life assessments for patients with limb salvage is scanty. Sugarbaker was the first to make this sort of assessment in patients who had undergone limb salvage as opposed to amputation for soft tissue sarcomas.[23] The limb salvage group had undergone surgical excision of the tumour followed by high dose radiotherapy, whereas the amputees had undergone the appropriate level of amputation. All the patients had had chemotherapy. The study concluded that there was remarkably little difference between the two groups. The only significant difference was in sexual functioning, which was worse in the limb salvage group. It was thought that this may have been due to decreased spermatogenesis or possibly limited lower limb mobility, both following radiotherapy.

Weddington *et al* have looked specifically at psychological outcome in survivors of extremity sarcoma treated by amputation or limb salvage.[24] Overall there was remarkably little difference between the two groups, and it was concluded that no statistical advantage of limb salvage surgery could be shown compared to amputation.

Postma *et al* looked at 33 patients with lower extremity bone cancer and compared the 14 with limb salvage to the 19 with amputation.[25] They were looking at a much younger group than Sugarbaker, with a median age of 26, and were reviewing them at a median of 10 years from treatment. After extensive testing, Postma's group could also find no significant difference between the two groups but the patients with limb salvage reported more physical complaints (job resettlement, for example) whilst the amputees showed a trend towards lower self esteem and isolation in their social life. It was concluded that limb salvage had a cosmetic advantage over amputation if no other.

Finally, Harris's paper looked specifically at function after surgery for tumours above the knee and analysed walking speed and oxygen consumption in patients who had had amputation, arthrodesis, or arthroplasty.[26] He found no difference between the three groups but identified that patients who had undergone amputation were the most active and least concerned about damaging their limb, whilst patients with arthrodesis performed more demanding physical work but had difficulty sitting. The patients with arthroplasties were more sedentary and protective of their limb but were least self conscious. Harris concluded that either there was no psychological or physical difference between the three groups or that the means of assessing it simply were not sensitive enough.

It is interesting to mention two studies which have looked specifically at the problems of adjustment to amputation in adolescents. Boyle's paper of 1982[27] compared patients with amputation due to malignancy with a group who underwent amputation for trauma. On the whole the group with malignancy had adjusted better to their disability and were leading full and productive lives. They were not without problems, however, with difficulties being experienced in mobility and sport and with 34% experiencing regular discomfort from their artificial limb. Forty-six percent found that the limb needed frequent repair and 33% stated that the artificial limb did not meet their expectations, often limiting their choice of clothing or making them unsightly.

Tebbi in 1989[28] assessed a different group and found that only 58% wore their artificial limb. Most patients had adjusted their lifestyle to match their disability, and overall their approach to their amputation was positive.

The overall conclusion from this group of studies is that patients with musculoskeletal tumours of the limbs will adjust well no matter whether they have limb salvage surgery or amputation. It is constantly surprising that no significant difference can be shown between the two groups on quality of life scores. This may indeed be because there is no difference between the two groups or because the instruments used to assess this are not sensitive enough. It is most probably a combination of these and the fact that most survivors of childhood cancer are on the whole fairly stoical and accept their lot.

The overall conclusion of this review is that:
- there is no convincing evidence that the oncological outcome is worse following limb salvage surgery
- there is no convincing evidence that the quality of life is better following limb salvage surgery

Costs of limb salvage

The costs of treating patients are becoming increasingly important to quantify and in some circumstances to assess the cost/benefit ratio.

Some of the costs are easy to quantify, some virtually impossible. Some will be identical whether the patient undergoes limb salvage or amputation. The costs of staging, biopsy, chemotherapy, and oncological follow up will be the same for both groups. At current prices this will amount to about £10 000. The costs for all the other aspects will be different and will depend partly on the site of the tumour and the age of the patient. The following calculations are made for a skeletally mature adult with a tumour of the lower femur.

Costs involved in treating a patient with osteosarcoma

- Staging
- Biopsy
- Chemotherapy
- Surgical treatment of tumour
- Prosthesis costs (internal or external)
- Rehabilitation
- Oncological follow up
- Treatment of complications
- Alterations to lifestyle

Surgical treatment

The costs of this will be related to length of stay in hospital and theatre time. An amputation on average will require two hours of theatre time (£250 an hour) and 12 days in hospital (£250 a day). A limb salvage operation needs 4 hours of theatre time and 14 days in hospital. On average an amputation costs £3500 and limb salvage £4500.

Prosthesis costs

The custom-made prostheses used at our centre are all manufactured at the Department of Biomedical Engineering in Stanmore, part of the University of London. They have many years of experience and their products are in fact cheaper than many commercially available and less well tried implants. The costs of the relevant implant should be added to the surgical costs.

The cost of artificial limbs is not so readily available. An approximation (personal communication) suggests that a below-knee prosthesis costs £1000 (but these are virtually never adequate for patients with osteo-sarcoma); an above-knee one costs about £2000, and a hip disarticulation prosthesis may be as much as £4000. For servicing, an allowance of £1000 per year will cover the repair and replacement of an above-knee prosthesis. Most patients will have two prostheses supplied within the first year and for an above-knee amputation the cost is thus £4000 in the first year with servicing being £1000 per year. In the private sector costs are easier to come by. For a below-knee amputee a commercial company will charge £3500 with further servicing costs being 50% in the second year, 30% in the third, and 50% in the fourth; then a completely new prosthesis will be

---

Costs of implants

• Proximal femoral replacement	£1650
• Distal femoral replacement	£2600
• Total femoral replacement	£3310
• Extensible distal femur	£3750

---

needed. Thus, for a below-knee amputation the costs would be £8050 over a four year period. For an above-knee prosthesis the original cost is nearer £5000 with similar servicing charges making a total of £10 500 over four years.

Rehabilitation

Following limb salvage with a prosthesis the patient is walking with crutches at 48 hours and will leave hospital at 14 days walking safely on sticks. After six weeks the patient is readmitted for a week of intensive physiotherapy when all walking aids are discarded. No further physiotherapy is required, although the patient continues with a strict exercise programme. In patients not receiving chemotherapy it would be normal to return to work after three months.

Following amputation it is current practice to see the patient for a first assessment at the limb fitting centre after six weeks. It will often be three months until a satisfactory artificial limb is provided, all of which time must be spent on crutches. The patient will then need several weeks of outpatient physiotherapy to learn to walk again. In an otherwise fit person four months off work or school would be expected.

After the first year the costs will be those of follow-up and treatment of complications. A figure of £1000 per year is said to cover the costs of the average amputee.

Follow up

The costs of oncological follow-up will be the same for both groups. For patients with an artificial limb the extra follow up is included in the £1000 per year. For patients with limb salvage an extra annual visit will usually be needed, currently costed in our centre at £120, which includes all radiological investigations.

Complications

For limb salvage the costs of ensuing years will depend upon the incidence of complications. The ideal endoprosthetic replacement causes no further problems to the patient after insertion. Unfortunately most patients will require further surgery at some stage.

Balance sheet for the first year		
	Limb salvage	Amputation
Surgery	£4500	£3500
Prosthesis	£2600	£4000
Rehabilitation	£1000	£1000
Time off work or school	3 months	4 months
Total	£8100	£8500

Minor complications	**Major complications**
• Lengthening procedure	• Local recurrence
• Resurfacing patella	• Infection
• Soft tissue reconstruction	• Mechanical loosening
• Rebushing prosthesis	• Fracture of prosthesis

The minor complications usually require little more than a few days in hospital and are of low cost. The major complications may lead to amputation or revision of the prosthesis to a new one.

The cost of a revision procedure is currently £8000, to include the cost of a new endoprosthesis. Knowing the risk of failure it is now possible to calculate the additional costs of limb salvage surgery. For example, after eight years approximately 50% of distal femoral implants will have failed resulting in an average additional cost of £4000 per patient.

Knowing all these costs it is now possible to calculate the relative costs of follow-up for patients with amputation and with limb salvage. It is necessary to include a factor for the decreasing survival of the patients (35% mortality by five years) and also for re-revision of endoprostheses (estimated at 5%/year). Using the above figures the costs shown in Figure 8.2 are obtained.

It can be seen that for the distal femur the cost of limb salvage in the long term is dramatically less than for amputation but for proximal tibial replacements (which have historically had a high failure rate) there is no

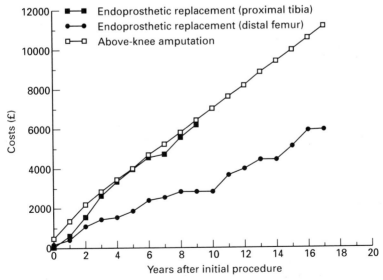

Fig 8.2 Costs of maintaining a patient with an above-knee amputation (NHS prices) against the likely costs of further surgery in a patient with an endoprosthesis

133

cost difference. Recent modifications to the design of the prosthesis and to surgical technique should lower the complication rate significantly and thus decrease the costs of limb salvage in comparison with amputation.

In the proximal femur the costings are different in that although the artificial limb is very expensive it is on the whole rarely used and thus the servicing costs will be less. Equally, replacements of the proximal femur fare well. The functional difference, however, is dramatically in favour of the limb salvage procedure. Similarly in the upper limb, the functional advantage of saving the hand is so great that the cost of the implant and limb salvage surgery far outweighs the alternative of shoulder disarticulation or forequarter amputation.

Conclusion

Remarkably little work has been done on the costs and benefits of limb salvage surgery for patients with primary bone tumours. Despite the fact that limb preservation seems to be an essential goal of treating musculoskeletal tumours, the results available to date have shown no convincing functional or psychological advantage for limb salvage in patients with tumours around the knee. The overall costs of limb salvage and amputation are similar in the short term, but over a lifetime limb salvage will be cheaper providing the failure rate leading to major revision surgery is low. With improvements in prosthetic design this should be the case.

It is obviously vitally important to fully inform the patient and his or her family, and to advise them appropriately before embarking upon limb salvage with its potential for lifelong servicing requirements.

1 Price CHG. Primary bone forming tumours and their relationship to skeletal growth. *J Bone Joint Surg* 1958; **40B**: 574–93.
2 Rosen G, Murphy ML, Huvos AG *et al.* Chemotherapy, en bloc resection and prosthetic bone replacement in the treatment of osteogenic sarcoma. *Cancer* 1976; **37**: 1–11.
3 Goorin AM, Abelson HT and Frei E. Osteosarcoma: Fifteen years later. *N Engl J Med* 1985; **313**: 1637–45.
4 Link M, Goorin AM, Horowitz M *et al.* Adjuvant chemotherapy of high grade osteosarcoma of the extremity. Updated results of the multi-institutional osteosarcoma study (1991). *Clin Orthop* 1991; **270**: 8–14.
5 Bramwell VHC, Burgess M, Sneath RS *et al.* A comparison of two short intensive adjuvant chemotherapy regimens in operable osteosarcoma of limbs in children and young adults: the first study of the European Osteosarcoma Intergroup. *J Clin Oncol* 1992; **10**: 1579–91.
6 Enneking WF, Spanier SS, Goodman MA. A system for the surgical staging of musculoskeletal sarcoma. *Clin Orthop* 1980; **153**: 106–20.
7 Simon MA, Aschliman MA, Thomas N, Mankin HJ. Limb-salvage treatment versus amputation for osteosarcoma of the distal end of the femur. *J Bone Joint Surg* 1986; **68A**: 1331–7.
8 Picci P, Capanna R, Bacci G *et al.* Margins, necrosis and local recurrence after conservative surgery in osteosarcoma. *Chir Organi Mov* 1990; **75**: 82–85.
9 Enneking WF, Shirley PD. Resection arthrodesis for malignant and potentially malignant lesions about the knee using an intramedulary rod and local bone grafts. *J Bone Joint Surg* 1977; **59A**: 223–36.
10 Kotz R, Salzer M. Rotation-plasty for childhood osteosarcoma of the distal part of the

femur. *J Bone Joint Surg* 1982; **64A**: 959–69.

11 Mankin HJ, Lange TA, Spanier SS. The hazards of biopsy in patients with primary bone and soft tissue tumours. *J Bone Joint Surg* 1982; **64A**: 1121–7.

12 Berrey BH, Lord F, Gebhardt MC, Mankin HJ. Fractures of allografts. *J Bone Joint Surg* 1990; **72A**: 825–33.

13 Lord CF, Gebhardt MC, Tomford WW, Mankin HJ. Infections in bone allografts. *J Bone Joint Surg* 1988; **70A**: 369–76.

14 Burrows HJ, Wilson JN, Scales JT. Excision of tumours of humerus and femur, with restoration by internal prostheses. *J Bone Joint Surg,* 1975; **57B**: 148–59.

15 Dobbs HS, Scales JT, Wilson JN *et al*. Endoprosthetic replacement of the proximal femur and acetabulum. *J Bone Joint Surg* 1981; **63B**: 219–24.

16 Roberts P, Chan D, Grimer RJ *et al*. Prosthetic replacement of the distal femur for primary bone tumours. *J Bone Joint Surg* 1991; **73B**: 762–9.

17 Chandler HP, Reineck FT, Wixson RL, McCarthy JC. Total hip replacement in patients younger than 30 years old. *J Bone Joint Surg* 1981; **63A**: 1426–34.

18 Dorr LD, Luckett M, Pierce Conaty J. Total hip arthroplasties in patients younger than 45 years. *Clin Orthop* 1990; **260**: 215–19.

19 Gordon-Taylor G, Wiles P. Interinnomino-abdominal (hind-quarter) amputation. *Br J Surg* 1935; **22**: 671–95.

20 Enneking WF. Modification of the system of functional evaluation of surgical management of musculoskeletal tumours. In: WF Enneking, ed., *Limb salvage in musculoskeletal oncology.* New York: Churchilll Livingstone, 1987, 626–39.

21 Aaronson NK, Ahmedzai SA, Bergman B *et al*. The EORTC QLQ-C30: A quality of life instrument for use in international clinical trials in oncology. *J Natl Canc Inst* 1990; **85**: 365–76.

22 Aaronson NK, Ahmedzai SA, Bullinger M *et al*. The EORTC Cor Quality of Life Questionnaire: interim results of an international field study. In: Osoba D (ed.), *The effect of cancer on quality of life.* Boston: CRC Press, 1991, 185–204.

23 Sugarbaker PH, Barofsky I, Rosenberg SA, Gionola FJ. Quality of life assessment of patients in extremity sarcoma clinical trials. *Surgery* 1982; **91**: 17–23.

24 Weddington WW, Segraves KB, Simon MA. Psychological outcome of extremity sarcoma survivors undergoing amputation or limb salvage. *J Clin Oncol* 1985; **3**: 1393–9.

25 Postma A, Kingma A, de Ruiter *et al*. Quality of life in bone tumour patients comparing limb salvage and amputation of the lower extremity. *J Surg Oncol* 1992; **51**: 47–51.

26 Harris IE, Leff AR, Gitelis G, Simon MA. Function after amputation, arthrodesis or anthroplasty for tumours about the knee. *J Bone Joint Surg* 1990; **72A**: 1477–85.

27 Boyle M, Tebbi CK, Mindell ER, Mettlin CJ. Adolescent adjustment to amputation. *Med Paed Oncol* 1982; **10**: 301–12.

28 Tebbi CK, Petrilli AS, Richards ME. Adjustment to amputation among adolescent amputation patients. *Am J Paed Haematol/Oncol* 1989; **11**: 276–280.

9: Psychological and psychiatric morbidity

PETER MAGUIRE

Introduction

If adolescents are to come to terms with the diagnosis and treatment of cancer, certain specific hurdles have to be overcome. They also have to manage general issues concerned with their personal development. Parents have to cope with hurdles relating to the adolescent's illness and treatment and fulfil their responsibilities for rearing their children and maintaining a constructive relationship with each other. The nature of these hurdles will be reviewed briefly before the nature and extent of the psychological and psychiatric morbidity associated with the diagnosis and treatment of cancer in adolescence is described, problems of recognition are highlighted, and possible solutions are discussed.

Hurdles for the adolescent due to diagnosis

Uncertainty

Adolescents have to come to terms with the fact that they have a disease for which the outcome is often uncertain. It is likely that the disease may recur and cause a premature death even after they have had intense and unpleasant treatments. So, a key question is whether they can put concerns about this uncertainty to the back of their minds or whether it begins to plague them and seriously impedes their day to day functioning. Any uncertainty will be compounded by frequent visits to hospital for the necessary treatments, witnessing other patients with similar diseases doing badly, and adverse reports in the newspapers and television.

Contributing to survival

Adolescents cope better if they feel there is something they can do to contribute to their physical survival. In the absence of known risk factors it is hard for them to adopt particular behaviours that may enhance the prospects of recovery. However, if they can adopt measures like a healthy diet, relaxation, or meditation, without allowing these to become an overriding obsession, they are likely to cope better psychologically.

Search for meaning

It is difficult for cancer patients to explain why they should have contracted cancer at a given point of time. It is especially hard for adolescents at the threshold of adult life to find any sensible explanation for why they have been struck down with it. Those who fail to find a meaning or cannot tolerate the absence of a satisfactory explanation find it harder to adjust psychologically.

Stigma

Cancer is still viewed as a disease which is almost as stigmatising as mental illness, partly because people still believe it is contagious and can become uncontrollable. Adolescents may, therefore, feel of less value as persons having contracted the disease, especially if they feel they have been singled out for such misfortune. Should they feel stigmatised there is a danger they will avoid their normal social relationships for fear of rejection.

Isolation

It is hard to justify why any adolescent should develop cancer. So, friends and relatives can find it hard to relate to them normally. They fear that asking how the adolescent is faring in terms of his or her response to treatment will produce replies that are hard to handle, for example, explaining that treatment is "horrendous". Relatives and friends may then begin to avoid the adolescent and this will intensify any isolation that had developed because of feelings of stigma. Adolescents are then at risk of psychological and psychiatric morbidity because they are not receiving the necessary emotional and practical support.

Openness

Adolescents who are able to be open about their illness and treatment with others fare better psychologically in both the short and longer term. So, a key question is whether they feel able to be honest about their predicament with those close to them.

Support

Those who perceive they are receiving sufficient practical and emotional support fare better than those who perceive that support is inadequate to their needs. This is true of the support they receive both from friends and relatives and from health professionals. If they perceive that support is inadequate a key question is whether they can assert their needs and remedy this.

Hurdles due to adverse effects of treatment

In addition to the hurdles relating to the diagnosis of cancer, the adolescent has to come to terms with serious adverse effects of treatment. Thus, the patient may have to come to terms with losing an important part of the body, for example, a limb as a result of treatment for a sarcoma. The adolescent may also have to come to terms with the loss of an important body function, for example, as after the fashioning of an ileostomy following treatment for colon cancer. The patient may then have difficulty adjusting both to the stoma itself and to managing the bag.

Problems adjusting to the loss of a body part or function may lead to profound body image problems including an intolerance of feeling less than whole, a lowering of self esteem, feeling self conscious, and worry that other people must somehow guess that they have lost a body part or function. According to the body parts affected, it may threaten their sexual identity and make them feel less masculine or feminine.

Chemotherapy in combination is often used to try to eradicate cancer. Unfortunately, such treatment can have adverse effects, particularly nausea and vomiting and the development of conditioned responses. Here, patients experience nausea and vomiting within the first two or three treatments. Any stimulus that reminds them of treatment, be it visual, auditory, or olfactory, triggers the same adverse effects as the treatment. This may make the adolescent feel that the only solution is to opt out of what might otherwise have been a life-saving treatment. Chemotherapy can also cause the patient's hair to fall out and provoke body image problems. It may adversely affect sexual functioning and lead to infertility and sterility.

Radiotherapy can also cause adverse effects, particularly exhaustion and tiredness and interfere with daily functioning. When the adolescent is suffering from a brain tumour the need to remove this surgically and/or the need to treat the affected part with radiotherapy may result in brain damage and cognitive impairment. This may lead to impairment of short term memory, attention, and concentration and affect psychological adjustment adversely and interfere with education or work.

Hurdles related to personal development

As if these hurdles related to diagnosis and treatment are not enough, the adolescent has to try and continue to develop normally as a person.[1] Particular hurdles include the ability to separate from parents while maintaining a healthy dependence on them. They also have to strive to achieve a personal identity so that they can answer questions like "who am I?" and "where am I going?". They need to develop realistic plans for the future, education, and work.

It is particularly important that adolescents make effective relationships with their peers and develop a positive self image and confidence in their ability to control their destiny. The nature of their illness and treatment can thwart their ability to manage these hurdles and result in psychological and psychiatric morbidity.

Additional hurdles for parents

Parents of an adolescent with cancer have to cope with certain additional hurdles. First, they have to try and accept that their child has contracted a potentially fatal illness despite their best efforts to ensure that the child reaches a healthy adulthood. If they fail to accept the situation they can become plagued by a sense of failure and guilt feelings.[2]

It is difficult for parents to treat their child as normal given the problems associated with the diagnosis and treatment of cancer. Yet, they must do this if the child's psychological development and adjustment is to be normal. A particular problem for the parents of an adolescent with cancer is how to do justice to the sick child's needs during active treatment, and yet meet the needs of each other and their other children. Problems in balancing needs can be hindered by the need to visit the sick adolescent regularly and by financial problems that arise if they have to travel a considerable distance or take time off work.

These hurdles are considerable, parents cope well providing they can agree on a strategy for dealing with them or can tolerate differences between them in how they attempt to cope. Where parents disagree in how these problems should be managed but cannot tolerate their disagreement this can lead to serious psychological consequences and make it very difficult for the child and parents to maintain a healthy psychological adjustment.[2]

Psychological morbidity

In a study funded by the Leukaemia Research Fund, 184 children with leukaemia, their siblings, and parents were assessed. Participating centres included Birmingham, Leeds, Liverpool, Manchester, Nottingham, and Sheffield. Assessments were based on in depth interviews with the parents. They were interviewed 2 and 12 months after the diagnosis of the child with leukaemia by trained interviewers. The interviewers elicited a history of the child's illness using a semi-structured interview and a Social Interview Schedule to establish the nature and extent of any social morbidity. The Present State Examination was used to determine whether the parents had suffered from an anxiety state or depressive illness.[3] The Rutter Behaviour Schedule was administered to parents to indicate whether the adolescents with cancer and their siblings had developed any behaviour disorders during the first year after diagnosis.[4] The parents reported that 51% of the children with cancer had experienced four or more behavioural problems to a mild, moderate or severe degree during the 12–18 months follow-up period. This compared with the teachers' assessments of 17%. Importantly, there was no difference in the prevalence of behaviour problems in those aged 12–15 compared with those aged 5–11. Temper tantrums were the most common (27%), followed by generalised irritability (21%), and continued complaints of aches and pains (16%).

Other studies have suggested that up to one fifth of adolescents may develop an anxiety state or depressive illness in the period of active treatment.[5] While it is clear that a number of adolescents develop body image problems, for example, following the loss of a limb or hair loss, it is not clear how many of these problems become persistent and further studies are needed to clarify this. Up to a fifth of adolescents develop conditioned responses in relation to chemotherapy. Thus, the impact of diagnosis and treatment in the short term in terms of psychological and psychiatric morbidity is considerable and affects a substantial minority of adolescents.

In the multicentre study mothers were especially at risk of developing an anxiety state and/or depressive illness within 12–18 months of the child's diagnosis; 30% of mothers had an episode of an anxiety state or depressive illness. These became chronic in most mothers since the provoking and maintaining factors were not dealt with. This prevalence represents a relative risk of five times the expected rate in a matched group of mothers whose children are free of disease. Fathers were less prone to develop affective disorders (13%), but the relative risk was still two to three times that of a comparable population.

The data on the psychological and psychiatric morbidity concerning the adolescents have been derived from indirect reports from parents. Longitudinal studies are needed which include interviewing adolescents using standardised instruments to determine the true prevalence of psychological and psychiatric morbidity.

Impact of survivorship

The literature suggests that up to a fifth of adolescents who survive their cancer develop a psychiatric or psychological disorder.[6] These may include a depressive illness, generalised anxiety disorder, panic disorder, low self esteem, persisting body image problems, and somatisation where the adolescent continues to complain of physical symptoms even though they are free of disease and off active treatment. Further longitudinal controlled studies are needed to clarify this.

Parents continue to have considerable concerns about the adolescents' health in general, the risk of relapse, their social development, and their ability to develop relationships, and continue to feel that they need support from health professionals. Since a clear link has been found between the number of unresolved concerns a person has and the risk of a later affective disorder, these findings are important.[7] However, the incidence of anxiety and depression in parents of survivors has not yet been properly estimated.

Several studies have suggested they are no more prone than a comparable population of parents to develop psychopathology.

Problems of recognition

Whatever subsequent studies show, there is no doubt that a substantial minority of adolescents and their parents develop psychological and psychiatric morbidity. However, it is evident from the Manchester study and previous studies that the majority (50–80%) of problems which develop in patients, parents and siblings are not detected. Even if they are detected they tend to be dismissed as understandable or self limiting and so treatment is not usually undertaken.

Reasons for poor recognition

A major reason for the poor recognition of problems is that adolescents do not disclose them. They believe these problems are an inevitable consequence of having cancer and cancer treatment and so feel they cannot be alleviated. They do not wish to burden health professionals who are clearly doing their best to help them and ensure their physical survival. They are particularly concerned about their self image and do not wish to be judged inadequate or poor copers. Since they do not recall being asked specific questions about their psychological welfare by health professionals, they do not believe it is legitimate to discuss such issues. If they do try and give verbal or non-verbal cues they report that they are met by distancing strategies, for example, "you are bound to be upset, everybody is when they first know they have got leukaemia, but we will sort it out for you".

Parents also believe that it is not legitimate to mention psychological problems. They also keep them hidden because they wish to protect their child and partner from distress and further burden. Moreover, they feel they have no right to express a need for help themselves since all the attention should be on the sick child.[2]

Health professionals also contribute to this hidden morbidity in three ways. They avoid focusing on psychosocial aspects. Thus, for example, they do not ask screening questions like "how have you felt about losing a leg?" When an adolescent or parent offers cues about the physical welfare of the adolescent and psychological matters, the health professional selectively attends to physical aspects. Adolescents and their parents then try to give cues about their distress or problems. They are likely to be met by distancing strategies.[8]

Distancing strategies

These include normalisation (I can see you are upset, you are bound to be, everybody is at first), premature reassurance (I am sure we will get you better in no time), premature advice (let me tell you what we plan to do),

141

false reassurance (I am certain you are going to get better, I am sure the tests will prove that), passing the buck (I am afraid I am not in a position to tell you, you will have to ask your consultant), switching the subject (here the topic is moved directly away from the psychological to safer waters by switching of the topic by the health professional), and jollying along ('come on John, there is no need to look so glum, the sun is shining'). A key question is why health professionals dedicated to the care of adolescents with cancer use such distancing strategies. For example, Wilkinson[9] found that cancer nurses working in cancer hospitals use such blocking tactics in over 50% of their utterances when assessing patients' problems. There appear to be several reasons for this.

In depth interviews reveal that doctors and nurses involved in cancer care are well aware that the nature of the cancer and treatment outcomes is uncertain at the best of times. Getting close to patients' predicaments and concerns would remind them of this uncertainty and might hinder their ability to make key decisions. It could also remind them of the limitations of modern high technology medicine.

They perceive cancer patients and relatives as vulnerable psychologically. This particularly applies to their view of adolescents and children. Thus, they believe that any psychological enquiry might "unhinge" the patient and cause psychological damage. It is better, therefore, to avoid such enquiry and ignore key cues.

They feel ill equipped to make such psychological enquiry because they have not been taught how to enquire about patients' emotions and help them express them without getting into difficulty. They fear that if emotions do emerge they won't be able to handle them or help the patient talk them through. They also believe it might take up too much time.

These doctors and nurses also feel ill equipped to deal with common but important communication tasks like how to break bad news, how to challenge denial, and how to break collusion. They have profound worries about whether they could work in a psychological way and survive emotionally at the same time. This concern about emotional survival is illustrated by two anecdotes from a study conducted by Rosser and Maguire (1982).[10]

> If you actually have to go and talk to somebody about your failure to cure them that is also putting you, yourself, in a different position that is difficult to cope with. It takes time and it does burn me up and I come away exhausted.

> Young people who seem to apparently die unjustifiably, have diseases which they have no justification in getting. They don't deserve them and one has to see the agonies of suffering for some time before they die. I think these are the more draining.

There are then formidable barriers in the way of patient disclosure and recognition by the health professional of the psychological and psychiatric morbidity that develops in adolescents and their parents. Ways need to be found, therefore, to improve their ability of health professionals to promote disclosure.

Promoting disclosure

Studies of health professionals caring for cancer patients who attended residential workshops to help them improve their communication, assessment and counselling skills have confirmed that certain skills promote the disclosure of concern by patients. These include the use of open directive questions designed to encourage a patient to talk about issues like losing a leg ("how have you felt about losing a leg?").[11] Questions that indicate a definite interest in psychological aspects also promote disclosure ("How do you see your illness working out?", "what do you make of what's been happening?"). Open directive questions and questions with a psychological focus prompt the patient to give important cues like "I have been feeling upset" or "I am worried about the future". Clarification of these cues ("in what way have you felt upset?", "what are your worries about the future?") promote further disclosure. Once a number of cues have been offered, summarising them lets the patient know that these have been heard and acknowledged. Being genuinely empathic ("so, you felt devastated then") prompts both disclosure and the mention and expression of the feelings associated with specific concerns.

As health professionals talk with adolescents and parents, they often get a hunch about what the patient or parent is concerned about or what they are feeling. However, then tend to keep these to themselves rather than risk making a guess that could be wrong. In reality, making such a guess educates the patient or parent to believe that the health professional is trying to understand their predicament even if the guess is wrong. This also promotes the disclosure of concerns and the mention and expression of feelings.

In contrast, there are behaviours which inhibit disclosure. These include leading questions ("so chemotherapy has gone very well, hasn't it?") and multiple questions where several questions are asked at once. Here the patient answers the first or last question in the sequence and ignores those in the middle.

The longer the doctor or nurse spends asking questions about physical aspects the more likely the adolescent or parent is to believe that they are only interested in physical aspects. Then if they ask about psychological aspects the patient will consider, albeit wrongly, that they are not interested in the answer. The key is to integrate questions about physical and psychological aspects.

One of the most effective ways of preventing patients' disclosure of concerns is to offer advice or reassurance immediately after hearing the patient volunteer his or her initial concerns. When such advice or reassurance is offered prematurely, that is before the initial and other concerns have been properly evaluated, it is even more likely to block disclosure.

When health professionals are assessed in terms of the extent to which they possess these positive and inhibitory behaviours, it has been found that for every positive behaviour they use in an assessment interview they use three which inhibit patient disclosure. Only if health professionals are trained to ask the right kinds of questions and relinquish these inhibitory behaviours and distancing strategies will adolescents' and parents' concerns and any associated psychological and psychiatric morbidity be disclosed.

Training specialist nurses

Specialist nurses who have had training in key assessment skills are successful in detecting those adult cancer patients who develop psychological and psychiatric problems after surgery for breast cancer.[12] While 75% of those who developed psychological or psychiatric morbidity were recognised and referred for help in the group monitored by a specialist nurse, only 15% of those so affected in a control group were referred. Since subsequent psychological and psychiatric treatment is effective, this results in a fourfold reduction in psychological and psychiatric morbidity in women monitored after mastectomy for breast cancer.

The monitoring involved assessing each patient every two months at home. This sensitised some patients to worry more than they would otherwise have done about their cancer predicament. It created an increasing load for the nurse, promoted dependency, and encouraged some patients to turn to the nurse for help with problems unrelated to the cancer.

A limited intervention scheme was therefore developed and was compared with the original regular monitoring system and a system in which ward nurses and health visitors were trained to do the psychological assessment.[13] In the limited intervention each woman was seen once at home by a trained specialist nurse. Only if there were problems was contact continued or the patient was referred to the psychiatrist for help. Otherwise, patients were instructed that they would not be followed up but should contact the specialist nurse should any problems arise later on.

They heeded this offer, and most patients who developed problems did contact the nurse subsequently. Consequently, the psychiatric and psychological morbidity evident in this group 12–18 months after surgery was no greater than that found in the group that had received regular two-monthly monitoring. Those patients allocated to the ward and community arm fared much worse. Little of the morbidity was recognised and treated. Nurses on the ward failed to achieve the necessary level of competence in assessing anxiety and depression, while health visitors and district nurses generally were reluctant to carry out the necessary psychological assessments.

Similar schemes were implemented in the Manchester Childrens Hospital in relation to the use of specialist nurses to detect problems in adolescents with leukaemia and their parents, and were found to be much more effective than systems that relied on non-specialist nurses or specialist nurses without this specific training in assessment skills.

The necessary skills can be acquired through attendance at residential courses that teach communication and counselling skills.[14] Alternatively, training may be on a more regular basis. Supervision and support are necessary if health professionals are to maintain and apply these assessment skills within their daily practice.

Prevention

Prevention should be possible since it has been established that there are factors that increase the likelihood that an adolescent or parent will develop psychological or psychiatric morbidity. These factors include the number of unresolved concerns about the cancer diagnosis and treatment, closed communication within the family, lack of perceived support from family and health professionals, the development of a skew relationship between a parent and a sick child where this relationship becomes over-riding and all important, persisting body image problems, a stormy illness, and severe adverse effects of treatment.

The more health professionals are able to identify and meet the information needs of individual patients and then elicit and resolve their concerns the less likely it is that they will develop psychological or psychiatric problems.

The promotion of open communication in the family and ensuring they have sufficient support to meet their needs should reduce morbidity.[15] However, when discussing the possibility of practical and emotional support it is important that health professionals emphasise the importance of families using their own resources. Otherwise, mothers in particular and some adolescents will lean on the health professional rather than maintain healthy links with their own family. The parent and adolescent can then be detached from the rest of the family and this can lead to profound friction.

Though it is difficult, it is also important for health professionals to encourage parents from an early stage to take time out from visiting the hospital and from being present during treatments. Otherwise they may use up all their emotional and physical energy and then be much more vulnerable to psychiatric breakdown if the adolescent has a recurrence of illness or dies.

Prevention might also be successful if specialist nurses focused on those who are most at risk of developing psychological and psychiatric morbidity. Thus, it might be prudent to concentrate the monitoring on those who fail to surmount one or more of the hurdles related to disease and treatment, and exhibit one or more of the general risk factors. This monitoring could be carried out by these specialist nurses or health visitors who have been trained in the relevant assessment skills discussed earlier.

Other approaches

It has been claimed that providing support by running groups for adolescents with cancer, their siblings, and/or their parents can prevent psychological and psychiatric morbidity. However, controlled studies are needed to confirm this. Otherwise, health professionals will remain sceptical about the value of these endeavours. Similarly, the value of family meetings to try and encourage common policy between family members and promote openness may have a place but remain to be evaluated.

1 Rowland JH. Developmental stage and adaptation: Child and adolescent model. In: Holland J, Massie J. eds, *Handbook of psychosocial oncology.* Oxford: Oxford University Press, 1991: 519–43.

2 Maguire P. Can the parental psychological morbidity associated with childhood leukaemia be reduced. *Cancer Surveys* 1984; **3**: 617–31.

3 |Wing JK, Cooper JE, Sartorius N. *Measurement and classification of psychiatric symptoms.* Cambridge: Cambridge University Press, 1974.

4 Rutter M, Tizard J, Whitmore K. *Education, health and behaviour.* London: Longman, 1970.

5 Kashani J, Hakami N. Depression in children and adolescents with malignancy. *Can J Psych* 1982; **27**: 474–7.

6 Koocher GP, O'Malley JE, Gogan JL, Foster DJ. Psychosocial adjustment among paediatric cancer survivors. *J Child Psychol* 1980; **21**: 163–73.

7 Parle M, Maguire P. Exploring relationships between cancer, coping and mental health. *J Psych Oncol* 1995; **13**, 1/2, 27–50.

8 Maguire P. Improving the recognition and treatment of affective disorders in cancer patients. In: Granville-Grossman K ed., *Recent advances in clinical psychiatry.* Edinburgh: Churchill Livingstone; 1992; 15–30.

9 Wilkinson S. Factors affecting communication with patients with cancer. *J Adv Nursing,* 1991; **16**: 677–88.

10 Rosser J, Maguire P. Dilemmas in general practice: The care of the cancer patient. *Soc Sci Med* 1982; **16**: 315–22.

11 Maguire P, Booth K, Elliott C, Hillier V. Helping cancer patients disclose their concerns. *Eur J Cancer.* In press.

12 Maguire GP, Tait A, Brooke M *et al.* The effect of counselling on psychiatric morbidity associated with mastectomy. *Br Med J* 1980; **281**: 1454–6.

13 Wilkinson S, Maguire P, Tait A. Life after breast cancer. *Nursing Times,* 1986; **84**: 34–7.

14 Maguire P, Faulkner A. How to improve the counselling skills of doctors and nurses involved in cancer care. *Br Med J* 1988; **297**: 847–9.

15 Slavin LA, O'Malley JE, Koocher GP, Foster DJ. Communication of the cancer diagnosis to paediatric patients: Impact on long term adjustment. *Am J Psychiatry* 1982; **139**: 179–82.

10: Cytotoxic-induced damage to the gonad during childhood

SM SHALET

The impact of combination cytotoxic chemotherapy on gonadal function is dependent on the nature and dosage of the drugs received by the child. Drugs that have been shown to cause gonadal damage include the alkylating agents such as cyclophosphamide, chlorambucil, and the nitrosoureas, in addition to procarbazine, vinblastine, cytarabine, and cisplatinum.

It is known that the normal adult testis is extremely sensitive to the effects of external irradiation. However, neither the threshold dose of irradiation required to damage the germinal epithelium in childhood, nor the dose above which irreversible damage occurs, is known. In irradiated girls, the response of the ovary involves a fixed pool of oocytes which once destroyed cannot be replaced. The dose of radiation which will kill 50% of oocytes (LD_{50}) for the human ovary has recently been estimated not to exceed 400 cGy.[1]

The germinal epithelium of the testis is far more vulnerable than the Leydig cells to cytotoxic-induced damage. Thus, in the adolescent boy, puberty is usually completed spontaneously but the testes are pathologically small for the stage of puberty. In girls fertility prospects are less frequently affected than in boys by cytotoxic-induced damage, but if severe ovarian damage has occurred then steroidogenesis as well as fertility is likely to be affected and hormone replacement therapy will be required.

It used to be thought that the prepubertal testis was less vulnerable than the pubertal testis to cytotoxic-induced damage. This has never been confirmed, but it is now clear that the testicular germinal epithelium of both prepubertal and pubertal boys may be irreversibly obliterated by gonadotoxic chemotherapy or irradiation.

Acute lymphoblastic leukaemia

Combination chemotherapy and the testis

Lendon et al.[2] studied testicular histology in 44 boys treated with combination chemotherapy for acute lymphoblastic leukaemia (ALL). At the time of testicular biopsy, 21 boys were still receiving cytotoxic drugs and 23 had completed their chemotherapy some time earlier. Based on a count of at least 100 cross-sections of tubules per biopsy, the tubular fertility index (TFI) was calculated as the percentage of seminiferous tubules containing identifiable spermatogonia. The mean TFI in the 44 biopsies was 50% of that in age-matched controls and 18 of the biopsies showed a severely depressed TFI of 40% or less. Three variables had a highly significant effect on the TFI. Previous chemotherapy with cyclophosphamide or cytarabine (total dose > 1 g/m^2) depressed the TFI, whereas with increasing time after completion of chemotherapy the TFI improved. These conclusions were supported by the findings of Uderzo et al.[3]

Shalet et al.[4] studied testicular function in the 44 boys whose testicular biopsies were reported by Lendon et al.[2] They reported normal Leydig cell function as assessed by the testosterone response to human chorionic gonadotrophin (HCG) but described abnormalities of follicle stimulating hormone (FSH) secretion, consistent with germ cell damage, in the pubertal boys. In this study, all the boys achieved normal adult secondary sex characteristics subsequently and had a serum testosterone concentration within the normal adult range consistent with normal Leydig cell function.

Supportive evidence of germ cell damage in 25 leukaemic boys was seen following treatment with a modified LSA$_2$L$_2$ protocol,[5] which consisted of 10 cytotoxic agents including cyclophosphamide and cytarabine, given for 3–4 years. In 24 testicular biopsies assessed at the time of completion of chemotherapy, there was an absence of germ cells in 13 and in the remaining 11 the germ cells were markedly depleted. Raised basal FSH levels and an exaggerated FSH response to an acute bolus of gonadotrophin releasing hormone (GnRH) were reported in the majority of boys who were pubertal at assessment.

To assess the reversibility of documented germ cell damage after chemotherapy for ALL in childhood, our group[6] has studied testicular function in 37 male long term survivors. This study was conducted at two separate time points; initially a wedge testicular biopsy was performed at or near completion of chemotherapy to assess the incidence of occult testicular relapse. The TFI was calculated as described earlier,[2] and subsequently, at a median time of 10·7 years after stopping chemotherapy, the patients were reassessed by clinical examination, measurement of gonadotrophins and testosterone levels and, in 19, by semen analysis. The median TFI for all 37 biopsies was 74%, and at reassessment six men had evidence of severe damage to the germinal epithelium. Five of these men had azoospermia and one, who did not provide semen for analysis, had a reduced mean testicular volume and a raised basal FSH consistent with severe germ cell damage.

Of 11 males who had a TFI below 50% at testicular biopsy, five recovered normal germ cell function at a median of 10·1 years after completing chemotherapy. Of the 26 males who had a TFI above 50%, 23 showed completely normal testicular function when reassessed subsequently, and in the remaining 3 the results were inconclusive. Clearly, with increasing time after completion of treatment, germ cell function can improve so that normal fertility may be a possibility for some patients who have sustained damage to the germinal epithelium. Nonetheless, the long term prognosis for fertility may remain poor for at least 10 years in those most severely affected.

Combination chemotherapy and the ovary

Ovarian damage following combination chemotherapy for ALL has been reported only rarely.[7] In contrast, morphological studies have shown that the ovaries from girls treated for ALL between 1 and 12 years of age and studied one week to four years after diagnosis, demonstrated inhibition of follicular development.[8] The girls who had received chemotherapy for only a short period of time had normal ovaries with ample follicular growth and many small non-growing follicles. This implied that cytotoxic drugs rather than the disease itself had disrupted ovarian morphology.

To evaluate ovarian function and pregnancy outcome after treatment of ALL, Green et al.[9] reported 27 pregnancies in 12 out of 39 women who had been treated for ALL during childhood or adolescence. There were four spontaneous abortions, one stillbirth, and 22 liveborn infants. Two of the liveborn infants had congenital anomalies (one heart murmur, one epidermal naevus) and none of the children (ages 1 month to 10 years) had developed childhood cancer.

Two studies emphasise that the prevalence of ovarian dysfunction partly reflects the length of follow up. Quigley et al.[5] described a high incidence of ovarian damage in 20 girls treated with a modified LSA_2L_2 protocol. Basal and peak FSH levels after administration of GnRH were significantly higher in both the prepubertal and pubertal girls than in the comparable control groups. Further evidence of ovarian damage was the undetectable serum inhibin, a granulosa cell product, in a high proportion of the girls. Despite clear evidence of primary ovarian damage, none of the girls had a delay in reaching puberty and oestradiol levels were normal.

In contrast, Wallace et al.[10] studied ovarian function in 40 women who had remained in first remission following combination chemotherapy for childhood leukaemia over 10 years earlier. All achieved adult sexual development and 37 had regular menses. Ten patients had 14 live births and evidence of ovulation was obtained in a further 11 patients. Four showed biochemical evidence of ovarian damage, three of whom received craniospinal irradiation and one cyclophosphamide. Thus, the long term outlook for ovarian function is good for the majority of childhood ALL survivors. A premature menopause, however, remains a possibility if significant follicular depletion has occurred at the time of cytotoxic treatment.

Testicular irradiation

Brauner et al.[11] studied 12 boys with ALL who had received direct testicular irradiation (2400 cGy in 12 fractions over 18 days) between 10 months and 8·5 years earlier for a testicular relapse (in 9) and as testicular prophylaxis (in 3). Leydig cell dysfunction, manifested by a low or absent testosterone response to human chorionic gonadotrophin, or an increased basal level of plasma LH or both, was present in 10 of the 12 boys. Similar findings were reported by Leiper et al.[12] who studied 11 prepubertal boys who had received 2400 cGy in 10–12 fractions over 14–16 days.

Subsequently it has been shown that severe Leydig cell damage was present fairly soon after irradiation, often within the first year, and that there is no evidence of Leydig cell recovery up to five years after irradiation.[13]

A recent study by Castillo et al.[14] has examined the effect of "intermediate" doses of testicular irradiation on Leydig cell function in boys treated for ALL. Of the 15 boys studied, 12 received 1200 cGy "prophylactic" testicular irradiation in six 200 cGy fractions over eight days, and the other three were treated for overt testicular relapse with 2400 cGy (in two patients) and 1500 cGy (in one patient). The seven patients old enough to provide semen for analysis were azoospermic. Eleven of the 12 patients who received 1200 cGy, as well as the patients who received 1500 cGy, had normal pubertal development for their age, with an appropriate basal testosterone level and response to hCG. Elevated basal or post-GnRH stimulation LH levels in the pubertal boys suggests that subclinical Leydig cell damage is common after this dose of testicular irradiation.

All boys who have received direct testicular irradiation for ALL will require a biochemical assessment of testicular function. In the presence of results that indicate Leydig cell failure, if there are no signs of puberty by 13–14 years of age, or if there is failure to progress through puberty, then androgen replacement therapy should be initiated.

Brain tumours

Both the adjuvant cytotoxic chemotherapy and the spinal fields of irradiation may damage the gonads in children treated for brain tumours. Ahmed et al.[15] studied gonadal function in children previously treated for medulloblastoma with surgery, followed by postoperative craniospinal irradiation. The nine children in the group that received adjuvant chemotherapy with nitrosoureas (carmustine [BCNU] or lomustine [CCNU]) plus procarbazine (in three patients) showed clinical and biochemical evidence of gonadal damage with elevated FSH concentrations and, in the boys, small testes for their stage of pubertal development. There was no evidence of gonadal damage in the group that did not receive

150

chemotherapy, all eight children completed pubertal development normally; the boys had adult-size testes and the girls regular menses. Ahmed *et al.*[15] concluded that nitrosoureas were responsible for the gonadal damage, with procarbazine contributing to the damage in the three children who received this drug.

Subsequently, long-term follow up in 21 girls and 29 boys who had received a nitrosourea (carmustine or lomustine) with or without procarbazine has shown that there is a high prevalence of primary gonadal dysfunction.[16 17] Both sexes progressed through puberty normally, with consistently raised basal concentrations of FSH and, occasionally, increased concentrations of LH. The girls achieved menarche at an appropriate age. As adults, most of the boys had inappropriately small testicular volumes, which are likely to be associated with severe oligospermia or azoospermia, and infertility. A sex difference in the reversibility of damage was observed. The boys showed no evidence of recovery of germinal epithelial function and no deterioration in Leydig cell function in a follow up extended to 11 years. In contrast, several girls who had previously been shown to have ovarian damage have continued with regular menses and normal FSH and oestradiol concentrations. Although it was not known whether these cycles are ovulatory, it is likely that these girls had recovered from the ovarian damage. The prospect of fertility among such girls is good in the early child-bearing years, but a premature menopause remains a possibility. Many of these children also received spinal irradiation, which results in a scattered irradiation dose to the gonad. In the boys, this results in a small dose to the testis estimated at 46–120 cGy (following a fractionated course of radiotherapy delivering a total dose of 3500 cGy to the whole spine in the Manchester centre). This small radiation dose is likely to contribute to the observed testicular damage. At other centres, individual boys who were treated with craniospinal irradiation but no chemotherapy have developed testicular dysfunction, but the scattered testicular irradiation dose is unknown.

In girls, the dose of irradiation received by the ovary may show greater variation. In the Manchester centre, a total dose in the range 90–1000 cGy has been estimated to reach the ovaries. The position of the ovaries in relation to the spinal field, and therefore the radiation dose received, can be difficult to estimate as the ovaries are mobile and their position may vary throughout the course of treatment. Nonetheless, the radiation dose received may contribute appreciably to ovarian dysfunction and this may be irreversible.

The scattered dose to the ovary will vary depending on the radiotherapy technique used at different centres. In a large study of gonadal dysfunction following treatment of intracranial tumours,[18] 18 of 42 girls (43%) showed evidence of primary ovarian dysfunction. Seven out of 11 girls who received craniospinal irradiation but no chemotherapy, and 9 out of 14 who had both craniospinal radiotherapy and adjuvant chemotherapy, had ovarian dysfunction. The authors concluded that spinal irradiation was the dominant gonadotoxic treatment. Hence the individual contributions of spinal irradiation and cytotoxic chemotherapy to ovarian damage following the treatment of intracranial tumours will vary depending on the radiotherapy techniques used and the nature of the adjuvant chemotherapy.

Abdominal tumours

Radiation damage to the ovary

There have been few studies of ovarian function following ovarian radiation, uncomplicated by the effects of other cytotoxic agents, in humans. Ovarian morphology following whole abdominal radiation (2000–3000 cGy) has been studied by Himmelstein-Braw et al.[19] in seven girls who died from malignant disease. They found that follicle growth was inhibited and, in the majority, the number of oocytes was markedly reduced.

The natural history of radiation-induced ovarian failure[20] was studied in 53 patients treated in childhood for an abdominal malignancy by surgery and radiotherapy. Of 38 patients who received whole abdominal irradiation (2000–3000 cGy), 27 failed to undergo or complete pubertal development (pubertal failure), and a premature menopause (median age 23·5 years) occurred in a further 10. Of 15 girls who received flank irradiation (2000–3000 cGy), ovarian function was normal in all but one in whom pubertal failure occurred. The median age at last assessment of this latter group is only 15 years. In only one patient, who developed pubertal failure after whole abdominal irradiation and required sex steroid replacement therapy to achieve normal secondary sex characteristics, has there been evidence of reversibility of ovarian function with a documented conception at the age of 22·7 years.

It is clear that the outlook for normal ovarian function following whole abdominal irradiation is poor. Flank irradiation, which was introduced intermittently from 1972, has resulted in less pubertal failure but the possibility of a premature menopause still exists. By further study of the 18 of these girls who received megavoltage whole abdominal radiotherapy (3000 cGy), and developed pubertal failure, the LD_{50} for the human oocyte has been estimated not to exceed 400 cGy as discussed above. Knowledge of the radiosensitivity of the human oocyte provides a more factual basis on which to provide fertility counselling for such patients. The dose of irradiation received by an ovary is dependent on the position in relation to the radiation field; this can be determined by pelvic ultrasound examination. If the dose received by the ovary furthest from the radiation field is calculated, then the surviving fraction of oocytes can be estimated and the predicted age at ovarian failure determined assuming an average complement of oocytes for age at the time of irradiation. With knowledge of the relationship between radiation dose and ovarian function, oophoropexy can be performed in carefully selected individuals with Hodgkin's disease or other pelvic tumours, thereby reducing the subsequent incidence of ovarian failure.[21][22]

Radiation and the uterus

In women in whom ovarian function is preserved, but in whom the uterus has been involved in the radiation field, there is evidence that radiation to the uterus often results in failure to carry a pregnancy. In 38 women who received whole abdominal irradiation (2000–3000 cGy) during childhood, studied by Wallace et al.[20] there were six conceptions in four patients, all ending in second trimester miscarriages. The majority of these 38 developed radiation-induced ovarian failure following whole abdominal irradiation. The uterine physical characteristics and blood flow were evaluated in 10 women, as was the functional uterine response to exogenous sex steroid replacement.[23] Those who received whole abdominal irradiation in childhood had uteri significantly smaller in length than women with premature ovarian failure not attributable to irradiation. This implies that prepubertal exposure to irradiation may have an irreversible effect on uterine development and vasculature. In addition, the endometrium was unresponsive to physiologic serum levels of oestradiol and progesterone, which were given by exogenous administration. Doppler signals from the uterine arteries were absent in most. It is unclear whether there is damage to the vasculature of the uterus, although this is possible as appropriate vascularisation and subsequent growth of the endometrium are essential for implantation and successful continuation of pregnancy. In summary, it is unlikely that women receiving a significant dose of abdominal irradiation in childhood will be able to sustain a pregnancy to term.

Radiation damage to the testis

There remain very few studies of testicular function following relatively low dose irradiation to the testes in childhood. Shalet et al.[24] studied testicular function in 10 men aged between 17 and 36 years who had received irradiation for a Wilm's tumour in childhood. The dose of scattered irradiation to the testes was 270–980 cGy (20 fractions over 4 weeks). Eight men had either oligo- or azoospermia (sperm count 0 to 5·6 million/ml) and seven of these had an elevated FSH level. All patients progressed through puberty spontaneously.

The impact of larger doses of testicular irradiation has been described in the ALL section. Additional comparative studies examining the age-dependency of radiation-induced Leydig cell damage have shown a much greater vulnerability to Leydig cell failure following the same dose of testicular irradiation in the prepubertal boy compared with the adult male.[25]

Bone marrow transplantation

The testis

Sklar et al.[26] examined eight males aged between 10 and 17 years at the time of transplant who were followed up for between 13 and 77 months after the bone marrow transplant. Therapy before bone marrow transplant consisted of high dose cyclophosphamide alone (two patients), high dose cyclophosphamide plus total lymphoid irradiation (one patient); the remaining five patients received total body irradiation (TBI) and either high dose cyclophosphamide or a combination of carmustine, cyclophosphamide, and cytarabine. Total lymphoid irradiation was given as a single dose of 750 cGy; the calculated dose of irradiation to the testis was 35–99 cGy. Total body irradiation was delivered as a single dose of 750 cGy. The basal serum FSH was elevated in six patients, and small testes were noted in four. Of the six with abnormal FSH levels, four, who were followed serially, showed a return of the basal FSH level to the normal range. Semen analysis, performed in one patient, revealed oligospermia despite normal basal gonadotrophins. Leydig cell function was less impaired in that seven of the eight patients had normal adult male levels of testosterone and all eight progressed through puberty normally.

The largest study to date of growth and development following bone marrow transplantation in childhood is from the Seattle group.[27] They studied 142 patients, aged between 1 and 17 years at the time of transplantation, who have survived disease free for more than one year after marrow transplantation for haematological malignancies. Before transplant all children received multiagent chemotherapy and 55 also received central nervous system irradiation given as a single dose of 920–1000 cGy (79 patients) or as fractionated doses of 200–225 cGy/day for 6–7 days (63 patients).

Sixty-three boys between the ages of 1 and 13 years were prepubertal at transplant. At study, 31 of these boys were between 13 and 22 years of age and 21 showed delayed development of secondary sexual characteristics. Biochemical investigations in 25 of the 31 boys who had entered puberty revealed isolated elevation of FSH concentration in 7 boys and both FSH and LH levels raised in 10 of the remainder, 4 of whom had an undetectable testosterone level. All 10 showed delayed development.

Biochemical investigations in 25 of 27 boys who were postpubertal at the time of transplant revealed raised FSH levels in 23, raised LH in 10, and a normal testosterone level in all. Semen analysis in four boys revealed azoospermia, thereby confirming the severe damage to the testicular germinal epithelium.

These results are in agreement with earlier conclusions on radiation-induced testicular damage. The Leydig cells of the prepubertal testis appear more vulnerable than those of the postpubertal testis to damage induced by total body irradiation. Severe damage to the germinal epithelium after TBI is inevitable and the chances of reversibility remain to be quantified.

The high incidence of delayed pubertal development and requirement for exogenous androgens to promote pubertal development[27][28] was surprising. These patients had received either 920–1000 cGy single exposure or 1200–1575 cGy fractionated TBI. In contrast Castillo et al.[14] had shown that after direct testicular irradiation used in the treatment of ALL, Leydig cell function is unimpaired with irradiation doses less than 1500 cGy given in eight fractions to prepubertal boys.

A recent collaborative study by Ogilvy-Stuart et al. between the Manchester and Glasgow Centres has shed some light on this controversy.[29] Testicular function was studied in 22 boys previously treated with fractionated TBI (1200–1500 cGy) in preparation for a bone marrow transplant. In addition four boys had received direct testicular irradiation (600–1000 cGy). Pubertal boys exhibited damage to the germinal epithelium with elevated FSH levels and small testicular volumes for pubertal stage. Nine of 12 pubertal boys entered and progressed through puberty spontaneously; the remaining three, who all received testicular irradiation in addition to TBI, required androgen therapy to induce puberty. Two had sufficient Leydig cell function on completion of puberty for androgens to be discontinued. Blunted testosterone responses to HCG stimulation were seen in all but four boys but did not accurately predict the potential for natural puberty. In conclusion, after fractionated TBI in childhood, Leydig cell damage is almost universal but often subtle. The requirement and timing of androgen replacement therapy needs clinical rather than biochemical determination.

The ovary

In view of the radiosensitivity of the human oocyte ($LD_{50} < 400$ cGy)[1] it is not surprising that a high prevalence of primary ovarian failure is found after TBI. In the large study by Saunders et al.[27] 35 girls were prepubertal at transplant (age 2–12 years), and 16 of the 35 were progressing through puberty at the time of the study. Six girls achieved menarche at an appropriate age (four of these six had received fractionated TBI) but the remaining ten girls showed delayed development of secondary sexual characteristics. Gonadotrophin and oestradiol levels in 11 of the 16 girls over the age of 12 years showed very high FSH and LH levels and an oestradiol level in the prepubertal range in seven, with transiently abnormal results in two of the remaining four girls.

Of the 17 girls who were postpubertal at the time of transplant, all had amenorrhoea with elevated FSH and LH levels and low oestradiol levels for the first two years post-transplant. Among 14 girls followed up between 3 and 14 years after transplant, four have shown recovery of ovarian function between three and five years after transplant. In conclusion, the majority of girls who have received high dose chemotherapy and total body irradiation before bone marrow transplantation are likely to develop irreversible ovarian failure. Appropriate sex steroid replacement therapy may be necessary to induce secondary sexual characteristics, alleviate symptoms of oestrogen deficiency, prevent osteoporosis, and decrease the risk of ischaemic heart disease in these patients.

Hodgkin's disease

Combination chemotherapy has greatly improved the prognosis for patients treated for Hodgkin's disease. This has resulted in the survival of an increasing number of young patients, cured of this cancer, but at risk from the late effects of the treatment.

Combination chemotherapy and the testis

Sherins et al.[30] were the first to report chemotherapy-induced testicular damage in patients treated for Hodgkin's disease in childhood. They studied 19 Ugandan boys who had been treated for Hodgkin's disease with mustine, vincristine, procarbazine, and prednisolone (MOPP) and were at least two years out from treatment. Eight out of nine pubertal boys had a raised basal FSH level, and in all six boys biopsied, testicular histology revealed germinal aplasia. Whitehead et al.[31] also found evidence of severe damage to the germinal epithelium in patients who received MOPP in childhood. Six patients, two of whom had also received a small dose of testicular irradiation, provided semen analysis between 2·4 and 8 years after completion of chemotherapy and were found to be azoospermic. Four boys studied whilst still prepubertal showed normal basal gonadotrophin levels and gonadotrophin responses to GnRH. However, several subjects treated when prepubertal showed normal serum gonadotrophin levels in pre-pubertal life but an evolving pattern of abnormally elevated gonadotrophin levels in early puberty, despite the increasing length of time since completion of chemotherapy. Despite the gloomy prognosis over the first 10 years after completion of chemotherapy, recovery of spermatogenesis has been described but only in a minority of subjects.[21 32]

There is no doubt that the cytotoxic drugs which damage the testis predominantly affect the germinal epithelium. However, subtle impairment of Leydig cell function has been suggested in adult men and boys treated with a regimen called MVPP in which vinblastine replaces the vincristine used in the MOPP regimen, for Hodgkin's disease. While the circulating testosterone concentration and response to hCG are normal, the basal LH concentration is frequently elevated and the LH response to a GnRH test exaggerated. The bioactive to immunoactive LH ratio is normal and there is no disturbance of LH pulse frequency; however, the amplitude of the LH pulses is significantly elevated. Due to this compensatory process, androgen replacement therapy is rarely indicated following chemotherapy-induced testicular damage[33] in adult life, whilst all boys treated with MVPP for Hodgkin's disease progress through puberty unaided.

Combination chemotherapy and the ovary

There are very few reports of ovarian function in girls treated for Hodgkin's disease with combination chemotherapy alone but the prognosis appear reasonable for the majority.[21][34]

In adulthood, the age of a woman is an important factor is determining if ovarian failure is likely to follow MOPP or MVPP for Hodgkin's disease. As the number of oocytes decreases steadily with increasing age, it is likely that ovarian function in prepubertal and pubertal girls may be less susceptible to cytotoxic-induced damage than in adult life.

Conclusion

In this review I have concentrated on the potential outcome for gonadal function following therapy for the common malignancies of childhood and adolescence such as ALL, brain tumours, Hodgkin's disease and Wilm's tumour. Clearly, however, a child or adolescent with any form of malignancy is at risk of infertility in adult life if he or she receives gonadotoxic chemotherapy or a radiation field which includes the gonad. Apart from inducing puberty in those in whom gonadal steroidogenesis has been damaged, there are risks of infertility and the possibility of recovery of fertility which must be discussed. Thus these teenagers and young adults require regular monitoring of their gonadal status and advice from a member of the medical team trained in reproductive endocrinology, usually a gynaecologist or an endocrinologist. The latter is a crucial member of the combined team responsible for dealing with the "late problems" amongst the increasing number of survivors of childhood malignancy.

1 Wallace WHB, Shalet SM, Hendry JH *et al.* Ovarian failure following abdominal irradiation in childhood: the radiosensitivity of the human oocyte. *Br J Radiol* 1989; **62**: 995–8.
2 Lendon M, Hann IM, Palmer MK *et al.* Testicular histology after combination chemotherapy in childhood for acute lymphoblastic leukaemia. *Lancet* 1978; **ii**: 439–41.
3 Uderzo C, Locasciulli A, Marzorati R *et al.* Correlation of gonadal function with histology of testicular biopsies at treatment discontinuation in childhood acute leukaemia. *Med Pediatr Oncol* 1984; **12**: 97–100.
4 Shalet SM, Hann IM, Lendon M *et al.* Testicular function after combination chemotherapy in childhood for acute lymphoblastic leukaemia. *Arch Dis Child* 1981; **56**: 275–8.
5 Quigley C, Cowell C, Jimenez M *et al.* Normal or early development of puberty despite gonadal damage in children treated for acute lymphoblastic leukaemia. *N Engl J Med* 1989; **321**: 143–51.
6 Wallace WHB, Shalet SM, Lendon M, Morris-Jones PH. Male fertility in long-term survivors of childhood acute lymphoblastic leukaemia. *Int J Androl* 1991; **14**: 312–19.
7 Siris ES, Leventhal BG, Vaitukaitis JL. Effects of childhood leukaemia and chemotherapy on puberty and reproductive function in girls. *N Engl J Med* 1976; **294**: 1143–6.
8 Himmelstein-Braw R, Peters H, Faber M. Morphological study of the ovaries of leukaemic children. *Br J Cancer* 1978; **38**: 82–7.
9 Green DM, Hall B, Zevon A. Pregnancy outcome after treatment for acute lymphoblastic leukaemia during childhood or adolescence. *Cancer* 1989; **64**: 2335–9.
10 Wallace WHB, Shalet SM, Tetlow LJ, Morris-Jones PH. Ovarian function following the treatment of childhood acute lymphoblastic leukaemia. *Med Pediatr Oncol* 1993; **21**: 333–9.

11 Brauner R, Czernichow P, Cramer P et al. Leydig cell function in children after direct testicular irradiation for acute lymphoblastic leukaemia. N Engl J Med 1983; 309: 25–8.

12 Leiper AD, Grant DB, Chessells JM. The effect of testicular irradiation on Leydig cell function in prepubertal boys with acute lymphoblastic leukaemia. Arch Dis Child 1983; 58: 906–10.

13 Shalet SM, Horner A, Ahmed SR, Morris-Jones PH. Leydig cell damage after testicular irradiation for lymphoblastic leukaemia. Med Pediatr Oncol 1985; 13: 65–8.

14 Castillo LA, Craft AW, Kernahan J et al. Gonadal function after 12-Gy testicular irradiation in childhood acute lymphoblastic leukaemia. Med Pediatr Oncol 1990; 18: 185–9.

15 Ahmed SR, Shalet SM, Campbell RHA, Deakin RHA. Primary gonadal damage following treatment of brain tumours in childhood. J Pediatr 1983; 103: 562–5.

16 Clayton PE, Shalet SM, Price DA, Morris-Jones PH. Ovarian function following chemotherapy for childhood brain tumours. Med Pediatr Oncol 1989; 17: 92–6.

17 Clayton P, Shalet SM, Price DA, Campbell RHA. Testicular damage after chemotherapy for childhood brain tumors. J Pediatr 1988; 112: 922–6.

18 Livesey EA, Brook CGD. Gonadal dysfunction after treatment of intracranial tumours. Arch Dis Child 1988; 63: 495–500.

19 Himmelstein-Braw R, Peters H, Faber M. Influence of irradiation and chemotherapy on the ovaries of children with abdominal tumours. Br J Cancer 1977; 36: 269–75.

20 Wallace WHB, Shalet SM, Crowne EC, Morris-Jones PH, Gattamaneni HR. Ovarian function following abdominal irradiation in childhood: Natural history and prognosis. Clin Oncol 1989; 1: 75–9.

21 Ortin TTS, Shostak CA, Donaldson SA. Gonadal status and reproductive function following treatment for Hodgkin's disease in childhood: the Stanford experience. Int J Radiat Oncol Biol Phys 1990; 19: 873–80.

22 Thibaud E, Ramirez M, Brauner R et al. Preservation of ovarian function by ovarian transposition performed before pelvic irradiation during childhood. J Pediatr 1992; 121: 880–4.

23 Critchley MOD, Wallace WHB, Shalet SM et al. Abdominal irradiation in childhood; the potential for pregnancy. Br J Obstet 1992; 99: 392–4.

24 Shalet SM, Beardwell CG, Jacobs HS, Pearson D. Testicular function following irradiation of the human prepubertal testis. Clin Endocrinol 1978; 9: 483–90.

25 Shalet SM, Tsatsoulis A, Whitehead E, Read G. Vulnerability of the human Leydig cell to radiation damage is dependent upon age. J Endocrinol 1989; 120: 161–5.

26 Sklar CA, Kim TH, Ramsay KC. Testicular function following bone marrow transplantation performed during or after puberty. Cancer 1984; 53: 1498–1501.

27 Sanders JE, Pritchard S, Mahoney P et al. Growth and development following marrow transplantation for leukaemia. Blood 1986; 68: 1129–35.

28 Sanders JE, Buckner CD, Sullivan KM et al. Growth and development in children after bone marrow transplantation. Horm Res 1988; 30: 92–7.

29 Ogilvy-Stuart AL, El-Abiary W, Clark DJ et al. Gonadal function after fractionated total body irradiation (TBI). J Endocrinol 1993; 137(suppl): 190.

30 Sherins RJ, Olweny CLM, Ziegler JL. Gynecomastia and gonadal dysfunction in adolescent boys treated with combination chemotherapy for Hodgkin's disease. N Engl J Med 1978; 299: 12–16.

31 Whitehead E, Shalet SM, Morris-Jones PH et al. Gonadal function after combination chemotherapy for Hodgkin's disease in childhood. Arch Dis Child 1982; 57: 287–91.

32 Shafford EA, Kingston JE, Malpas JS et al. Testicular function following the treatment of Hodgkin's disease in childhood. Br J Cancer 1993; 68: 1199–204.

33 Talbot JA, Shalet SM, Tsatsoulis A et al. Lutenizing hormone pulsatility in men with damage to the germinal epithelium. Int J Androl 1990; 13: 223–31.

34 Bramswig JH, Heiermann E, Heimes U et al. Ovarian function in 63 girls treated for Hodgkin's disease (HD) according to the West German DAL-HD-78 and DAL-HD-82 therapy study. Med Ped Oncol 1989; 17: 344.

11: Quality of life in Hodgkin's disease and lymphomas

JENNIFER DEVLEN

Recent advances in treatment, especially combination chemotherapy, have meant that certain previously fatal cancers can now be successfully treated. One might therefore reasonably predict that cancers with such optimistic prognoses might be associated with less psychological and social morbidity than those of a poorer prognosis or whose treatment entails the loss of a body part or function. Hodgkin's disease and the non-Hodgkin's lymphomas, although comparatively rare, are particularly interesting in this respect. They occur in relatively young patients, including both males and females, curative treatments are now available, and disfiguring surgery is not usually required. Yet, despite these favourable criteria, clinicians involved in treating this group of patients were aware that many had not regained their previous levels of functioning and psychological adjustment. These observations prompted the detailed study of the effects of diagnosis and treatment on these patients and their subsequent long-term adjustment. In the absence of any specific investigations of the impact of lymphomas on adolescents this chapter will review what is known from adult studies of Hodgkin's disease and non-Hodgkin's lymphomas which have often included teenage subjects in their sample.

Much of the data, both quantitative and qualitative, will be drawn from two studies that colleagues and I conducted in Manchester in the 1980s. We completed in depth interviews with a total of 210 patients, 10% of whom were aged 16–20 years. Our results will be compared to, and supplemented with, data reported by others who have studied this patient group.

There are three distinct stages in the progression from healthy individual to diagnosed cancer patient and then to cancer survivor, each posing specific problems, challenges, and concerns.

Becoming a cancer patient: the impact of diagnosis

Despite the optimism of the medial profession in relation to certain cancers, pessimistic attitudes of the general public still prevail and the diagnosis of cancer is still perceived with dread. In our investigations we were interested to find out what symptoms or signs patients first noticed, their subsequent route through the medical referral system, and their associated feelings as they made the transition to being a cancer patient.[1] Patients most commonly (78%) presented with an enlarged, palpable gland, either with (55%) or without (23%) other symptoms of tiredness, night sweats, weight loss, and pruritus. The delay between noticing signs or symptoms and seeking medical attention was generally short. Almost 50% claimed to have contacted their doctor within one week, while a percentage (13%) delayed more than three months, and a few (8%) as long as a year or more.

The onset of disease, or discovery of an enlarged gland, and progression from general practitioner to a specialist cancer centre has been found to be associated with a great deal of emotional distress. Over one third of patients suffer clinically significant anxiety or depression, or both, during this time.[2 3] These levels are equivalent to those found in subjects diagnosed with cancer of the breast[4] or lung.[5]

In our studies conducted in the Manchester area, the widespread reputation throughout the region of the Christie Hospital as a cancer hospital caused significant anxiety and worry in patients on learning of their own referral there.

> No one really told me. I knew I had something up with me—I had cancer or something when I got the letter [of an appointment to attend the Christie Hospital].

Often they were not given much information but nonetheless sensed the severity of the situation. Consultants at other local hospitals are no doubt aware of this and, not wanting to alarm the patient, were often very cautious in reporting results of preliminary investigations until they were certain.

> I kept asking what it was they'd done and what was the lump, and I kept being told 'we're waiting for a path lab report'. Well, then straight away my mind was on another wavelength—they've got something they don't want to tell me, which more or less proved so.

Changes in attitude toward more open communication about the diagnosis of cancer are reflected in patients' increased awareness of their cancer compared with several decades ago. Only 2% of patients in one study appeared to have no idea about their diagnosis[1] and another sample of patients were unanimous in their approval of having been told their diagnosis.[3]

Enduring treatment

Consultation with doctors and commencement of treatment resolves much of patients' anxiety and depression. Over one third of those who were anxious or depressed during this initial period improved significantly once treatment started.[2] Being given a clear diagnosis and a prognosis which was, for the most part, not as terrible as they had feared, undoubtedly does much to reassure patients. Those who had endured months of pain or vague physical symptoms were relieved that something was being done at last.

The mainstay of treatment for the lymphomas is combination chemotherapy, with or without radiation to site of disease. The treatment most commonly given to Hodgkin's disease patients is a cocktail comprising mustine, vincristine, prednisolone, and procarbazine (MOPP, or MVPP where vinblastine is substituted for vincristine). One cycle consists of mustine and vinblastine/vincristine given intravenously on days 1 and 8, with procarbazine and prednisolone taken orally for 14 days. Cycles are repeated at six-weekly intervals, and patients received usually 6–8 cycles over a period of 8–12 months. The majority of non-Hodgkin's lymphoma patients received vincristine, doxorubicin, and prednisolone or cyclophosphamide, vincristine, and prednisolone.[2]

Side effects

The use of chemotherapy in the treatment of Hodgkin's disease is noted as one of the successes of oncology,[6] but it is an aggressive treatment programme and severe side effects are associated with almost all of the cytotoxic agents used. Surveys of patients have catalogued up to 20 different treatment effects.[2 7 8]

Loss of hair is one of the most common adverse effects and, judging by patients' comments, the most devastating. Up to 28% become bald and a further 42% experienced hair loss to varying degrees. Although MVPP does not generally cause alopecia, hair loss from slight thinning to the extent of requiring a wig has been reported.[2] The significance of hair loss brought a deeper realisation for at least one patient. The following describes her reaction on being told she would lose her hair:

> That to me was even worse than telling me I had a tumour. That made me realise there was something wrong with me. It was something physical that I could see.

It was also the first outwardly visible sign, and patients who had wanted to keep their cancer private were now obliged to field questions from other people.

The other major side effects are nausea and vomiting. Vomiting is more severe during, and in many cases limited to, the afternoon or evening following an injection/infusion, when patients would vomit regularly, often every 10 minutes for several hours. Subsequent days were characteristically accompanied by feelings of nausea but this was comparatively mild.

Patients' appetites were also affected, varying in severity and duration. Loss of appetite was a consequence of either nausea or the experience of taste loss, associated with certain specific foods or with all food and drinks. This latter group would often increase their use of salt or spices in an attempt to provide some taste to otherwise bland food. Appetites for specific foods also altered, with some patients developing a "sweet tooth" while others found they uncharacteristically abhorred sweet foods. A few patients found they were eating more than normal, often with an insatiable appetite, due largely to the steroids given.

In spite of the fact that the cycles may be pharmacologically identical, patients' experiences of side effects, both in terms of their presence and severity, varies considerably from one cycle to the next[8] and this unpredictability enhances feelings of helplessness.[9]

It is important to note that these studies were carried out when chemotherapy for Hodgkin's disease consisted largely of mustine and vinca alkaloids, procarbazine, and prednisolone. New regimens with different or reduced toxicity now exist, but these studies remain relevant to the evaluation of young people undergoing toxic chemotherapy.

Conditioned responses

The dramatic emetogenic properties of the cytotoxic agents have caused patients to develop a conditioned response such that they become nauseous or even vomit before the administration of their chemotherapy. This phenomenon has been recorded in 21–34% of patients.[2 7 8 10] As the course of treatment progressed 7% would feel nauseous at the sight, smell, or thought of treatment.[2] A further 12·5% actually vomited on seeing the hospital and 7·5% would vomit at the mere thought of treatment. Conditioning also occurred with a variety of other stimuli, including travelling along the particular motorway leading to the hospital, or the chemotherapy nurse herself. Even outside the hospital context patients could experience severe nausea on a chance sighting of the nurse. These conditioned responses can be firmly developed by the fourth or fifth treatment cycle, putting patients in a severe dilemma. The treatment was becoming intolerable but their survival might be compromised if they opted out. They are particularly resistant to antiemetic medication although there is evidence that psychological interventions, such as relaxation training, systematic desensitisation, and hypnosis are effective.[11]

Psychiatric morbidity on treatment

Once treatment commences, the levels of depression and anxiety are never as high as during the initial period surrounding the onset and diagnosis of lymphoma. Prevalence figures vary depending on the criteria used to define morbidity and the length of the assessment period. Data from questionnaires reveal that 61% of a sample of lymphoma patients receiving chemotherapy rated themselves as having been depressed.[7] Using a standardised psychiatric interview Lloyd and colleagues[3] report 26% of their sample to have scores in the morbid range at the time of second assessment, 4–6 months after starting treatment. In a 12 month prospective study of 120 patients the month by month prevalence of anxiety and depression were assessed using a standardized psychiatric interview schedule.[12] Monthly levels of depression were in the range 8·3–15% and those for anxiety were 5–12·5%.[1] In total, 51% of patients had clinical levels of psychiatric morbidity at some time during the first year postdiagnosis: 26% suffered an anxiety state, depressive illness or mixed affective disorder, and a further 25% experienced borderline anxiety and/or depression. While the majority of this morbidity occurred in the first three months of treatment, patients were still likely to develop an affective disorder, especially depression at later times. Episodes of severe anxiety or depression lasted on average four months, while borderline cases lasted two months.

While as many lymphoma patients experience an episode of depression as do women after mastectomy, the overall prevalence of anxiety within lymphoma patients is less.[4] The duration of episodes of morbidity is shorter when compared with mastectomy patients.[4] Women with breast cancer face a more uncertain future and a higher risk of relapse and death, which may account for the higher levels of anxiety. Another critical difference is that mastectomy patients have to cope with the altered body image as a consequence of the removal of their breast. With the exception of the relatively few Hodgkin's disease patients who have a diagnostic laparotomy or splenectomy, surgery is limited to nodal biopsy. While a number of lymphoma patients are severely affected by surgery, permanent altered body image is less relevant to this group of patients.

In addition there was evidence of transient episodes of depression specifically related to treatment reported by one in five patients.[2] These episodes, ranging in length from one hour to three days, did not last long enough to be rated using the strict criteria of the psychiatric interview schedule. They occurred at the same point in the treatment schedule and, despite their subclinical nature, were quite distinct and caused patients a great deal of worry.

In addition to the above physically related effects, treatments caused distress for various other reasons. Patients who coped with the chemotherapy by looking forward to its completion and counted off each course were distressed if told they needed additional courses. Patients often became upset if they could not receive treatment on schedule because of a low blood count, for example, while on the other hand, those who were told that their disease had responded rapidly were perplexed and resentful by the need to continue treatment.

Identifying psychiatric morbidity

One third of lymphoma patients who suffered a depressive illness or anxiety state were referred to a psychiatrist,[2] a higher detection and referral rate than that previously found in mastectomy patients.[12] Open communication between clinicians and patients clearly assisted in the detection of psychological problems. The doctors regularly asked patients how they were feeling on treatment, but what patients were prepared to reveal varied:

> I don't talk [to the doctors] much about the illness because there isn't a lot to talk about. I know what the situation is . . . I go and if I'm alright I'm very happy and I leave. I don't mention problems and side effects.

Specifically asking patients about treatment or psychological problems would improve the early detection of morbidity.

Memory difficulties

In our initial retrospective study of 90 patients who had completed treatment,[13] one third of patients complained of difficulty in remembering names, addresses, or shopping lists without writing them down. In each case patients emphasised that this was a deterioration from their normal state before diagnosis. This was often rationalised as a sign of advancing years, but even patients in their early twenties were attributing this change to age.

Prompted by this finding, objective tests of memory[14] were included in a prospective study.[2] Baseline assessments were made before patients commenced treatment, against which assessments at six and twelve months were compared. Scores for the Hodgkin's disease/non-Hodgkin's lymphoma patient sample were within the normal range[14] and showed little change over time. Despite the evidence of little objective change, 39% of the sample complained of subjective memory impairment. These complaints were made at several assessment interviews, indicating that it was not a transient condition. Patients who reported subjective impairments had consistently and significantly lower scores than those who did not report any such impairment.

Insufficient numbers receiving individual treatment regimens prevented any analysis of treatment as a possible predictor of these cognitive impairments. Similar testing by Oxman and Silberfarb[15] failed to find any direct relationship between impairment and chemotherapy, implying that it may be wrong to view chemotherapy as a direct cause of organic brain damage. However, there are other possible explanations. Organic brain damage may have been caused by the disease itself, either directly or indirectly from metabolic changes. Alternatively, it may have been produced by a secondary effect of chemotherapy, through viral infections when patients were immunosuppressed. Memory impairment could also have been due to disturbances of mood, particularly depression. This may explain some of the subjective impairment in the later stages of treatment, when a relationship with mood disorder was found,[1] but it is unlikely to be a sufficient explanation because few of those who complained of impairment some two to three years postdiagnosis had an affective disorder.[13]

Social and occupational functioning

In the first few months after diagnosis, it is perhaps expected that there will be some disruption to work and social life.[8] Patients are feeling unwell with the side effects of treatment, and so would be unlikely to be as active as they had been before. However, there is evidence to suggest that while some patients return to normal activities relatively quickly, others are unwilling to attempt too much activity too soon in case their illness returns.

Many previously active patients appeared to be content to take a passive role and be looked after by a caring relative.

Many of those employed at the time of diagnosis preferred to stay off work until all treatment was finished. This was perceived as preferable to taking several days "off sick" after each course of chemotherapy, which might disrupt or upset their employer. This pattern might also jeopardise their eligibility for sickness benefit, with its consequent financial implications. Those who returned to work almost immediately and those who delayed returning for more than one year were more likely to be depressed when compared with those who stayed off work for 3–12 months. One could hypothesise that the benefits of re-attaining the work role may be outweighed by the burden of taking on too much when patients are not physically strong enough, and returning too soon may be a causal factor in the onset of depression. For those patients who continued working or returned fairly quickly, it was often not to their previous position but to a different one within the firm, usually with less responsibility, and this may be the source of the discontent.

Younger patients still at school had difficulties keeping up with existing course work and simultaneously catching up on work missed while they were off sick. This added further pressures upon them at a time in their lives when they were taking important examinations and making applications for further education or employment.

Finances

Major illness carries with it a variety of hidden expenses, over and above what is covered by national or private health insurance and these can mount up to a substantial proportion of the annual family income.[16] Regional centres treat patients from far and wide, and with 20% travelling more than 50 miles to attend one such centre[1] families may incur substantial travel costs. Coupled with possible loss of earnings through not working, there may well be financial problems to contend with.

Relationships

With the exception of two investigations[2 13] few of the studies of lymphoma patients during treatment have provided much information about social or relationship problems. Much of what we know has come from the research on survivors who are often asked retrospectively about possible difficulties while they were on treatment. The evidence suggests that the illness brings most patients and their families closer together, but there are some notable difficulties. Some patients report that they had to be supportive to their families and not vice versa. This role reversal can be true for teenagers who sometimes have to take on very mature responsibilities.

> I tried to keep calm because I knew if I panicked others would, especially my parents . . . I talked a lot with my parents . . . I had to convince them that I wasn't going to die.

165

A small proportion (12·5%) of married patients report a decline in communication and 30% said that there were areas they could not discuss with their spouses.[17] Some feel that their spouse cannot cope and often turn to another family member for support[1] as these quotes suggest:

> I felt closer to my mother. My husband won't think of anything bad happening. He tells me not to be so stupid. I can't seem to get close to him on that subject.

> I can discuss everything with my mother. I don't talk to my wife much because I seem to depress her most times.

This apparent inability to cope with the situation on the part of spouses hints at what may be real problems in communication which may have ultimately negative consequences for the partnership, as we shall see when we consider the long term effects.

Termination of therapy

While only 1% of patients actually discontinue treatment, almost half contemplate doing so.[8] Patients complained that they found it very difficult to make themselves attend for chemotherapy and this got progressively worse with each cycle. Rather than rejoicing at reaching the last cycle, they may find this the hardest to face:

> The last 7 tablets I had to take, I couldn't have taken them if you'd given me £100, I was heaving so much just looking at them.

Yet, despite the complications of chemotherapy and radiotherapy, finishing treatment could be distressing. This may be especially so if treatment is terminated prematurely, when the patient may feel a sense of "failure" and personally responsible should a recurrence develop for not having completed the advised protocol.[9] While the clinicians may feel their goal has been achieved, patients may not feel prepared to take sole responsibility for their health. The change in status from patient to convalescing cancer survivor is accompanied by various social expectations for which the patient/survivor may not yet have the physical and psychological resources to manage.[9]

Surviving cancer

The five-year survival rate for all cancer sites has been estimated to have improved from 10% earlier this century to more than 50% now.[18] The picture for certain cancers, notably Hodgkin's disease, is even better and the majority of patients can consider cure. With the increasing number of cancer survivors, research has directed attention to describing the quality of life in this group who have come close to the prospect of death and suffered the ordeals of cancer treatment. This has been not merely an academic exercise, but prompted by the experience of clinicians who were concerned about the levels of adjustment in this group.

There have been several studies specifically investigating the psychosocial adjustment in Hodgkin's disease and/or non-Hodgkin's lymphoma survivors at differing points after the completion of treatment[13 19 20 21] so providing important information highlighting the problems and their likely trajectories over time.

Physical effects

Both radiotherapy and chemotherapy have carcinogenic effects and this oncogenic impact is thought to be enhanced when combined modality treatment is used as is often the case in the treatment of lymphomas. Survivors of Hodgkin's disease have been shown to have an increased risk of developing leukaemia, non-Hodgkin's lymphoma, and, less strongly, solid tumours,[18] although the actual incidence is still very modest and the value of current treatments is considered to far outweigh the risk.[22] More immediately, one study reports that 45% of Hodgkin's disease survivors had a serious medical problem after completing treatment.[23] The details were not given, but 22% were judged likely to have been related directly to the Hodgkin's disease or its treatment.

In addition to these more serious late medical complications and general poor health, substantial numbers of survivors complain of specific physical symptoms, similar in kind to the B symptoms,[19] low energy,[13 21] and lack of stamina.[19] Energy levels may be low for well over a year after finishing treatment and even nine years later 37% felt their energy had not fully returned.[21] These are problematic in themselves, as well as interfering with functioning, and are implicated in inducing depression.[21] Younger patients remained more active and had a quicker return of energy than older patients.

Continuing fears about health

An 80% cure rate may be interpreted very optimistically by clinicians and epidemiologists, but the patient may focus instead on the 20% chance of recurrence and death. At the time of diagnosis patients' concerns are centred around the results of tests, and then, once treatment starts, they worry about predicted side effects and how well they are responding to treatment. Once remission is attained, the perspective changes to concerns about the possibility of recurrence. Even years after completing treatment, the disease is still an inseparable part of survivors' lives. Such fears are certainly not allayed by being refused health or life insurance, a not uncommon occurrence.

Conditioned nausea and vomiting

Unfortunately, the conditioned responses developed during chemotherapy appear not to be so easily extinguishable once treatment ceases. In the following two years 61% are still experiencing nausea with a very small percentage (5%) actually vomiting[24] in response to a number of stimuli associated with the hospital. Extinction does gradually occur with time, but nonetheless, 39% still continue to be affected[20 24] making attendance for

167

follow up appointments problematic. Psychological interventions have proved successful at this time as well as during chemotherapy (MacLeod, personal communication) but the difficulty may lie in identifying which individuals are still suffering.

Sexual problems

The effects of advanced disease, radiotherapy, and chemotherapy on gonadal function are now well documented (Sutcliffe[25] and Shalet, this volume) which is unfortunate given that Hodgkin's disease affects patients in a younger age group where gender role, sexual function, and fertility are major concerns. In the first two years after completing treatment one third of men had confirmed evidence or considered themselves infertile[23] and sexual problems in the form of decreased interest, activity or satisfaction are present in 20–25% of both men and women.[13 19] The prevalence of sexual problems remains at this level even seven years later.[21] It is important to appreciate that patients do not readily interpret these changes as due to gonadal function and so their physiological origins should be made explicit by the health care team in order to avoid any further distress.

Psychological morbidity

Levels of anxiety and depression gradually decrease over the first year after diagnosis[2] but estimates of the long-term prevalence of psychiatric morbidity vary considerably between different studies. Clinical levels of morbidity have ranged from 14% at approximately three years post-diagnosis[13] to 22% six years post-treatment.[20] Psychological symptoms are generally higher than those given for normative samples, but Cella and Tross found equally high levels in age-matched male friends of their 60 male survivors.[19] Six years after completing treatment, clinical depression in survivors was reported to be no more common than in a community sample[21] or in healthy controls.[19] It would appear that major psychopathology is rare but there is some consensus about the existence of a small subgroup of survivors who continue to suffer psychiatric problems.

Neuropsychological problems

As we have seen, formal prospective testing of memory before and during treatment failed to identify deficits outside the normal range, although those who noted difficulties had significantly lower test scores. Persistent impairment of memory and concentration with prevalence of 27–33% have been noted in more than one study,[13 19] but the precise origins are as yet unclear.

Relationship difficulties

The closeness that patients and their spouses reported during treatment may not last, and the long-term outcome for relationships appears less good. In one sample, one half of those who were married at the time of diagnosis and who subsequently divorced attributed their marriage breakdown directly to their Hodgkin's disease.[21] In those who do stay together, both partners note a decline in supportiveness and communication after treatment finishes. For survivors their prominent concerns are now focused on the fear of recurrence, but their wives avoided talking about problems, fears, and concerns in order to "protect" their spouse.[17] The authors underscore the negative effects on relationships and the need to devise ways of intervening with couples to enhance long-term marital functioning and to resolve this conspiracy of silence.

Occupational limitations

As discussed earlier, the illness and treatment required patients to take time off work, but one quarter of those who were employed at the time of their diagnosis did not subsequently return to work at all.[13] A number took early retirement, some very reluctantly. In contrast, one woman gave up her job saying:

> I'm not working and having cancer as well. If I've got to die I might as well die happy.

Others were no longer physically able to work and expressed guilt when their spouse was subsequently obliged to seek work. Illness, tiredness, and difficulties in concentrating affected those still at school and some teenage patients had to repeat their national exams or gave up studying altogether. Career aspirations of some were also dashed, as the following quote of a teenage boy illustrates:

> My first two career choices [of the army and the police] have both been wiped out because I'm not A1 fit any more.

Whether or not these individuals find satisfying alternative careers is not known. There are reported incidences of direct discrimination at work, including subjects being fired, demoted, or encouraged to leave their job[23] and, looking back, up to one third feel their cancer has had a negative effect on their career, income or educational achievements.[19 23]

Predicting psychological morbidity

While minor degrees of depression and anxiety are very common, and natural reactions at times of crises, these must be distinguished from emotional states of sufficient intensity or persistence to be considered morbid and justifying psychiatric or psychological treatment. Being able to identify which patients might be at risk of developing clinically significant morbidity would enable health care professionals to monitor these more closely and permit earlier intervention. To this end, attempts have been made to identify variables and characteristics which distinguish those patients who experience psychological disturbance from those who do not, with somewhat inconsistent results.

169

Impact of Hodgkin's disease and non-Hodgkin's lymphoma on the quality of life of survivors

Medical
 physical discomfort, poor general health
 major medical problems
 second malignancy
 sleep disruption
 poor appetite
 loss of energy
 poor stamina
 persisting nausea/vomiting
Sexual
 infertility
 decreased interest, activity, satisfaction
Psychological
 anxiety
 depression
 irritability
 negative body image
 fears of recurrence
Neuropsychological
 poor concentration
 memory impairment
Relationship
 separation, divorced, never marrying
 communication difficulties with partner
Occupational
 discrimination at work
 decreased earning potential
 exclusion from certain professions
 decreased educational achievement
 denial of health and life insurance

During treatment

Lloyd and colleagues report that women had significantly higher morbidity scores than men,[3] but no sex difference during treatment was found by others.[2] There is no evidence from any source to date that the patient's age is relevant. Neither the type of tumour nor more advanced disease seem to have any relationship with psychological problems during this time.

Both depression and anxiety are highly correlated with the number[2][7][8] and severity of side effects[2] experienced. Those consistently found to be correlated with morbidity are those involving the gastrointestinal tract which render eating difficult, like nausea, vomiting, appetite loss, sore mouth, and changes in the taste of food. Patients often stressed the importance of eating well to maintain their strength in order to endure treatment and combat the disease, and the prevention of this may explain some of this association with psychiatric morbidity.

The exact causal relationship between treatment side effects and psychological morbidity is hard to disentangle. The unpleasant side effects wear patients down over time, and anxiety and depression may be a consequence of continually experiencing these adverse effects. Conversely, mood disturbance may have lowered patients' tolerance of treatment and particularly any adverse effects.

Social theories of depression, useful in other populations,[26] have received little support in studies of lymphoma patients. The presence or absence of a close confiding tie was not found to be a predictor of psychiatric morbidity.[1] However, lymphoma patients who were married or cohabiting were found to be more at risk for depression during treatment than those who were single, divorced, or widowed. Information from interviews suggests that patients may have avoided disclosing their concerns because they did not want to distress their loved ones. If this is true, research should be directed toward investigating not the absence or presence of a confiding relationship in general, but whether patients can utilise and disclose their concerns about their cancer to this person. The fact that many patients talk more freely and fully to a research interviewer than to anyone else is worrying.

For lymphoma patients presenting with a palpable lymph node, the effectiveness of treatment can be monitored by the accompanying reduction in size of their node(s). Indeed, patients who notice a gradual diminution of their nodes over several cycles of treatment have been found to be less distressed or depressed when compared with those who have either a rapid, dramatic response or a late response in node size.[7]

After completing treatment

Overall treatment toxicity and the same specific gastrointestinal effects found to be associated with morbidity during treatment are also related to psychiatric problems later on.[13] Lack of energy has also been noted as a significant variable.[21] The authors suggest a knock-on effect of persisting symptoms leading to inability to perform usual activities and resultant loss of social contact and self esteem which inhibits normal recovery and possibly leads to depression. A number of studies have found levels of psychological morbidity to be inversely related to time since completing treatment,[19 21] and it may be that psychological wellbeing improves in conjunction with physical status.

Other demographic and disease variables have been investigated with contradicting results. Kornblith et al.[23] note that the highest distress scores two years after treatment for advanced Hodgkin's disease were more likely in men, but record no gender differences at six years.[20] Again, there is no evidence of any relationship between adjustment and age and this can be tentatively interpreted as adolescent patients having an equal risk of becoming anxious or depressed as older adults, but clearly more research needs to be conducted on this particular group.

Conclusions

Those with Hodgkin's disease or non-Hodgkin's lymphoma suffer considerable physical, psychological, and social problems directly related to the diagnosis and treatment of their disease, at levels similar to those found in patients with worse prognosis cancers. The use of aggressive treatment has resulted in very good five year survival figures, but the cost to survivors' long term quality of life has been shown to be high. Major psychopathology and functional disruption appear to be rare, but subtle residual effects are common. Specifically asking patients at routine follow-up visits about persisting conditioned nausea/vomiting, depression, sexual problems, and relationship difficulties will help to identify those who could benefit from intervention.

There is a general policy of greater openness about diagnosis, prognosis, and general patient education. Yet researchers still report that patients express a desire to be better informed about the potential side effects and disruptions to their functioning. To be forewarned is to be forearmed, and many patients gain comfort from hearing that the feelings and impairments they are experiencing are not uncommon and, usually, reversible. Having a realistic understanding allows patients to modify their expectations and minimise frustration and helplessness. As more information about these long-term difficulties becomes available this should be passed on to patients.

To date there is little information about how Hodgkin's disease/non-Hodgkin's lymphoma affects individuals at different stages in the life cycle, and therefore research could profitably be turned to investigating the impact on adolescents in relation to their specific physical, psychological and social developmental tasks and their long-term quality of life.

1 Devlen J. *Psychological and social aspects of Hodgkin's disease and non-Hodgkin's lymphoma.* PhD thesis, University of Manchester, 1984.
2 Devlen J, Maguire P, Phillips P, Crowther D. Psychological problems associated with diagnosis and treatment of lymphomas. II: Prospective study. *Br Med J* 1987; **295**: 955–7.
3 Lloyd GG, Parker AC, Ludlam CA, McGuire RJ. Emotional impact of diagnosis and early treatment of lymphomas. *J Psychosom Res* 1984; **28**: 157–62.
4 Maguire GP, Lee EG, Bevington DJ *et al.* Psychiatric problems in the first year after mastectomy. *Br Med J* 1978; **1**: 963–5.
5 Hughes J. *Cancer and emotion. Psychological preludes and reactions to cancer.* Chichester: Wiley, 1987.
6 Selby P, McElwain TJ, Canellos G. Chemotherapy for Hodgkin's disease. In: Selby P, McElwain TJ, eds, *Hodgkin's disease.* Oxford: Blackwell, 1987.
7 Nerenz DR, Leventhal H, Love RR. Factors contributing to emotional distress during cancer chemotherapy. *Cancer* 1982; **50**: 1020–7.
8 Love RR, Leventhal H, Easterling DV, Nerenz DR. Side effects and emotional distress during cancer chemotherapy. *Cancer* 1989; **63**(3): 604–12.
9 Cohn KH. Chemotherapy from an insider's perspective. *Lancet* 1982; **1**: 1006–9.
10 Morrow GR. Prevalence and correlates of anticipatory nausea and vomiting in chemotherapy patients. *J Natl Cancer Inst* 1982; **68**: 585–8.
11 Watson M, Marvell C. Anticipatory nausea and vomiting among cancer patients: a review. *Psychology and Health* 1992; **6**: 97–106.
12 Maguire P, Tait A, Brooke M. Emotional aspects of mastectomy: a conspiracy of pretence.

Nursing Mirror 1980; Jan 10; 17–19.

13 Devlen J, Maguire P, Phillips P *et al.* Psychological problems associated with diagnosis and treatment of lymphomas. I: Retrospective study. *Br Med J* 1987; **295**: 953–4.

14 Wechsler D. A standardized memory scale for clinical use. *J Psychol* 1945; **19**: 87–95.

15 Oxman TE, Silberfarb PM. Serial cognitive testing in cancer patients receiving chemotherapy. *Am J Psychiatr* 1980; **137**: 1263–5.

16 Lesko LM. Hematological malignancies. In: J C Holland, JH Rowland, eds, *Handbook of psychooncology: psychological care of the patient with cancer.* New York: Oxford University Press, 1990.

17 Hannah MT, Gritz ER, Wellisch DK *et al.* Changes in marital and sexual functioning in long-term survivors and their spouses: testicular cancer versus Hodgkin's disease. *Psycho-Oncology* 1992; **1**: 89–103.

18 Tross S, Holland JC. Psychological sequelae in cancer survivors. In: JC Holland, JH Rowland, eds, *Handbook of psychooncology psychological care of the patient with cancer.* New York: Oxford University Press, 1990.

19 Cella D, Tross S. Psychological adjustment to survival from Hodgkin's disease. *J Consult Clin Psychol* 1986; **5**: 616–22.

20 Kornblith AB, Anderson J, Cella DF *et al.* Hodgkin Disease survivors at increased risk for problems in psychosocial adaptation. *Cancer* 1992; **70**: 2214–24.

21 Fobair P, Hoppe RT, Bloom J *et al.* Psychosocial problems among survivors of Hodgkin's disease. *J Clin Oncol* 1986; **4**: 805–14.

22 Colman M, Selby P. Second malignancies and Hodgkin's disease. In: Selby P, McElwain TJ, eds, *Hodgkin's disease.* Oxford: Blackwell, 1987.

23 Kornblith AB, Anderson J, Cella DF *et al.* Comparison of psychosocial adaptation and sexual function of survivors of advanced Hodgkin disease treated by MOPP, ABVD, or MOPP alternating with ABVD. *Cancer* 1992; **70**: 2508–16.

24 Cella DR, Pratt A, Holland JC. Persistent anticipatory nausea, vomiting, and anxiety in cured Hodgkin's disease patients after completion of chemotherapy. *Am J Psychiatry* 1986; **143**: 641–3.

25 Sutcliffe SB. Infertility and gonadal function in Hodgkin's disease. In: Selby P, McElwain TJ, eds, *Hodgkin's disease.* Oxford: Blackwell, 1987.

26 Brown GW, Harris T. *Social origins of depression.* London: Tavistock, 1978.

12: Management of testicular cancer

DP DEARNALEY and A HORWICH

Introduction

Testicular cancer is a relatively rare malignancy, accounting for approximately 1% of all male tumours. However, it is the most common form of cancer in men 15–35 years of age, and the white male has a 1 in 500 chance of developing testicular cancer.[1] The considerable majority of tumours are of germ cell origin. The peak incidence of seminoma at a medium of 37 years is 10 years more than for malignant teratoma (median 27 years), and seminoma in the adolescent age group is extraordinarily uncommon. The age incidence of patients with germ cell tumours presenting to the Royal Marsden Hospital is shown in Figure 12.1, approximately 11% of men presenting with teratoma were under 20 and a further 27% between 20 and 24. There has been a continuing rise in the incidence of testicular cancer during the century in the majority of Western countries. For example, an approximate doubling in registrations for men aged 15–44 years was recorded in England and Wales between 1963 and 1981.[2] It is particularly of interest that cryptorchidism which is present in about 10% of testicular cancer patients is also increasing in incidence. Studies from the Oxford

---

Risk factors for testicular cancer

Age—High risk 24 years

Upper social class

Race—white > black

Low birthweight

Cryptorchidism

Inguinal hernia

Prenatal oestrogen exposure

Familial syndromes

First degree family relative with testicular cancer

Group revealed a 65% increase between 1960 and 1984; as cryptorchidism and testicular cancer share etiological factors the rising incidence suggests that testicular cancers will continue to become more common over the next 20 years.[3]

It is, therefore, perhaps fortunate that teratoma has become a model for curable cancer, and that treatment approaches have been revolutionised since the introduction of effective cisplatin-containing chemotherapy in the 1970s. About 85–90% of patients with disseminated germ cell tumours can now be successfully cured: a dramatic change from the early 1970s when less than 20% of men would have been successfully treated. The role of surgery remains essential both for removal of the primary tumour and resection of any postchemotherapy residual masses. A further important feature of testicular cancer which distinguishes it from other neoplasms is the availability of accurate serum markers—human chorionic gonadotrophin (βHCG) and α-fetoprotein (AFP)—which are essential aids to the diagnosis, staging, follow-up (particularly during surveillance), and monitoring of response to chemotherapy treatment. The Royal Marsden Hospital staging system is shown in Table 12.1, and Table 12.2 shows the stage distribution of patients with malignant teratoma presenting at the Royal Marsden Hospital between 1980 and 1989. The treatment of each stage has evolved over the last decade and has become refined as careful analysis of multicentre series has determined the factors predicting outcome.

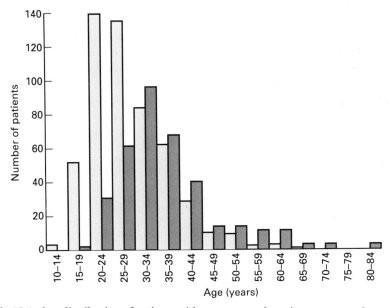

Fig 12.1 Age distribution of patients with teratoma and seminoma presenting to the Royal Marsden Hospital between 1980 and 1988. Dark bars, teratoma; light bars, seminoma

Table 12.1   Royal Marsden Hospital Staging classification

Stage		Definition
I	M	Rising postorchidectomy markers only
II		Abdominal lymphadenopathy
	A	<2 cm
	B	2–5 cm
	C	>5 cm
III		Supradiaphragmatic lymphadenopathy
	O	No abdominal disease
	ABC	Abdominal node size as in stage II
IV		Extralymphatic metastases
	L1	≤3 lung metastases
	L2	>3 lung metastases all <2 cm diameter
	L3	>3 lung metastases, 1 or more >2 cm
	H+	Liver involvement

Management of stage I teratoma

Prior to the introduction of cisplatin-containing chemotherapy, adjuvant radiation to the retroperitoneal and pelvic lymph nodes or retroperitoneal lymph node dissection were the standardly employed treatment options. Radiotherapy is now principally of historical interest but in a randomised study carried out by the Danish Testicular Cancer Study Group[4] 11 of 67 patients randomised to receive radiotherapy developed recurrent disease but all but one were salvaged by chemotherapy. There were no retroperitoneal relapses. Although this policy had some merit, treatment toxicity included an increased risk of gastrointestinal and bone marrow complications if salvage chemotherapy was required and additional toxic effects of radiotherapy include peptic ulceration.[5] At this time the debate between radiotherapy and surgery revolved around the unwanted effects of these treatments. The classic bilateral retroperitoneal lymph node dissection is associated with loss of autonomic enervation affecting seminal emission in the majority of cases.[6] Subsequently, on the basis of detailed description by Donohue and colleagues of the distribution of retroperitoneal metastases in early stage non-seminoma, modified surgical procedures have been adopted.[7][8] Approximately 90% of patients submitted to unilateral retroperitoneal lymph node dissection have been reported to maintain or recover antegrade ejaculation postoperatively.[9] Retroperitoneal recurrence is extremely uncommon (reported at 0·7% by Rorth et al. 1989.[10] Although the procedure demands an expert surgeon, in experienced hands there should be negligible postoperative mortality. This approach of nerve-sparing retroperitoneal lymph node dissection has gained wide acceptance in many parts of North America and Europe. However, in the United

Table 12.2   Stage distribution of testicular teratoma, Royal Marsden Hospital 1980–9

Stage	I	Im	II	III	IV
Percentage of patients	46	2	23	3	26

Table 12.3. Testicular tumours Teratoma Stage I surveillance

Month	0	1	2	3	4	5	6	7	8	9	10	11	12
CPD		+		+		+		+		+		+	
Markers		+	+	+	+	+	+	+	+	+	+	+	+
CXR		+	+		+	+		+	+		+	+	+
CT chest, abdomen, and pelvis				+			+			+			+

Year 2	OPD q 3/12 (CT abdomen and pelvis @ 24/12)
Year 3	OPD q 4/12
Year 4	OPD q 6/12

Then annually (markers and CXR each visit, no routine CT)
Teratoma post-chemotherapy F/U

Year 1	q 2/12
Year 2	q 3/12
Year 3	q 6/12

Then annually (markers and CXR each visit, no routine CT)

Kingdom a different philosophy has been adopted. The successful treatment of disseminated germ cell tumours with cisplatin-containing chemotherapy led to the introduction of surveillance as an initial management policy with salvage chemotherapy for relapsing patients.[11] In the 1980s many other centres in the United Kingdom followed this lead and the Medical Research Council (MRC) initiated two prospective studies of "surveillance" which have shown that approximately 30% of men with stage I teratoma go on to develop metastatic disease—which of course means that 70% of patients avoid further treatment after initial orchidectomy. From the total of 632 men entered into these studies, only 5 have died from recurrent teratoma.[12] Detailed and rigorous follow-up is required to ensure that recurrence is detected as soon as possible so that the probability of cure will not be compromised. The follow-up schedule adopted at the Royal Marsden Hospital is shown in Table 12.3, although there remains some debate concerning the optimal frequency of follow-up investigations.[12]

The MRC Testicular Tumour Working Party has reviewed histology from the orchidectomy specimens of men in these surveillance studies and developed prognostic models which predict the risk of developing recurrent disease. Data from the first MRC study showed that teratoma recurred in 70 of 233 men; the overall recurrence rate was 32% at five years with 95% confidence intervals of 25–40%. Multivariate analysis determined four factors which were related to the risk of recurrence (box).

Recurrence risk factors

- tumour invasion of testicular veins
- tumour invasion of testicular lymphatics
- the presence of undifferentiated cells
- the absence of yolk sac elements

If three or four of these factors were present, then the five year relapse-free rate was 42%.[13] This high risk group of patients comprised 25% of the total patient population. Subsequently, this model was validated in the second prospective MRC study which included 373 patients.[14] The 83 patients (22% of the study group) with three or four risk factors had a 53% two year relapse-free rate compared to 80% for patients with two risk factors or fewer. On univariate analysis venous or lymphatic invasion were the most important predictive factors and using these criteria alone defined a high risk subgroup (venous or lymphatic invasion positive) which comprised 190 patients (51% of the study group) who had a 62% relapse-free rate compared to 85% for patients without venous or lymphatic invasion. The value of these observations is firstly, that it enables more accurate information to be given to patients and secondly, that definition of a high risk subgroup permits selection of patients for adjuvant chemotherapy.

The first study of adjuvant chemotherapy was performed by the Testicular Cancer Intergroup Study reported by Williams et al (1987).[15] In this study 195 men with stage II disease (determined by retroperitoneal lymph dissection) were randomised to surveillance or adjuvant chemotherapy using two courses of bleomycin, etoposide, and cisplatin (BEP). The recurrence rate in the surveillance arm was 40% with three deaths from disease. In the adjuvant chemotherapy arm there were six recurrences (6%), but five of these patients recurred before receiving their cytotoxic treatment; in this arm of the study there was one death from disease. The second study has been performed by the MRC Testicular Tumour Working Party. Patients with three out of four of the high risk factors defined above were treated in an open phase II study with two courses of BEP chemotherapy. Preliminary results (data from MRC Testicular Tumour Working Party) shows that 2 out of 115 eligible patients have developed recurrent disease but no disease-related deaths have been reported.[16]

It is now clear that there are a number of different treatment approaches which achieve near 100% cure rates for men with stage I teratoma. The choice between the options depends on the physician's and patient's perceptions of the relative toxicities and hazards of each treatment approach, but decisions may be significantly helped by the use of the MRC pathological risk factors. Surveillance gives the best chance of avoiding any further treatment, and is particularly appropriate for patients with low pathological risk factors. Disadvantages include the requirement for close meticulous follow up which may generate anxiety. As the probability of recurrence rises, the option of adjuvant chemotherapy may become more attractive to the patient who needs to balance the risk of relapse with treatment toxicity. Ideally any overall management strategy should not significantly increase the use of chemotherapy, and it can be argued that the most appropriate place for adjuvant therapy is in a group of patients with an approximately 50% chance or greater of developing recurrence. For this group the overall use of cytotoxic would be similar for either a surveillance or an adjuvant chemotherapy policy. For the surveillance policy half the patients would be treated with the standard four courses of chemotherapy at the time of relapse whilst the policy of adjuvant chemotherapy gives all of the patients in this subgroup two courses. The toxicity of chemotherapy at least in part relates to the number of courses given, but with the standard BEP regimen patients can expect alopecia, temporary infertility, and a degree of gastrointestinal upset and myelosuppression during therapy.

In order to make a reasonable comparison between the results of retroperitoneal lymph node dissection with approaches using surveillance (with or without adjuvant chemotherapy), it is necessary to look at the results in patients who were initially classified as having clinical stage I disease prior to surgery. A total of three series has assessed 787 patients in this way.[17-19] Between 24 and 30% of men had pathological stage B disease (mean 28%), and 12% of patients with pathological stage A disease subsequently relapsed compared to 34% with pathological stage B disease. In the largest series of Donohue and colleagues[19] out of 378 men there were two cancer deaths and one operative death, but no recurrences within the retroperitoneal area following selective retroperitoneal lymph node dissection. These figures allow comparisons between different management strategies to be made (Table 12.4). Following the policy of surveillance approximately one third of patients will need a full four courses of chemotherapy and approximately 30% of these men will additionally need lymph node dissection for residual masses.[20] Using pathological risk factors to stratify patients reduces the number relapsing to approximately 9%, the overall use of chemotherapy increases a little (from 128 to 136 courses per 100 patients), but the need for lymph node dissection might be anticipated to drop to approximately 3%. A policy of primary lymph node dissection alone will still be associated with an approximate 17% relapse rate, although the total amount of chemotherapy given will be approximately halved at the cost of retroperitoneal lymph node dissection in all patients. The use of adjuvant chemotherapy in stage B disease reduces the relapse rate to approximately 10%, with a slight increase in the overall use of chemotherapy. The final option of stratifying patients on the basis of histopathological risk factors using surveillance in good risk patients, and surgery with or without adjuvant chemotherapy for poor risk patients might be anticipated to halve the need for lymph node dissection and is associated with only a small rise in the use of chemotherapy. All of these five different strategies should be associated with near 100% cure rates, and the balances to be made are between the total use of chemotherapy and number of patients treated with either chemotherapy or lymph node dissection. If chemotherapy is to be used in an adjuvant setting morbidity should be as low as possible, and the next MRC study will evaluate the use of vincristine instead of etoposide in combination with bleomycin and cisplatin in an attempt to reduce the incidence of alopecia. This study will include a quality of life assessment using the EORTC QLQ–C30 assessment with an additional module designed for testicular cancer patients. It is to be hoped

179

Table 12.4 Use of chemotherapy and surgery in stage I teratoma: a comparison of treatment strategies

		Number of patients	Number relapsing (%)	Courses of chemotherapy	Number of patients treated with chemotherapy†	Number of patients treated surgically‡
1.	Surveillance	100	32 (32)	128	32	10
2.	Surveillance Good risk§	50	8 (15)	32	8	3
	Poor risk§	50	1 (2)	104	50	—
	Adj CT Total	100	9	136	58	3
3.	RPLND + observation p Stage A¶	77	9 (12)	36	9	77
	RPLND + observation p Stage B¶	23	8 (34)	32	8	23
	Total	100	17	68	17	100
4.	RPLND + observation p Stage A¶	77	9 (12)	36	9	77
	RPLND + Adj CT p Stage B¶	23	1 (6)	48	23	23
	Total	100	10	84	31	100
5.	Surveillance Good risk§	50	8 (15)	32	8	3
	Poor risk§					
	RPLND + observation p Stage A¶	27	3 (12)	12	3	27
	RPLND + Adj CT p Stage B¶	23	1 (6)	48	23	23
	Total	100	12	92	34	53

RPLND, retroperitoneal lymph node dissection; Adj CT, adjuvant chemotherapy
† Assumes four courses of BEP for relapse: two courses for adjuvant therapy.
‡ Assumes approximately 30% of relapsing patients will need postchemotherapy lymph node dissection.[20]
§ Good risk, no vascular or lymphatic; poor risk, vascular or lymphatic invasion present.
¶ Recurrences from p Stage A/p Stage B adjusted from surgical series so that relapses from p Stage A + No. of recurrences after surveillance (32%).

when such instruments are fully validated that we will gain useful information which may further guide patients' choice of appropriate treatment strategies. Such assessments need to take into account mens' worries about their health and fears of relapse, and concerns about finance, employment and insurance as well as treatment effects which may impact on body image, sexual function and fertility.[21]

Management of metastatic disease

Chemotherapy of testicular teratoma during the 1960s and early 1970s consisted of for example actinomycin as single agent therapy or in combination with methotrexate and chlorambucil.[22] Although partial responses or complete responses were seen they were approximately 50% and 10–20% respectively; long-term disease-free survival was seen in only 5–10% of patients. In the 1970s Samuels and colleagues[23] introduced a high dose combination of vinblastine and bleomycin which although extremely toxic produced response rates of 70–95% and complete remissions of 33–65%.[24 25] The remarkable activity of cisplatin in germ cell tumours was appreciated for the first time in the mid 1970s and in the first phase II trials in combination with vinblastine and bleomycin (PVB) a 70% complete remission rate was achieved.[26] The PVB schedule was associated with severe neuromuscular toxicity associated with the high dose of vinblastine employed (0·4 mg/m^2)and a high rate of neutropenic sepsis. Further studies[27 28] showed it was possible to reduce the dose of vinblastine decreasing toxicity, but remaining with similar therapeutic efficacy. Additionally etoposide was found to be active against cisplatin resistant tumours. Williams et al.[29] demonstrated that cisplatin–etoposide combinations achieved long term disease-free survival in 25% of 30 patients refractory to prior chemotherapy. It had been noted that PVB chemotherapy caused particularly marked bowel toxicity in patients who had prior radiotherapy for stage I disease, and Peckham and colleagues[30] substituted etoposide for vinblastine to produce the BEP chemotherapy schedule. BEP was subsequently compared in a randomised study with PVB by Williams and colleagues.[31] There was a superior complete response rate in 123 patients treated with BEP (83%) compared to 74% in 121 patients receiving PVB and a statistically significant improvement in survival for patients with advanced disease. The substitution of etoposide for vinblastine produced less parasthesia, abdominal cramps, and myalgias although the incidence of myelosuppression and pulmonary toxicity was similar. BEP has subsequently become the standard schedule for treatment of all stages of testicular teratoma. It must be noted, however, that there are a number of varieties of the BEP schedule. In the Royal Marsden Hospital schedule cisplatin was given at a dose of 20 mg/m^2 for 5 days (total dose 100 mg/m^2), etoposide at 120 mg/m^2 days 1–3 (total dose 360 mg/m^2), and bleomycin 30 units on days 2, 9, and 15.[30] The standard regimen used in North America studied by the South Eastern Cancer Study Group

(SECSG) gave etoposide at a dose of 100 mg/m² days 1–5 (total dose 500 mg/m²) with a similar schedule of cisplatin and bleomycin. Subsequently there have been variations in the scheduling of cisplatin and bleomycin dosage has been reduced in an attempt to decrease the incidence of bleomycin lung damage. The Royal Marsden Hospital schedule gives excellent long term results for patients with small volume disease according to the 1985 MRC Classification,[32] but poorer outcomes with increasing volume of disease, and for patients with high marker levels (AFP > 500 international units/l, HCG > 1000 international units/l (Figure 12.2). The side effects of BEP chemotherapy are shown in Table 12.5. Subsequent developments of chemotherapy have attempted to reduce toxicity for good risk patients whereas the aim for patients with a poorer prognosis has been to increase treatment efficacy. It is generally agreed that measures of tumour volume and extent of disease together with serum levels of β-human chorionic gonadotrophin (HCG), AFP, and lactate dehydrogenase (LDH) can be used to predict outcome. However, consensus has not yet been reached on the most appropriate way of dividing patients into prognostic categories. The various systems used are tabulated in Table 12.6

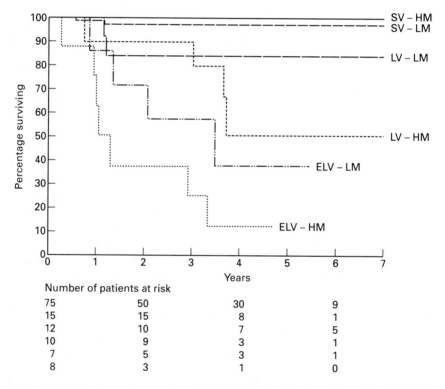

Fig 12.2 BEP chemotherapy in NSGCT, Royal Marsden Hospital 1979–88. Survival by tumour volume and marker levels. SV, small volume; LV, large volume; ELV, extra large volume; LM, low markers; HM, high markers

Table 12.5   Side effects of BEP chemotherapy

Cisplatin	Nausea and vomiting
	Nephrotoxicity
	Ototoxicity
	Peripheral neuropathy
Etoposide	Bone marrow suppression
	Alopecia
	Leukaemogenesis (dose related)
Bleomycin	Pneumonitis and pulmonary fibrosis
	Raynaud's phenomenon
	Fever
	Skin pigmentation
	Infertility

but this lack of uniformity has made it difficult to compare the results from different groups of investigators.[33]

Chemotherapy for good risk patients

Several modifications of treatment have been explored (box). Cisplatin causes approximately a 20–25% reduction in glomerular filtration rate after four courses of BEP chemotherapy and there has been a suggestion that there is an increased risk of subsequent hypertension.[34] Carboplatin causes little renal toxicity at conventional dosage and does not cause neurotoxicity or ototoxicity. There is also less emesis than with cisplatin. The drug is therefore considerably easier to give and does not require intravenous hydration or inpatient treatment. A phase II study of CEB (carboplatin, etoposide, bleomycin) was performed in 112 patients at the Royal Marsden Hospital between 1983 and 1989. Carboplatin was given according to the Calvert formula[35] to achieve a target carboplatin plasma concentration $\times$ time (AUC) of 5. After a median follow up of 30 months, cause specific survival was 98·5%. Six patients relapsed but 110 remained alive and disease free after salvage treatment, there being one toxic death due to bleomycin pneumonitis and one coincidental death. This study was undertaken in patients with small volume disease (MRC 1985)[32] or large volume disease provided serum markers were low. Etoposide was delivered at a dose of 120 mg/m^2 days 1–3 and bleomycin 30 units given on days 2, 9, and 15 in each of four cycles of treatment given at 21 day intervals. Subsequently two randomised studies have compared regimens containing

---

Modification of treatment for good risk patients

- substitution of carboplatin for cisplatin to reduce the renal, oto- and neurotoxicity as well as acute gastrointestinal toxicity associated with cisplatin
- reduction in dose of bleomycin to avoid bleomycin pneumonitis
- reduction in the standard number of courses of treatment from four to three

Table 12.6 Different classification systems for defining high risk groups

	Abdomen	Lung	Mediastinum	Liver/brain	Extragonadal primary	HCG	AFP	LDH	Reference
Medical Research Council	—	L3	—	+	No	>1000	>500	NE	MRC (1985)[32]
Medical Research Council	—	>20	>5 cm	+	No	>10000	>1000	NE	Mead et al. (1992)[41]
Indiana	>10 cm +pulmonary metastases	>10/lung	>50%	+	No	No	No	No	Birch et al. (1986)[66]
National Cancer Institute	>10 cm or obstructive uropathy	>5/lung field	>5 cm	+	Yes	>10000	>2000	NE	Ozols et al. (1988)[65]
Memorial Sloane-Kettering	(number of sites)	No	No		Yes	Probability of CR <0·5*			Bosl et al. (1983)[67]
Institut Gustave Roussy	No	No	No	No	NE	Probability of CR <0·7**			Droz et al. (1989)[68]

* Probability CR = exp h/(1 + exp h) where h = 8·514 − 1·973 log (LDH + 1) − 0·53 (log HCG + 1) − 1·111 TOTMET, where TOTMET = 0,1,2 depending on the number of sites of metastases.

** Probability CR = exp h/(1 + exp h) where h = 1·90 − 0·033 or (AFP$^{1/2}$) − 0·021 (HCT$^{1/2}$) + 0·033 (HCG).

Table 12.7 Dose and dose intensity of chemotherapy regimens for high risk non-seminomatous germ cell tumours

Regimen	Duration (weeks)	Total dose in 12 weeks P (mg/m⁻²)	E (mg/m⁻²)	B (mg)	Mean dose/week, week 1–4 P (mg/m⁻²)	E (mg/m⁻²)	B (mg)	Overall mean dose/week P (mg/m⁻²)	E (mg/m⁻²)	B (mg)	Reference
BEP	10	400	2000	360	50	250	30	40	200	30	Pizzocaro et al. 1985[8] / Williams et al. 1987[15]
Intensive induction											
BOP/BEP	13	540	1080	345	70	0	45	42	83	25	Dearnaley (1991)[41]
C BOP-BEP	13	660*	1500	345	100*	0	45	51*	115	25	Horwich et al. (1991)[51]
BOP	7	440	0	480	80	0	90	63	0	69	Wettlaufer et al. (1984)[53]
HIPE	9	486	21314	210	54	146	23	54	146	23	Murray et al. (1986)[54]
Alternating											
POMP/ACE	13+	480	1500	120	60	0	15	37	115	9	Newlands et al. (1983)[60]
CISCA/VB	13+	360	1000**	300	30	250**	38	28	77*	23	Logothetis et al. (1986)[61]
BOP/VIP	12	600	900	90	75	0	18	50	75	8	Kaye et al. (1989)[48]
PVB/BEP	10	400	1720**	360	50	215**	30	40	172*	30	Stroter et al. (1986)[28]
VAB-6/EP	20	600	2600**	450	44	150**	30	33	75	23	Bosl et al. (1987)[62]
High dose											
PEB	7	600	3000	270	100	500	38	86	428	30	Daugaard and Rorth (1986)[63]
PEB	10	700	2400	360	88	300	38	70	240	30	Schmoll et al. (1987)[64]
PVeBV	7	600	2490**	270	100	415**			355*		Ozols et al. (1988)[65]

P, cisplatin; B, bleomycin; VCR, vincristine; MTX, methotrexate; Act D, actinomycin; IF, ifosfamide; F, etoposide; HI, high intensity; VAB, PVeBV, CISCA/VB

Additional drugs, total/mean weekly doses m⁻² (*total doses). BOP/BEP, VCR 12 mg/1 mg*; BOP, BCR 14 mg/2mg*; HIPE, VCR 7 mg/0.8 mg; POMB/ACE, VCR 4 mg/0.3 mg, MTX 1200 mg/160, Act D 2.25 mg/0.18 mg*, CY 1500 mg/125 mg; CISCA/VB, Adr 240 mg/20 mg, CY 3000 mg/250 mg; BOP/VIP, VCR 6 mg/0.5 mg, IF 15 g/1.25 mg; VAB-6/EP, Act D 3.0 mg/0.15 mg, CY 1800 mg/90 mg.

* Approximate equivalence taking carboplatin AUC 3 as similar to cisplatin 60 mg/m²
** Approximate equivalence taking 0.15 mg/kg⁻¹ vinblastine days 1–2 as similar to 100 mg/m⁻² VP16 days 1–5.

cisplatin and carboplatin. The first of these from the Memorial Sloan–Kettering Group[36] compared four courses of platinum/etoposide (EP) with carboplatin at a dose of 500 mg/m^2 together with etoposide at the same dose of 100 mg/m^2 for five days as in the comparator arm. The carboplatin schedule (EC) was given at four-weekly intervals due to increased bone marrow toxicity. The complete response and disease-free survival at a median follow up of 22 months were 90% and 87% respectively for EP and significantly less at 88% and 76% for EC. The MRC/EORTC have completed a joint study comparing four courses of BEP with CEB.[37] BEP was given using the Royal Marsden Hospital schedule (three days of etoposide at 120 mg/m^2), but with a reduced dose of bleomycin to 30 international units on day 2 only; in the comparator arm carboplatin was given at an AUC of 5 using the same doses of etoposide and bleomycin. Although the CEB arm was associated with significantly less renal, neuro- and ototoxicity and a reduction in inpatient days, there was a small increase in myelosuppression. However, the outcome was significantly less good for men in the CEB arm: the failure-free survival at one year was 80% and there have been 14 deaths in the CEB arm compared to 90% and 4 in the BEP group. Possible reasons for the poorer results than in the Royal Marsden Hospital phase II study include the reduction in dose of bleomycin and inclusion of poorer risk patients.

Bleomycin is associated with a small ($\leq 2\%$) incidence of fatal pneumonitis when given at a dose of 30 units per week to a total dose of 360 units in the standard four courses using the BEP chemotherapy. Other toxicities include Raynaud's phenomenon, hyperpigmentation, and stomatitis. A reduction of bleomycin dose is therefore a reasonable objective. A number of randomised studies have been performed. The EORTC directly compared four cycles of BEP chemotherapy to four cycles of EP in patients with good risk criteria (lymph node metastases <5 cm, lung metastases <2 cm, AFP <1000 ng/ml, HCG $<10\ 000$ international units/l). Of 393 patients entered into the study, 97% of BEP-treated and 91% of EP-treated patients achieved complete remission, and of the complete responders six receiving EP and seven receiving BEP relapsed. There was no statistical difference between the survival of the two arms of the study, although disease related deaths on the EP arm was slightly higher. An ECOG prospective randomised study comparing three courses of BEP with three courses of EP in patients with minimal or intermediate disease according to the Indiana Classification had a reduced complete remission rate with EP and disease-free survival of 85% with BEP compared to only 69% with EP.[38] An Australian study has additionally shown that four courses of platinum and vinblastine are less effective than the three drug combination of PVB. The SECSG have compared four versus three courses of BEP treatment chemotherapy in patients with good prognosis testicular teratoma. The BEP schedule was with five days of etoposide at a dose of 100 mg/m^2 per day and with bleomycin at a dose of 30 units on days 2, 9, and 15 of each cycle. Of the 184 patients who entered the study, 98%

achieved disease-free status with three courses compared to 97% following four courses of treatment. There were five recurrences on each arm of the study and after a median follow-up of 19 months, 92% of patients on each arm of the study remained disease free.[39]

It is clear from this combination of studies that there is a fine line to be defined between reducing treatment toxicity and losing therapeutic efficacy. It is perhaps not surprising that results are critically dependent on the selection criteria for patient entry, and these studies indicate that there should be considerable caution in deviating from well-defined standard schedules. Four cycles of BEP chemotherapy currently remains standard treatment for good prognosis patients. In the next EORTC/MRC protocol it is intended to compare three-day schedules versus five-day schedules of BEP and additionally in a 2×2 factorial design three courses will be compared against four courses of chemotherapy.

Chemotherapy for poor risk patients

The randomised trial performed by the Indiana Group in 1987 demonstrated clear superiority of the BEP regimen compared to PVB for poor risk patients.[40] Since then this BEP schedule using 30 units of bleomycin weekly for 12 weeks and etoposide at a dose of 100 mg/m^2 for five days in each of four courses has been accepted as the standard therapy for poor risk metastatic teratoma and is the treatment with which other therapies need to be compared. As discussed above the variety of prognostic criteria that have been used by different centres makes direct comparison of the results of phase II protocols inappropriate. Nevertheless, it is clear that the outcome for some patient groups is less than optimal, and new strategies need to be defined. This can be appreciated from the second MRC study of prognostic factors[41] in which four adverse prognostic groups were identified (box). If none of these features was present the five-year survival was 92%, 71% if one of the four risk factors was present, 48% if two were present, and 26% if there were three or four of the factors. For these groups attempts at improving treatment efficacy are required and four main methods for modifying standard chemotherapy are possible (box).

The rationale for intensive induction chemotherapy is that the proliferation rate of testicular tumours may be very rapid with calculated potential doubling time as low as 0·6 days.[42] This will potentially allow rapidly dividing germ cell tumours to recover and proliferate between standard

---

Adverse prognostic factors

- The presence of liver bone or brain metastases
- Elevated markers (AFP > 1000 kU/l and HCG > 10 000 international units/l)
- ≥ 20 lung metastases
- > 5 cm mediastinal mass

Modification of standard chemotherapy for high risk patients

- Introduction of additional chemotherapy agents: for example, ifosfamide, cyclophosphamide, adriamycin, actinomycin-D, or methotrexate or taxanes
- Use of alternating potentially non-cross-resistant drug combinations
- Increased doses of chemotherapy either given conventionally or with bone marrow support factors
- Chemotherapy schedules using drugs given at increased frequency—intensive induction therapy

---

three-weekly courses of chemotherapy leading to at best the need for an increased number of courses of treatment to gain adequate cell kill, but potentially permitting the development of drug resistance clones.[43]

A relatively limited number of phase III studies have been completed in patients with adverse prognostic features. A randomised trial from the SECSG compared standard BEP with BEP using double dose (200 mg/m^2 of cisplatin).[44] Of the 159 patients included in this study, using standard dose chemotherapy, 73% of patients became disease free with chemotherapy alone or with surgery compared to 68% of patients receiving high dose cisplatin. After a median follow-up of 24 months 74% of patients were alive in each arm of the study. The toxicity of the double-dose cisplatin arm was markedly increased. This was a disappointing result, as it would seem to suggest that there may be a ceiling to the useful dose of cisplatin. Previous studies have shown an improved response rate for poor risk patients when comparing cisplatin at a dose of 120 mg/m^2 with 75 mg/m^2 in combination with vinblastine and bleomycin.[45] The SECSG has subsequently compared BEP with VIP chemotherapy (etoposide, ifosfamide and cisplatin) and a similar trial has been performed by the EORTC.[46 47] In the former study 304 patients were entered and with a median follow up at 16 months, 54% had become disease free with VIP compared to 49% with BEP, and 48% were continuously disease free after VIP compared to 42% after BEP (p=ns). There was significantly greater toxicity using VIP. In the European study 84 eligible patients were randomised; 78% of patients achieved a complete remission following VIP, compared to 82% with BEP and with a median follow up 2·5 years progression-free survival was 85% after VIP and 88% with BEP. Again VIP was found to be more myelotoxic. The results of two further studies comparing BEP with hybrid regimens is awaited. The MRC/EORTC have compared BEP with BOP/VIP[48] and the French Study Group are comparing the CISCA VB with BEP.

It has been proposed that chemotherapy dose and dose intensity are of major importance in determining the outcome of chemotherapy treatments.[49 50] Increases in dose intensity can be achieved either by increasing the dose by course and keeping the interval between treatment constant, or by increasing the frequency of courses and keeping the doses constant. If there is a steep dose–response curve then the former approach is attractive; however, if failure results from significant tumour proliferation and the dose–response curve is shallow then smaller frequent doses may provide a better strategy. The dose and dose intensity of regimens used for the treatment of high risk testicular teratoma are shown in Table 12.4. The approach using induction treatment with BOP achieves the same dose intensity as using double-dose cisplatin but without the associated increased toxicity.[43 51] For poor risk patients the BOP/BEP schedule gives 71% overall disease-free survival and in a retrospective comparison with previously treated patients at the Royal Marsden Hospital with high risk disease[32] a 61% compared to 27% survival was obtained.[52] The basis of this schedule is the regimen initially described by Wettlaufer and colleagues[53] and gives weekly treatment for the first month of the schedule using bleomycin given by continuous infusion, vincristine, and cisplatin. Vincristine is substituted for etoposide as if the latter is included myelosuppression prevents maintenance of an increased dose intensity.[54] Subsequently we have added carboplatin to the regimen with a relatively small increase in myelotoxicity and also increased the dose of etoposide to 100 mg/m^2 for five days rather than 120 mg/m^2 for three days in the BEP part of the schedule. A further 21 patients with high risk disease have been treated with CBOP/ BEP and with a median follow up of 18 months, 85% remained continuously disease free.[51] These results are encouraging and the regimen is under consideration for prospective evaluation in a phase III comparative study against standard BEP.

The principle new strategy to be explored is that of high dose chemotherapy using stem cell support. High dose carboplatin, etoposide, cyclophosphamide, and ifosfamide have been used in these approaches. Initial results were reported from patients who had relapsed after standard therapy and approximately 15% of patients achieved prolonged complete remission, but toxic deaths were not uncommon.[55 56] Such treatment appears better tolerated if given earlier in the course of disease, and phase II studies have piloted high dose chemotherapy as first line therapy in patients with poor risk germ cell tumours.[57] The correct evaluation of this technique is again by prospective randomised trial, and North American and European groups are developing such protocols for the treatment of very poor risk patients at initial presentation and in the salvage chemotherapy setting.

Conclusions

The introduction of cisplatin-containing chemotherapy has made dramatic changes in the management and outcome of patients presenting with all stages of testicular teratoma. However, there is no room for complacency in the treatment of these young men, and it is apparent that hospitals with the greatest experience of managing metastatic disease obtain the best results. In a Scandinavian study of over 200 patients, multivariate analysis showed that the Norwegian Radium Hospital which treated the largest number of patients obtained better results ($p < 0.04$) after taking other factors into account.[58] Similarly, analysis of 440 men treated in Scotland demonstrated the specialist Tertiary Referral Centre treating the majority of patients gave a higher proportion of chemotherapy according to nationally agreed protocols and that men who received protocol treatment obtained a better survival rate after adjusting for other important prognostic variables.[59] There is every reason to argue that men with testicular cancer should be treated in centres that have developed considerable expertise and experience in treating this disease. Such centres should be prepared to enter patients into national and international randomised studies so that further refinement of treatment strategies can be made and individual patients can be optimally treated.

1 Davies JM. Testicular cancer in England and Wales: some epidemiological aspects. *Lancet* 1981; **i**: 928–32.
2 Peckham MJ. Testicular cancer. *Rev Oncol* 1988; **I**: 439–53.
3 John Radcliffe Hospital Cryptorchidism Study Group. Cryptorchidism: an apparent substantial increase since 1960. *Br Med J* 1986; **293**: 1401–4.
4 Rorth M. Orchiectomy alone versus orchiectomy plus radiotherapy in stage I non-seminomatous testicular cancer. A randomized study by the Danish Testicular Carcinoma Study Group. *Int J Androl* 1987; **10**: 255–62.
5 Hamilton CAH, Easton A, Peckham MJ. Radiotherapy for stage I seminoma testis: Results of treatment and complications. *Radiother Oncol* 1986; **6**: 115–20.
6 Whitmore WFJ. Surgical treatment of clinical stage I non-seminomatous germ cell tumours of the testis. *Cancer Treat Rep* 1982; **66**: 5–10.
7 Donohue JP, Zachary JM, Maynard BR. Distribution of nodal metastases in non-seminomatous testis cancer. *Br J Urol* 1982; **128**: 315–20.
8 Pizzacaro G. Unilateral lymphadenectomy in intraoperative stage I non-seminomatous germinal testis cancer. *J Urol* 1985; **134**: 485–9.
9 Jewett MAS, Kong YS, Goldberg SD *et al.* Retroperitoneal lymphadenectomy for testis tumor with nerve sparing for ejaculation. *J Urol* 1988; **139**(6): 1220–4.
10 Rorth M. Management of patients with non-seminomatous germ cell tumours stage I. A position paper. Consensus Conference on Prostate and Testis Cancer. Hull, 12-15 April, 1989.
11 Peckham MJ, Barrett A, Husband JE, Hendry WF. Orchidectomy alone in testicular stage I non-seminomatous germ-cell tumours. *Lancet* 1982; **ii**: 678–80.
12 Cullen M. Management of stage I non-seminoma: Surveillance and chemotherapy. In: Horwich A, editor, *Testicular cancer—clinical investigation and management.* London: Chapman and Hall, 1991: 149–66.
13 Freedman LS, Parkinson MC, Jones WG *et al.* Histopathology in the prediction of relapse of patients with stage I testicular teratoma treated by orchidectomy alone. *Lancet* 1987; **ii**: 294–8.
14 Read G, Stenning SP, Cullen MH *et al.* Medical Research Council Prospective Study of Surveillance for Stage I Testicular Teratoma. *J Clin Oncol* 1992; **10**(11): 1762–8.
15 Williams SD, Stablein DM, Einhorn LH, *et al.* Immediate adjuvant chemotherapy versus observation with treatment at relapse in pathological stage II testicular cancer. *N Engl J Med* 1987; **317**(23): 1433–8.
16 Cullen MH, Stenning SP, Parkinson SP *et al.* Short course adjuvant chemotherapy in high risk stage I non-seminomatous germ cell tumours of the testis (NSGCTT): an MRC (UK) study report. *Proc Am Soc Clin Oncol* 1995; **14**: 244.
17 Klepp O, Olsson AM, Henrikson H *et al.* Predicting metastases in clinical stage I testicular teratoma: multivariate analysis of a large multicentric study (SWENOTECA). *Book of Abstracts, 2–7 September 1989 5th European Conference on Clinical Oncology (ECCO)* 1989; Abstract No. 0787.

18 Pizzocaro G. Management of stage I non-seminoma: Rationale for lymphadenectomy. In: Horwich A, editor, *Testicular cancer—clinical investigation and management*. London: Chapman and Hall, 1991: 167–73.

19 Donohue JP, Thornhill JA, Foster RS *et al*. Primary retroperitoneal lymph node dissection in clinical Stage A non-seminomatous germ cell testis cancer: Review of the Indiana University Experience 1965–1989. *Br J Urol* 1993; 71(3): 326–35.

20 Horwich A, Norman A, Fisher C *et al*. Primary chemotherapy for stage II non-seminomatous germ cell tumours of the testis. *J Urol* 1994; 151: 72–8.

21 Moynihan C. Psychosocial assessments and counselling of the patients with testicular cancer. In: Horwich A, editor, *Testicular cancer—clinical investigation and management*. London: Chapman and Hall, 1991: 353–68.

22 MacKenzie AR. Chemotherapy of metastatic testis cancer: results in 154 patients. *Cancer* 1966; 19: 1369–76.

23 Samuels ML, Lanzotti VJ, Holoye PY *et al*. Combination chemotherapy in germinal cell tumour. *Cancer Treat Rev* 1976; 3: 185–204.

24 Samuels ML, Johnson DE, Holoye PY. Continuous intravenous Bleomycin (NS-125066) therapy with Vinblastine (NSC-49842) in stage III testicular neoplasia. *Cancer Chemother Rep* 1975: 59: 563–70.

25 Nichols CR, Roth BJ. Management of metastatic non-seminoma: Development of effective chemotherapy. In: Horwich A, editor, *Testicular cancer—clinical investigation and management*. London: Chapman and Hall, 1991: 185–203.

26 Einhorn LH, Donohue J. Cis-diammine-dichloroplatinum, Vinblastine, and Bleomycin combination chemotherapy in disseminated testicular cancer. *Ann Intern Med* 1977; 87: 293–8.

27 Einhorn LH, Williams SD. Chemotherapy of disseminated testicular cancer: a random prospective study. *Cancer* 1980; 46(6): 1339–44.

28 Stoter G. High-dose versus low dose Vinblastine in Cisplatin–Vinblastine–Bleomycin combination chemotherapy of non-seminomatous testicular cancer: a randomized study of the EORTC Genitourinary Tract Cancer Group. *J Clin Oncol* 1986; 4: 1199–206.

29 Williams SD, Einhorn LH, Greco FA *et al*. VP16-213 salvage therapy for refractory germinal neoplasms. *Cancer* 1980; 46: 2154–8.

30 Peckham MJ, Barrett A, Liew K *et al*. The treatment of metastatic germ-cell testicular tumours with Bleomycin, Etoposide and Cis-platinum (BEP). *Br J Cancer* 1983; 47: 613–19.

31 Williams SD, Birch R, Einhorn LH *et al*. Treatment of disseminated germ-cell tumours: with Cisplatin, Bleomycin, and either Vinblastine or Etoposide. *N Engl J Med* 1987; 316(23): 1435–40.

32 MRC Working Party on Testicular Tumours, Peckham MJ. Prognostic factors in advanced non-seminomatous germ-cell testicular tumours: Results of a multicentre study. *Lancet* 1985; i: 8–12.

33 Bajorin DF. Prognostic classification in metastatic non-seminoma. In: Horwich A, editor, *Testicular cancer—clinical investigation and management*. London: Chapman and Hall, 1991: 69–82.

34 Hansen SW, Groth S, Daugaard G *et al*. Long-term effects on renal function and blood pressure of treatment with cisplatin, vinblastine and bleomycin in patients with germ cell cancer. *J Clin Oncol* 1988; 6(11): 1728–31.

35 Calvert AH, Newell DR, Gumbrell LA *et al*. Carboplatin dosage: prospective evaluation of a simple formula based on renal function. *J Clin Oncol* 1989; 7(11): 1748–56.

36 Bajorin DF, Sarosdy MF, Pfister DG *et al*. Randomised trial of Etoposide and Cisplatin versus Etoposide and Carboplatin in patients with good-risk germ cell tumours: A Multiinstitutional Study. *J Clin Oncol* 1993; 11(4): 598–606.

37 Horwich A, Sleifer D, Foss A *et al*. A trial of carboplatin-based combination chemotherapy in good prognosis metastatic testicular non seminoma. *Proc Am Soc Clin Oncol* 1994; 13: 231.

38 Loehrer PJ, Elson P, Johnson DH *et al*. A randomised trial of cisplatin plus etoposide with or without bleomycin in favorable prognosis disseminated germ cell tumours: ECOG study. *Proc Am Soc Clin Oncol* 1991; 10: 169.

39 Einhorn LH, Williams SD, Loehrer PJ *et al*. Evaluation of optimal duration of chemotherapy in favorable-prognosis disseminated germ cell tumours: A Southeastern Cancer Study Group Protocol. *J Clin Oncol* 1989; 7(3): 387–391.

40 Williams SD, Birch R, Greco FA *et al*. Disseminated germ cell tumours: superiority of a

VP-16 containing regimen in patients with high tumor volume. *Am Soc Clin Oncol* 1987; **6**: 98.

41 Mead GM, Stenning SP, Parkinson MC *et al.* The second Medical Research Council Study of prognostic factors in nonseminomatous germ cell tumours. *J Clin Oncol* 1992; **10**(1): 85–94.

42 Rabes HM. Proliferation of human testicular tumours. *Int J Androl* 1987; **10**: 127–37.

43 Dearnaley DP. Intensive induction treatment for poor risk patients. In: Horwich A, editor, *Testicular cancer—clinical investigation and management*. London: Chapman and Hall, 1991: 233–48.

44 Nichols CR, Williams SD, Loehrer PJ *et al.* Randomized study of cisplatin dose intensity in poor-risk germ cell tumours: A Southeastern Cancer Study Group and Southwest Oncology Group Protocol. *J Clin Oncol* 1991; **9**(7): 1163–72.

45 Samson MK, Rivkin SE, Jones SE *et al.* Dose-response and dose-survival advantage for high versus low-dose Cisplatin combined with Vinblastine and Bleomycin in disseminated testicular cancer. A Southwest Oncology Group Study. *Cancer* 1984; **53**: 1029–35.

46 Loehrer PJ, Einhorn LH, Elison P *et al.* Phase III study of cisplatin(P) plus etoposide(VP-16) with either bleomycin(B) or ifosfamide(I) in advanced stage germ cell tumours (GCT): An intergroup trial. *Proc Am Soc Clin Oncol* 1993; **12**: 261.

47 Stoter G, Sleijifer DT, Schormagel JH *et al.* BEP versus VIP in intermediate risk patients with disseminated non-seminomatous testicular cancer (NSTC). *Proc Am Soc Clin Oncol* 1993; **12**: 232.

48 Kaye S, Harding M, Stoter G *et al.* "BOP/VIP"—a new intensive regime for poor prognosis germ cell tumours. *Proc Am Soc Clin Oncol* 1989; **8**: 136.

49 Frei E, Canellos GP. Dose: a critical factor in cancer chemotherapy. *Am J Med* 1980; **69**: 585–94.

50 Hryniuk W, Bush H. The importance of dose intensity in chemotherapy of metastatic breast cancer. *J Clin Oncol* 1984; **2**: 1281–8.

51 Horwich A, Wilson C, Cornes P *et al.* Increasing the dose intensity of chemotherapy in poor-prognosis metastatic non-seminoma. *Eur Urol* 1993; **23**: 219–22.

52 Dearnaley DP, Horwich A, A'Hern R *et al.* Combination chemotherapy with bleomycin, etoposide and cisplatin (BEP) for metastatic testicular teratoma: long-term follow up. *Eur J Cancer* 1991; **27**(6): 684–91.

53 Wettlaufer JN, Feiner AS, Robinson WA. Vincristine, Cisplatin, and Bleomycin with surgery in the management of advanced netastatic nonseminomatous testis tumours. *Cancer* 1984; **53**: 203–9.

54 Murray N, Coppin C, Swenerton K. Weekly high intensity Cisplatin Etoposide (HIPE) for far advanced germ cell cancers (GCC). *Proc Am Soc Clin Oncol* 1987; **6**: 101.

55 Nichols CR, Andersen J, Lazarus HM *et al.* High-dose carboplatin and etoposide with autologous bone marrow transplantation in refractory germ cell cancer: An Eastern Cooperative Oncology Group Protocol. *J Clin Oncol* 1992; **10**(4): 558–63.

56 Motzer RJ, Geller NL, Tam CCY. Salvage chemotherapy for patients with germ cell tumours. The Memorial Sloan-Kettering Cancer Centre experience (1979–1989). *Cancer* 1991; **67**: 1305–10.

57 Motzer RJ, Mazumdar M, Gulati SC *et al.* Phase II trial of high-dose carboplatin and etoposide with autologous bone marrow transplantation in first-line therapy for patients with poor-risk germ cell tumours. *J Natl Cancer Inst* 1993; **85**(22): 1828–35.

58 Aass N, Kleep O, Cavallin-Stahl E *et al.* Prognostic factors in unselected patients with nonseminomatous metastatic testicular cancer: A multicenter experience. *J Clin Oncol* 1991; **9**(5): 818–26.

59 Harding MJ, Paul J, Gillis CR, Kaye SB. Management of malignant teratoma: does referral to a specialist unit matter? *Lancet* 1993; **314**: 999–1002.

60 Newlands ES, Begent RHJ, Rustin GJS *et al.* Further advances in the management of malignant teratomas of the testis and other sites. *Lancet* 1993; **i**: 948–51.

61 Logothetis CJ, Samuels MJ, Selig DE *et al.* Cyclic chemotherapy with Cyclophosphamide, Doxorubicin and Cisplatin plus Vinblastine and Bleomycin in advanced germinal tumors. Results with 100 patients. *Am J Med* 1986; **81**(2): 219–28.

62 Bosi GJ, Geller NL, Vogelzang NJ *et al.* Alternating cycles of Etoposide plus Cisplatin and VAB-6 in the treatment of poor-risk patients with germ cell tumours. *J Clin Oncol* 1987; **5**(3): 436–40.

63 Daugaard G, Rorth M. High-dose Cisplatin and VP-16 with Bleomycin, in the management of advanced metastatic germ cell tumors. *Eur J Cancer Clin Oncol* 1986;

22(4): 477–85.

64 Schmoll HJ, Schubert I, Arnold H *et al.* Disseminated testicular cancer with bulky disease: results of a phase II study with Cisplatin ultra high dose/VP-16/bleomycin. *Int J Androl* 1987; **10**(1): 311–17.

65 Ozols RF, C ID, Linehan WM, Jacob J *et al.* A randomized trial of standard chemotherapy v a high-dose chemotherapy regimen in the treatment of poor prognosis nonseminomatous germ-cell tumors. *J Clin Oncol* 1988; **6**(6): 1031–40.

66 Birch R, Williams S, Cone A *et al.* Prognostic factors for favorable outcome in disseminated germ cell tumours. *J Clin Oncol* 1986; **4**(3): 400–7.

67 Bosl GJ, Geller NL, Cirrincione C *et al.* Multivariate analysis of prognostic variables in patients with metastatic testicular cancer. *Cancer Res* 1983; **43**: 3403–7.

68 Droz JP, Pico JL, Ghosn M *et al.* High complete remission (CR) and survival rates in poor prognosis (PP) non seminomatous germ cell tumors (NSGCT) with high dose chemotherapy (HDCT) and autologous bone marrow transplantation (ABMT). *Proc Am Soc Clin Oncol* 1989; **8**: 130.

13: Treatment of acute myeloid leukaemia

JOHN REES

The incidence of acute myeloid leukaemia (AML) in the adolescent age group is low, representing only about 3–4% of all the new cases occurring in England and Wales in a year,[1] but it makes up 14% of all the patients entered into the United Kingdom Medical Research Council's (MRC's) tenth AML trial (AML 10) which is open to children and adults below the age of 55. This trial, which recruits about 300 patients each year, makes it possible to contribute to the extending body of experience in treating young adults with this disorder. It presents the haematologist and oncologist with a challenge, because expectations are relatively high and conservative management, a reasonable option in the elderly, is only rarely considered. In the United Kingdom and in the majority of European centres, treatment passes, at the age of 15, from the care of the paediatrician to the general haematologist or adult oncologist, and reports of paediatric trials reflect this policy. In other countries, including the United States, the paediatrician continues responsibility until patients pass the age of 18.

It has been possible to establish, certainly in the United Kingdom, that paediatric patients treated on a well organised national protocol, in specialist centres, have a better outcome than those treated in small hospitals lacking the necessary facilities and expertise to deal with acute problems. It is not feasible to provide such an arrangement for adults with AML, as the number of patients increases rapidly after the age of 50 to a maximum of approximately 450 patients per year in the 70–79 age group. The adolescent with AML is therefore in a transitional age group which presents the haematologist with some of the most difficult problems, not least because the majority of the patients in the group will be taking legal responsibility for their lives for the first time and may have a very different set of priorities from patients in their middle age or older.

Treatment

It is outside the province of this review to include a detailed analysis of all the aspects of treating AML, but remission rates obtained in some of recently reported studies are shown in Table 13.1.

194

Table 13.1 Recently reported response rates of children and young adults with AML

Reference	Age of patients (years)	Number of patients	Induction therapy	Complete remission rate (%)
Stevens et al.[2]	0–14	270	(D) 1,3,5 (A) 1–10 (T) 1–10 or (A)1–10 (D)1,3,5 (E)1–5	91
Goldstone et al.[3]	15–55	784	As above	80
Weinstein et al.[4]	0–21	353	(D)1,2 (A)1–7 (T)1–7	84
Ritter et al.[5]	0–16	210	(P), (T), (V), (Do) (A), (C), (M)	78
Mayer et al.[6]	16–40	1085	(D)1,2,3,(A)1–7	76
	40–60			69
Berman et al.[7]	17–60	120	(I)1,2,3,(A)1–5	80
			(D)1,2,3,(A)1–5	58
Vogler et al.[8]	>14	230	(L)1–3,(A)1–7	71
			(D)1–3,(A)1–7	58

(D), daunorubicin; (A), cytosine arabinoside; (T), 6-thioguanine; (E), etoposide; (P), prednisolone; (V), vincristine; (Do), doxorubicin; (C), cyclophosphamide; (M), methotrexate; (I), idarubicin.

The basis of these regimens have been combinations of cytarabine and an anthracycline, usually daunorubicin or idarubicin, or an anthracenedione such as mitozantrone. Etoposide has been included in the design of more recent protocols, partly due to the encouraging results from an Australian multicentre study[9] and the perceived possible advantage in the treatment of monocytic leukaemia which is rather more common in younger patients.

Randomised trials have shown a higher response with more intensive therapy[10 11] and there has been a progressive increase in the total doses of drugs given over the first three or four months following the diagnosis.

The largest randomised trial on the treatment of the children and young adults opened in 1988 under the auspices of the MRC (AML 10). Up to the end of April 1995, over 1857 patients had been entered in the trial from centres in the United Kingdom, the Republic of Ireland, and New Zealand.

The design of the trial (Figure 13.1) underlines the most important question which remains unresolved in the management of young patients with AML in the early 1990s; what is the role of bone marrow transplantation when complete remission has been achieved? The European organisation for Research and Treatment of Cancer (EORTC) study,[12] which opened before the MRC trial, ran concurrently with it for three years. Although there were some differences in detail the essential question was the same and provision for randomisation for autologous bone marrow transplantation after remission was made in both. The problems which arose in compiling adequate numbers for randomisation will be discussed later.

The remission rate in the adolescent age group in AML 10 is 85%, and nearly three quarters of responders achieve remission after one course. Although patients with secondary AML are eligible for the trial they represent only a small proportion of cases in this age group (<3%).

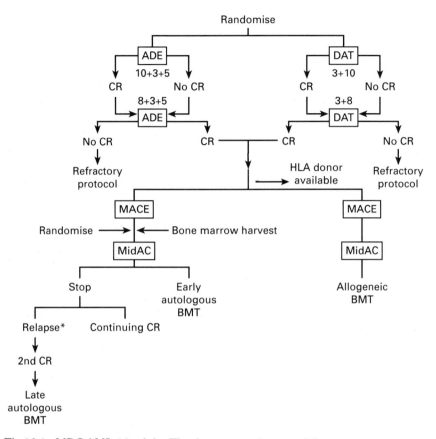

Fig 13.1. MRC AML 10-adults. The drug protocols are as follows.

DAT 3+10: daunorubicin 50 mg/m^2 intravenous push days 1, 3, 5; cytarabine 100 mg/m^2 12-hourly intravenous push days 1–10 inclusive; thioguanine 100 mg/m^2 12-hourly orally days 1–10 inclusive

DAT 3+8: daunorubicin 50 mg/m^2 intravenous push days 1, 3, 5; cytarabine 100 mg/m^2 12-hourly intravenous push days 1–8 inclusive; thioguanine 100 mg/m^2 12-hourly orally days 1–8 inclusive.

ADE 10+3+5: cytarabine 100 mg/m^2 12-hourly intravenous push days 1–10 inclusive; daunorubicin 50 mg/m^2 intravenous push days 1, 3, 5; etoposide 100 mg/m^2 12-hourly intravenously daily, days 1–5 inclusive

ADE 8+3+5: cytarabine 100 mg/m^2 12-hourly intravenous push days 1–8 inclusive; daunorubicin 50 mg/m^2 intravenous push days 1, 3, 5; etoposide 100 mg/m^2 12-hourly intravenously daily, days 1–5 inclusive

MACE: m-AMSA 100 mg/m^2 intravenously days 1–5; cytarabine 100 mg/m^2 intravenous continuous infusion days 1–5 inclusive; etoposide 100 mg/m^2 days 1–5

MidAc: mitozantrone 10 mg/m^2 intravenously days 1–5; cytarabine 1.0 mg/m^2 12-hourly days 1–3.

BMT, bone marrow transplant; CR, complete remission

The reasons for failure to achieve remission have been analysed extensively by Priesler[13] and have become particularly important in older patients where the failure rate is higher. In broad terms, early death due to infection and toxicity are matched by the percentage of patients with resistant disease but their proportions may vary among the age groups. It is very important to establish which factors play the dominant role in order to develop a more logical policy for future trial design.

The MRC's ninth AML trial (AML 9) showed that the more intensive 3 + 10 DAT regimen (daunorubicin, cytarabine, thioguanine) was slightly more effective in achieving remissions but was significantly more efficient in the demands placed on supportive care with antibiotics and blood products. Data from 567 patients achieving remission showed that the total number of days in hospital for induction therapy was 47 days for the 1 + 5 treatment and 39 days for the 3 + 10 ($p < 0.0001$).

The corresponding values for numbers of units of blood and platelets were 17 and 15 units of blood and 74 and 70 units of platelets for the 1 + 5 and 3 + 10 regimens respectively. The implications for financial savings are clear—more intensive chemotherapy is more efficient and cost effective and is particularly relevant in the adolescent age group not only because of their greater tolerance of higher doses of drugs but because a smooth, rapid passage into remission lays the foundation for a wider range of options to be discussed with the patient in the next phase of treatment. Reviews from the Royal Marsden Hospital[14] and L'hôtel Dieu, Paris,[15] have earlier shown that the major expenditure in the treatment of AML is the cost of supportive care, with cytotoxic drugs—when used in orthodox doses—playing a relatively minor role.

The attaining of remission in the young adult with AML is therefore not a major problem. The long term success or feature of the treatment program rests with the postremission therapy, although the intensity of the induction phase can influence the duration of remission as was shown in the AML 9 trial and by others.[6 11 12 16] Some of the recent reports are shown in Table 13.2.

The myelosuppressive effect of postremission therapy is gradually increasing and has led to a treatment-related mortality or death in remission of 8–15% in large collaborative trials and similar results are obtained in single institution studies. The overall death rate in remission in MRC's AML 10 is currently about 8% for the adults and children combined. However, it became clear, after the trial had been running for a year, that there was a close correlation between the time spent in hospital under close supervision following a course of consolidation treatment and the toxic death rate; only 1% for patients remaining in hospital more than two weeks, whereas 11% of patients discharged early had fatal infections or haemorrhage. Clearly there are important clinical and financial implications to these findings which may be influenced by the use of growth factors.

The central issue which has dominated policy for the postremission

Table 13.2 Postremission therapy and maintenance treatment of AML

Reference	Age of patients (years)	Induction therapy	Postremission therapy	Maintenance therapy	Results
Buchner et al.[11]	>16	TAD TAD+TAD or TAD+HAM	TAD X1 AMLG81 AMLG85	Cytar/Dauno, Cytar/6TG, Cytar/6TG, Cytar/Cyclo No therapy Cytar/Dauno, Cytar/6TG Cytar/6TG, Cytar/Cyclo or no therapy	24% continuous C/R 7% continuous C/R 34% continuous C/R (at 5 years)
Mayer et al.[6]	>16	Daunorubicin (3 d) with cytarbine (7 d) infusion	Cytar/Hidac (3 g/m² every 12d)×6 or Cytar infusion (400 mg/m²/d×5 or Cytar infusion (100 mg/m²/h)×5d (each treatment continued for four courses)	Cytarabine and daunorubicin	Improved outlook for Hidac group
Zittoun et al.[12]	45–60	Daunorubicin (3 d) and cytarbine (7 d)	Cytar (500 mg/m² every 12 h days 1–6)+AMSA (days 5–7) alternating with Cytar (2 g/m² every 12 h days 1–4) Dauno (days 5–7) or Dauno and Cytar (day 1 and 7)	None Dauno+Cytar (1+5, monthly)×6 or DAT (monthly)×4	26% disease-free survival at 3 years 22% disease-free survival at 3 years
Morrison et al.[16]	>15	Rubidazone and doxorubicin + vincristine, cytarbine and prednisone	Rubidazone and doxorubicin +vincristine, Cytar, and prednisone	Vincristine, Cytar, and prednisone×9±three courses POMP±levamisole	Median survival; for POMP, 34.5 months; for rest, +19·3 months

DAT, daunorubicin; cytarabine, and thioguanine; HAM, high dose cytosine arabinoside/mitozantrone; Hidac, high dose cytarabine; POMP, prednisone, vincristine, methotrexate, and mercaptopurine; TAD, thioguanine, cytarabine, and daunorubicin; Cytar, cytarabine; Dauno, daunorubicin; Cyclo, cyclophosphamide; C/R, complete remission.

treatment of AML has been the role of bone marrow transplantation (BMT).[17] It has been widely held that if a matched sibling donor is available, allogeneic BMT should be carried out in all patients under the age of 55. The Seattle group[18] has shown that patients in the adolescent age group do particularly well because of their tolerance of graft versus host disease.

The overwhelming problem hindering the adoption of allogeneic BMT is the availability of donors. A recent review by Berman[19] found that, of 350 patients with AML at the Memorial Sloan-Kettering Cancer Center from 1979 (when the policy of offering allogeneic transplantation was introduced) until 1990, 41% of patients were eligible by age; only 52 patients achieving complete remission had HLA-identical siblings and 30 of these patients (58%) underwent transplantation. These represented a small fraction (8.6%) of the original cohort in this time period.

Gray and Wheatley[20] have drawn attention to the risks of interpreting the results of bone marrow transplantation. The most common error is to compare the survival of transplanted patients with those of the entire chemotherapy-treated group, which includes patients with short remissions that make them ineligible for transplantation; data from AML 9 trial and other sources show that the median interval from remission to allogeneic BMT is six months. The interval from remission to autologous BMT is slightly longer, thereby exaggerating the degree of selection which occurred in the earlier reports. It became apparent therefore that the only method of establishing the place of autologous BMT was to conduct a randomised trial.

Studies have been set up by the EORTC/GIMEMA, MRC, and the HOVON groups in Europe, and the POG and combined SWOG/ECOG trials in the United States. The EORTC-GIMEMA collaboration has recently reported on their 8A trial in which autologous BMT was compared with chemotherapy or allogeneic BMT from matched siblings.[12] Between November 1986 and April 1993 992 adult patients were entered. Postremission chemotherapy included intermediate dose cytarabine and M-AMSA and either an autologous BMT or a second course of chemotherapy. Of the 619 patients who entered complete remission, 164 had matched donors and 4·7% died of toxicity associated with the first course of postremission therapy. A further 250 patients entered the randomisation for an autograft or further chemotherapy. The remainder of the patients were not randomised because of nonlethal excess toxicity in 57 patients, toxic deaths in 32, early relapse in 47, refusal to randomise by 80, protocol violations in 10 cases, and 7 who were lost to follow up. The result at four years, based on intention to treat, shows an advantage in disease-free survival in favour of those receiving an allogeneic or autologous BMT. However, the overall survival of remitters is no different in the three arms, with 59% of allogeneic BMT, 57% of autologous BMT, and 46% of chemotherapy treated patients being alive at four years.

The MRC study has faced similar problems with recruitment into the randomisation between an autologous bone marrow transplant and the alternative option, to stop treatment. The comparison remains coded as of May 1994 but an independent review by a monitoring committee shows no significant difference between the randomised arms at follow up intervals of up to five years on nearly 350 patients.

The Pediatric Oncology Group (POG) has recently published the findings of its trial in childhood AML (POG 8821).[21] Following induction therapy with DAT and by high dose cytarabine, 85% of 623 children and young adolescents achieved complete remission. Patients having a matched sibling donor, Down's syndrome, secondary AML, and isolated granulo-cytic sarcomas were not eligible for randomisation. Only 233 of the 382 that were eligible actually entered the randomisation process; 139 patients selected chemotherapy and 10 elected to have an autologous BMT. One hundred and eighteen patients were randomised to continue with a rotating combination of chemotherapy and 115 were assigned to autologous BMT with cyclophosphamide-purged autologous bone marrow. When the dis-ease-free survival at three years was assessed on the basis of intention to treat, the results were identical for the two groups at 37%. There was a lower leukaemia relapse rate but a higher treatment related mortality in the autologous BMT group compared with the group receiving chemotherapy (20% versus 3%).

Detection of the source of relapse after autologous BMT is obviously of great importance. Studies have already been carried out in St Jude's, Memphis, Tennessee to test the feasibility of using a neomycin gene marker which has been integrated into the genome of the donor cells.[22] In a report on preliminary experience with this technique, Brenner and his co-workers found that the reinfused autologous bone marrow cells were at least partially responsible for the subsequent relapse.

A great deal of interest has therefore developed in the role of peripheral blood stem cells (PBSCs) instead of bone marrow as a form of rescue from the potentially lethal effects of conditioning. Korbling[23][24] first developed this technique and was able to show a much more rapid reconstitution to safe neutrophil and platelet counts compared with autologous BMTs. The techniques for collecting peripheral blood stem cells have improved a great deal in the last few years and have become more widely available as increasing attention is focused on the cost of inpatient treatment. Indeed, the use of PBSCs has largely replaced autologous BMT as a source of stem cells.

A further alternative source of semipurified stem cells may be obtained by long-term bone marrow cultures. Leukaemia cells often fail to survive in such cultures, providing a mechanism of purging. This work has been developed at the Christie Hospital Manchester by Dexter and his colleagues.[25]

Prognostic factors

In an attempt to rationalise the treatment of acute leukaemia, many attempts have been made to establish whether individual groups of patients had a better or poorer chance of attaining and maintaining remission. The lead in this field came from analyses of childhood acute lymphatic leukaemia trials, due mainly to the spectacular improvement in the response rates which occurred in the 1970s and early 1980s. Apart from the risk of overtreating some patients, there was clearly a need for a different policy for a relatively small group of patients who did particularly badly.

The response rate in AML was, until recently, so poor—partly because of a high early toxic death rate—that reliable prognostic features were difficult to define in the face of overwhelming problems with adequate supportive care and a pessimistic outlook on the part of the physicians. Over the last 10 years, however, a plethora of prognostic factors have been reported; some are certainly epiphenomena and have achieved prominence following the analysis of relatively small groups of patients. A list of some of the newer factors reported in the last few years is included in Table 13.3.

Four consistently reliable pretreatment characteristics have been identified as playing a crucial role in the outcome for patients with AML. These are age, performance status, cytogenetic features and the presence of a pre-existing haematological disorder; to these may be added the response to treatment.

An analysis of the results of AML 10 trial has confirmed that the outcome is determined by a small group of factors but two stand out as of prime importance for the long term prospects; these are the response to the first course of treatment and the karyotype.[40 41]

Patients entering remission after the first course of treatment (and this applies to nearly three quarters of the patients in the trial) who also have one of the non-random chromosome changes which includes t(8;21), t(15;17), or inv(16), have a particularly good outlook.

Nearly 200 patients with one of these abnormalities have been identified among the first 1000 patients for whom cytogenetic data is available. The average age of this population is 25. The adolescent patients are therefore strongly represented in the most favourable prognostic groups. Of these patients, 75% are alive at five years, although only a relatively small proportion have undergone bone marrow transplantation. Comparison of the survival of transplanted patients with the chemotherapy treated group shows no significant difference. The question therefore arises, "Should we recommend BMT in first remission for patients with this group of cytogenetic abnormalities?". The body of evidence now mitigates against such a policy, and this option will not be recommended for prompt responders with favourable cytogenetic features in the next MRC AML trial (AML 12). This policy is very different from that adopted by the EORTC-GIMEMA group which proposes the incorporation of autologous transplants as an essential component in their future studies.

Table 13.3 Recently described prognostic factors in AML

Reference	Prognostic factor	Number of patients	Predictive value
Gucalp et al.[26]	Terminal transferase	114 adults	Not predictive
Gucalp et al.[26]	CDw65 antigen	114 adults	Good prognosis
Preisler et al.[27]	Interleukin-1β	22 all ages	Not predictive for achieving complete remission, but those with high interleukin-1β levels have short remissions
Hoyle et al.[28]	Sudan black positivity	1386 adults	Sudan black positivity ≥50% good prognosis for complete remission and for survival
Tidefelt et al.[29]	Glutathione transferase-π	60	For low expression of glutathione transferase-π, good prognosis for complete remission response and duration
Kornblau et al.[30]	Retinoblastoma protein	33	Low retinoblastoma protein was associated with low complete remission rate
Dinndorf et al.[31]	CD33 antigen	98 children	CD33+ have poor duration, complete remission, and survival
Willman et al.[32]	CD34 antigen	91 adults	CD34+ predicts poorer complete remission rate but not duration of complete remission
Geller et al.[33]	CD34 antigen	96 adults	CD34+ predicts poor complete remission rate
Myint and Lucie[34]	CD34 antigen	38	Relative risk of death >5× for CD34+
Urbano-Ispizua et al.[35]	CD7 antigen	60 adults	Complete remission rate higher and survival longer for CD7-patients
Ball et al.[36]	Lymphocyte markers, (CD2 and CD19)	170 adults	CD2+, better complete remission rate and duration; CD19+, did not predict
Marie et al.[37]	Multidrug resistance (MDR1) expression RNA levels	36	MDR1 >2 U had poorer complete remission rate, but MDR1 expression did not predict for complete remission duration
Pirker et al.[38]	MDR1 RNA levels	63 adults	Complete remission rate 89% for MDR1 messenger RNA negative compared with 53% for MDR1+
Campos et al.[39]	MDR1 expression (MRK-16 monoclonal antibody ± CD34 expression)	150 (by antibody method)	MDR1+ had a much lower complete remission rate as did CD34+; MDR1+ and CD34+ defined very poor prognosis
Walker et al.[40]	Cytogenetics	600 (in a collaborative study)	Remission rate for t(8;21), t(15;17), inv(16) was excellent Monosomy 7 has poor prognosis

A poor prognostic group has been defined for patients failing to enter remission after one course of treatment and cytogenetic abnormalities involving chromosomes 5 or 7.

Treatment of relapse

Reports on the response rates with salvage therapy in relapsed AML have often been difficult to interpret because details on the duration of first remission have not been included. Analysis of the second remission rates in AML 9 show that only 10% of patients relapsing within the first six months achieved complete remission, but the rate improves to 65% if treatment has been discontinued more than two years before the event. Younger patients have an additional advantage compared with the elderly at comparable stages of relapse. Hiddeman et al.[42] have reported encouraging results using the high dose cytarabine–mitoxantrone combination in Münster. They obtained a 47% second remission rate and the schedule has been successfully adopted by the German AML Cooperative Group which reported a 54% second remission rate in 65 patients.[43]

The purine analogue 2-chlorodeoxyadenosine showed improved results when used as a continuous infusion over 5 days at a dose of 9 mg/m^2 per day for the treatment of children with relapsed AML at St Jude Children's Hospital.[44]

An alternative approach to the management of relapsed disease is to proceed immediately to allogeneic BMT from a matched sibling if one is available, without attempting to induce a second remission. The chances of a prolonged disease-free survival appear to be the same (approximately 30%) whether a second remission is achieved before grafting or whether transplantation after conditioning is carried out immediately.[45-48] The latter policy requires more frequent supervision of a patient's progress with regular bone marrow examinations and a range of techniques available for the detection of minimal residual disease including morphology, cytogenetics in combination with fluorescent in situ hybridisation, and the use of molecular probes which are now available for t(8;21), t(15;17), and inv(16).

There is little doubt that the detection of minimal disease in acute promyelocytic leukaemia (APL) is a forerunner of relapse—usually within 3–6 months—and therapy with all-trans retinoic acid (tretinoin) or chemotherapy or both may prevent the appearance of florid relapse.[49 50] Resistance to tretinoin is, however, well documented and several mechanisms have been described. It has been possible to reverse the resistance with interferon.[51]

In young adults there is a strong case for not carrying out bone marrow transplants in first remission in APL but to monitor the disease carefully. The guidelines are not as clear cut with t(8;21) or inv(16) abnormalities. Although there is a slight increase in the incidence of chloromas (granulocytic sarcomas) in these two series of patients, the significance of detectable molecular abnormalities in bone marrow samples, which would otherwise fulfil the criteria of remission, is not known and at this stage of our knowledge it would be prudent to pursue a 'wait and see' policy supported by regular monitoring.

Biological response modifiers

There has been a resurgence of interest in the potential value of immunotherapy directed at the stimulation of lymphokine activated killer (LAK) cells. These have been shown to be absent or ineffective in killing leukaemia blast cells during the active phase of the disease.[52] LAK stimulation is therefore more feasible during remission when autologous LAK cells return to normal. Foa et al.[53 54] have reported on the results of using interleukin-2 on a group of patients in Milan and Turin. The patients were in relapse, but three of five patients entered second complete remission with escalating doses. Initial results with bolus injections of 1·5 million units/m^2 of interleukin-2 is effective in inducing LAK cells and high levels of tumour necrosis factor-α. Further studies have since been set up in France.

Arienti[55] has made the somewhat unusual observation that leukaemic blast cells from patients with AML or acute lymphoblastic leukaemias are more sensitive to allogeneic or autologous LAK cells at relapse than at diagnosis; furthermore, LAK cell mediated killing can be enhanced by pretreatment of myeloid leukaemia blasts with interleukin-3, but no effect was found on the killing of normal CD34 cells.[56]

An alternative method of enhancing natural killer cell production uses roquinimex (Linomide), a quinolone-3-carboxamide, following autologous BMT in second remission. Clinical trials in Europe and the United States are just being concluded and may support the initial encouraging results.

Other immunological approaches explore the potential of immunotoxins.[57] The anti-My9-blocked ricin immunotoxin is a hybrid material linking a monoclonal antibody to the ricin toxin, an extract from the castor bean. More recently a humanised antibody (HU M195) has been raised against the CD33 antigen and been used in the treatment of acute promyelocytic leukaemia.

Finally, interferon alfa has been very effective in the treatment of chronic myeloid leukaemia and myeloma and has recently entered clinical trials in the MRC's AML 11 trial for elderly patients. If an effect is demonstrated it may be applied to the treatment of younger patients in remission.

Supportive care

Improved quality of supportive care with antibiotics and blood products has made a major contribution to the improved outcome for patients with AML. It overshadows the relative merits of one form of anthracycline compared with another, and escalating doses of cytarabine.

The management of infections in acute leukaemia has again been reviewed recently in an authoritative account by Wade.[58]

Transfusion methods are constantly being refined; one interesting aspect of this work has been the introduction of filtration to reduce the level of leucocyte contamination and thereby the risk of alloimmunisation by HLA antigens. Three recent reports have approached the problem in slightly different ways.

Oskanen and his colleagues in Helsinki[59] studied, retrospectively, 115 patients with AML. Fifty patients received standard platelet concentrates and 65 patients were given platelets which were leucocyte depleted by filtration. Filtration mainly took place during the preparation stage in the Finnish Red Cross Blood Transfusion Service but, in a small percentage, it was carried out at the beside. Although the study was not randomised, the policy of using filtered or non-filtered platelets was maintained constant for each participating hospital. Refractoriness to platelets developed in 22% of the standard group and in 3% of the leucocyte depleted group. After the second and subsequent courses of chemotherapy there was a significant decrease in the number of platelets and red cells transfused in the leucocyte depleted patients. The duration of thrombocytopenia and neutropenia was also shorter and serious infections were less common (44% versus 59%). As a result, the patients receiving leucocyte-depleted platelets spent less time in hospital. The most interesting result of the study, however, was that patients receiving filtered platelets had a longer median relapse-free survival (23 months versus 10 months) although the remission rates in the two groups were virtually identical.

A multicentre study in the UK examined the efficacy of bedside filtration in the prevention of alloimmunisation using the Pall RC50 and RC100 red cell filters and PL50 and PL100 platelet filters;[60] there were 123 evaluable patients with a variety of haematologic disorders including 57 patients with AML of whom 27 were treated with the AML 10 protocol. Among the whole group, HLA antibodies developed in 21 out of 56 (37·5%) of patients receiving non-filtered products and in 15 out of 67 (22%) receiving filtered products. The patients with AML had higher alloimmunisation rates in both arms of the study and a greater effect of filtration (62·5% non-filtered versus 3% filtered).

Filtration did not affect the overall incidence of febrile transfusion reactions or of platelet refractoriness, and febrile reactions were also seen in 28 patients without HLA antibodies. There was no evidence from this study of a survival advantage for the patients receiving filtered blood products. One problem in the interpretation of the results lay in the difficulty in assessing the degree of leucocyte depletion which had been achieved in each case, as filter performance deteriorated during the procedure; isolated sampling was, therefore, a poor predictor of the number of leucocytes transfused into the patient. One explanation for the deterioration in filter performance has been provided by the studies of Sivakumaran and his colleagues in Leeds and Leicester.[61] They found that nearly one third of filters tested allowed substantial numbers of leucocytes to leak through towards the end of the transfusion of the second unit of blood. They were able to reproduce the defect by introducing as little as 2 ml of air into the RC100 filter; this can occur quite easily when an empty bag of blood is replaced by the next unit.

The quality of platelet transfusions is clearly of great importance in the management of AML but a recent review report from Edinburgh suggest that their beneficial effect are not determined by freshness, method of preparation, or increment achieved.[62]

The relative merits of techniques for platelet preparation will, however, soon be replaced by a choice of haemopoetic regulators which stimulate megakaryocyte proliferation. These include interleukin-3, interleukin-6, interleukin-11, and thrombopoietin. The action of each cytokine is rather slow, and side effects have proved troublesome. The most exciting development in efforts to promote platelet production came with the publication in *Nature* in June 1994 of four papers reporting the character-isation and cloning of thrombopoietin. Metcalf, in reviewing the papers, described the event as a "cause for celebration".[63] The potential contribu-tion of this spectacular advance to the quality of supportive care available to all patients with AML is incalculable and clinical trials have begun. Granulocyte colony stimulating factor (G-CSF) and granulocyte macro-phage stimulating factor (GM-CSF) are already licensed for certain neutrophenic states but their role in AML is now being explored in many randomised and non randomised studies.

The cost of treating AML in adolescents

Improvement in the results of treating AML in adolescents has made it possible and necessary to stand back a little from the original aims of clearing the disease to examine the intermediate and long-term conse-quences of the management of the patient's illness. This discipline is particularly important in the care of children and young adults who have a considerably higher expectation of long survival. The long term effects on children have been reviewed by Morris-Jones and others.[64] Adolescents present general and specific problems because of their stage of maturity when treatment is given. Some recent results on cardiac toxicity, ophthalmic problems, sexuality, and fertility will be discussed briefly.

Cardiac toxicity

Anthracycline antibiotics have become one of the principal components of drug combinations used in the treatment of AML. Their association with cardiac toxicity is well established[65] but the incidence of clinically significant cardiac impairment is difficult to establish, partly because evidence of cardiac failure in a very ill patient is often associated with severe infections and a generalised toxaemia. A high percentage of the few cases of cardiac-related deaths in the MRC AML 10 trial were found in association with overwhelming sepsis. Nevertheless, the problem is an important one and deserves serious consideration in the design of future trials for all ages. Hann[66] has reviewed the evidence from the paediatric patients entered into AML 10. On this regimen children receive 300 mg/m² of daunorubicin and 50 mg/m² of mitozantrone. Acute cardiac toxicity was rarely reported, with only 5 of 270 patients, at the time of the interim analysis, dying in remission of primary cardiac failure. A further 10 children had cardiotoxicity of WHO grade 3 or 4. Less severe toxicity could have been overlooked because detailed cardiac monitoring was not included in the trial protocol.

In a recent editorial in the *Lancet*, attention was drawn to a study of the treatment of children with anthracyclines for late stage solid tumours;[67] 201 children received 200–1725 mg/m² total dose of anthracyclines and 46 (23%) had abnormal cardiac function 4–20 years after treatment.[65] One technique which has been used to decrease the incidence of anthracycline-associated cardiac toxicity is the use of the bisdioxypiperazine compound (ICRF-187; ADR-529).[68-71] Its probable mechanism of action is that of an iron-chelating agent. It has been shown that ferrous ions increase the toxicity of anthracycline and withdrawal of "catalytic" ions reduces the rate of hydroxyl radical formation. Clinical trials have been carried out in adults with a variety of tumours, and the results will be of considerable interest to paediatricians.

Ophthalmic problems

Eye problems following bone marrow transplantation are providing increasing anxiety, as large numbers of cases with adequate follow up have now been reported. Two such series reviewed a total of 425 patients in Paris and in Basel. Among 228 assessable French patients over a minimum risk period of two years, the incidence was 18.4% after a median of 42 months (range 13–72 months). There was no difference in the incidence above or below the age of 20. The instantaneous dose rate was the only independent factor influencing the development of cataracts.[72]

In the Basel study[73] among 197 patients with follow-up of at least six months, the incidence was 69% for patients receiving single dose total body irradiation and the overall incidence was 36% for all total body irradiation dosing schedules. Of patients receiving single dose total body irradiation, 59% required surgery within 3·5 years of the transplant and all patients alive in this group had cataracts. In a parallel study in Basel the incidence of keratoconjunctivitis sicca was 19% at 10 years in a group of patients with haematological malignancies who had received BMT.[74] There was a close correlation between the incidence of graft versus host disease; 69% of patients with this disease developed the sicca syndrome.

Sexual problems

Perhaps the most intangible but profound consequences of the treatment of AML emerge from studies of the physical and mental wellbeing of the patient; their quality of life. This, again, has become relevant as the treatment of AML has improved and patients' expectations have changed dramatically over the last 10 years. Ropponen et al.[75] have analysed the psychosexual problems of male survivors following a childhood malignancy and found quite serious problems in adjusting to the changes normally experienced in the adolescent period. Baruch and colleagues[76] at the Royal Marsden Hospital have investigated the effect of bone marrow transplantation on sexual function in a group of 51 men who had been treated for haematological malignancies. They found a markedly raised prevalence of sexual dysfunction, but the clinical situation was often complex because of the contribution of general ill health and postural hypotension. Endocrine function was impaired, as indicated by raised gonadotrophins, but a functional element was also probably involved, because depression or anxiety was fairly common within the group.

The EORTC has drawn up a "quality of life" protocol for use in international clinical trials in oncology.[77] This has been modified and adopted for incorporation in the MRC AML 10 trial. The questionnaire, which is directed towards patients from 18 to 55 years of age, examines four aspects of life's qualities. There are 69 questions dealing with patients' current health condition, 9 about sexuality and fertility, and a further 9 dealing with disease-related modifications to a patient's life. A final section establishes a number of personal details, including marital status, which may have a bearing on the interpretation of the replies. Early results show some interesting differences between the three treatment groups of patients (chemotherapy only, allogeneic BMT, and autogeneic BMT) in respect to sexual function (M. Watson, personal communication). A significantly higher percentage of patients having a bone marrow transplant expressed decreased "interest" or "pleasure/satisfaction from sex" than in the chemotherapy group. The results of this and other components of the questionnaire will be analysed for a very lage group of patients and the conclusions will be of great interest.

1 Office of Population Consensus and Surveys. *Cancer Statistics: Registrations England and Wales 1987;* Series MBI, 20.

2 Stevens RF, Hann IM, Wheatley K, Gray RG. Intensive chemotherapy with or without additional bone marrow transplantation in paediatric AML: Progress report on the MRC AML 10 trial. *Leukaemia* 1992; 6(Suppl 2): 55–8.

3 Goldstone AH, Burnett AK, Rees JKH et al. MRC AML 10: A prospective randomised trial of autologous bone marrow transplantation versus no further chemotherapy in children and adults less than 55 years in first remission of acute myeloid leukaemia. *Proc Int Soc Haematol* 1992; 61:Abstr 238.

4 Weinstein H, Ravindranath Y, Krischer J et al. The impact of early intensive therapy on event-free survival (EFS) in children with acute myeloid leukaemia. *Leukaemia* 1992; 6 (Suppl 2): 52–4.

5 Ritter J, Creutzig U, Schellong G. Treatment results of three consecutive German childhood AML trials: BFM-78, -83 and -87. *Leukaemia* 1992; 6:(Suppl 2): 59–62.

6 Mayer R, Davis R, Schiffer C et al. Intensive post remission therapy with Ara-C in Adults with acute myeloid leukaemia and initial results of a CALGB phase III trial. *Leukaemia* 1992; 6:(Suppl 2): 66–7.

7 Berman E, Heller G, Stantorsa S et al. Results of a randomised trial comparing idarubicin and cytosine arabinoside with daunorubicin and cytosine arabinoside in adult patients with newly diagnosed acute meylogenous leukaemia. *Blood* 1991; 77: 1666–74.

8 Vogler WR, Velez-Garcia E, Weiner RS *et al.* A phase III trial comparing idarubicin and daunorubicin in combination with cytarabine in acute myelogenous leukaemia: A Southeastern Cancer Study Group study. *J Clin Oncol* 1992; **10**: 1102–11.

9 Bishop JF, Lowenthal RM, Joshua AD *et al.* Etoposide in acute nonlymphocytic leukaemia. *Blood* 1990; **75**: 27–32.

10 Rees JKH. Aspects of treatment of acute myeloid leukaemia in adults. *Curr Opin Oncol* 1993; **5**: 53–70.

11 Buchner T, Hiddemann W, Wormann B *et al.* Long term effects of prolonged maintenance and of very early intensification chemotherapy in AML: data from AML CG. *Leukaemia* 1992; **6**(Suppl 2): 68–71.

12 Zittoun R, Liso V, Mandelli F *et al.* Intensive consolidation chemotherapy versus standard consolidation maintenance in acute myelogenous leukaemia (AML) in first remission: an EORTC/Gimema phase III trial (AML 8b). *Leukaemia* 1992; **6**(Suppl 2): 76–7.

13 Preisler HD. Failure of remission induction in acute myelogenous leukaemia. *Med Pediatr Oncol* 1978; **4**: 275–6.

14 Lobo PJ, Powles R, Hanrahan A, Reynolds DK. Acute myeoblastic leukaemia—a model for assessing value for money for new treatment programmes. *Br Med J* 1991; **302**: 323–6.

15 Marie JP, Wdowik I, Bisserbe S, Zittoun R. Cost of complete remission induction in acute myeoblastic leukaemia: Evaluation of the cost effectiveness of a new drug. *Leukaemia* 1992; **6**: 720–2.

16 Morrison FS, Kopecky KJ, Head DR *et al.* Intensification with POMP chemotherapy prolongs survival in acute myelogenous leukaemia: results of a Southwest Oncology Group Study of rubidazone versus adriamycin for remission induction, prophylactic intrathecal therapy, late intensification and levamisole maintenance. *Leukaemia* 1992; **6**: 708–14.

17 Hurd DD. Post remission therapy for the younger adult patient with acute myelogenous leukaemia: Defining a role for transplantation. *J Clin Oncol* 1993; **11**: 1636–8.

18 Christiansen NP. Allogeneic bone marrow transplantation for the treatment of adult acute leukaemia. *Haematology/Oncology Clinics of North America* 1993; **7**: 177–200.

19 Berman E, Little C, Gee T *et al.* Reasons that patients with acute myelogenous leukaemia do not undergo allogeneic bone marrow transplantation. *N Engl J Med* 1992; **326**: 156–60.

20 Gray R, Wheatley K. How to avoid bias when comparing bone marrow transplantation with chemotherapy. *Bone Marrow Transplant* 1991; **7**(Suppl 13): 9–12.

21 Ravindranath Y, Yeager A, Krischer J *et al.* Intensive consolidation chemotherapy (ICC) vs purged autologous bone marrow transplantation (ABMT) early in remission for treatment of childhood acute myeloid leukaemia (AML): Preliminary results of Pediatric Oncology Group (POG) Study 8821. *Proc Am Soc Clin Oncol.* ASCO 1994; Abstr 1053.

22 Brenner MK, Rill DR, Moen RC *et al.* Gene-marking to trace origin of relapse after autologous bone marrow transplantation. *Lancet* 1993; **341**: 85–6.

23 Korbling M, Fuedner T, Holle R *et al.* Autologous blood stem cell (ABSCT) versus purged bone marrow transplantation (pABMT) in standard risk AML: Influence of source and cell composition of the autograft on haemopoietic reconstitution and disease-free survival. *Bone Marrow Transplant* 1991; **7**: 343–9.

24 Korbling M, Hunstein W, Fliedner TM *et al.* Disease-free survival after autologous bone marrow transplantation in patients with acute myelogenous leukaemia. *Blood* 1989; **74**: 1898–904.

25 Chang J, Allen TD, Dexter TM. Long-term bone marrow cultures: their use in autologous marrow transplantation. *Cancer Cells* 1989; **1**: 17–24.

26 Gucalp P, Paietta E, Weinberg V *et al.* Terminal transferase expression in acute myeloid leukaemia: biology and prognosis. *Br J Haematol* 1991; **78**: 48–54.

27 Preisler H, Raza A, Kukla C *et al.* Interleukin IB expression and treatment outcome in acute myelogenous leukaemia. *Blood* 1991; **78**: 849–50.

28 Hoyle CF, Gray RG, Wheatley K *et al.* Prognostic importance of Sudan black positivity: a study of bone marrow slides from 1386 patients with de novo acute myeloid leukaemia. *Cancer Res* 1992; **52**: 3281–5.

29 Tidefelt U, Elmhorn-Rosenborg A, Paul C *et al.* Expression of glutathione transferase-II as a predictor for treatment results at different stages of acute non lymphoblastic leukaemia. *Cancer Res* 1992; **52**: 3281–5.

30 Kornblau SM, Xu H-J, Del Giglio A *et al.* Clinical implications of decreased retinoblastoma protein expression in acute myelogenous leukaemia. *Cancer Res* 1992; **52**:

4587–90.

31 Dinndorf PA, Buckley JD, Nesbit ME *et al.* Expression of myeloid differentiation antigens in acute nonlymphocytic leukaemia: increased concentration of CD33 antigen predicts poor outcome—a report from the Children's Cancer Study Group. *Med Pediatr Oncol* 1992; **20**: 192–200.

32 Willman CL, Kopecky KJ, Weick J *et al.* Biologic parameters that predict treatment response in de novo acute myeloid leukaemia (AML): CD34, but not multidrug resistance (MDR) gene expression is associated with a decreased complete remission (C/R) rate and CD34+ patients more frequently achieve C/R rate with high dose cytosine arabinoside [abstract]. *Proc Am Soc Clin Oncol* 1992, **262**: 857.

33 Geller RB, Zahurak M, Hurwitz CA *et al.* Prognostic importance of immunophenotyping in adults with acute myelocytic leukaemia: the significance of the stem-cell glycoprotein CD34 (MY10). *Br J Haematol* 1990; **76**: 340–7.

34 Myint H, Lucie NP. The prognostic significance of the CD34 antigen in acute myeloid leukaemia. *Leuk Lymphoma* 1992; **7**: 425–8.

35 Urbano-Ispizua A, Matutes E, Villamor N *et al.* The value of detecting surface and cytoplasmic antigens in acute myeloid leukaemia. *Br J Haematol* 1992; **81**: 178–83.

36 Ball ED, Davis RB, Griffin JD *et al.* Prognostic value of lymphocyte surface markers in acute myeloid leukaemia. *Blood* 1991; **77**: 2242–50.

37 Marie J-P, Zittoun R, Sikic BI. Multidrug resistance (MDR) gene expression in adult acute leukaemias: correlations with treatment outcome an in vitro drug sensitivity. *Blood* 1991; **78**: 586–92.

38 Pirker R, Wallner J, Geissler K *et al.* Gene expression and treatment outcome in acute myeloid leukaemia. *J Natl Cancer Inst* 1991; **83**: 708–12.

39 Campos L, Guyotat D, Archimbaud E *et al.* Clinical significance of multidrug resistance P-glycoprotein expression on acute nonlymphoblastic leukaemia cells at diagnosis. *Blood* 1992; **79**: 473–6.

40 Walker H, Turker A, Goldstone AH *et al.* Cytogenetics as a prognostic indicator for acute myeloid leukaemia in the MRC AML 10 trial. *Proc Int Soc Haematol* 1992 Abstract 20.

41 Baer MR, Bloomfield CD, Cytogenetics and oncogenes in leukemia. *Curr Opin Oncol* 1992; **4**: 24–32.

42 Hiddeman W, Aul HC, Maschmeyer G *et al.* Proposal for the classification of relapsed and refractory acute myeloid leukaemias as the basis for an age-adjusted randomised comparison of sequentially applied highdose versus intermediate dose cytosine arabinoside in combination with mitozantrone (S-HAM). *Haematol Blood Trans* 1990; **33**: 604–9.

43 Buchner T. Acute leukaemia. *Curr Opin Haematol* 1993; 172–82.

44 Santana VM, Mirro J, Kearns C *et al.* 2-Chlorodeoxyadenosine produces a high rate of complete haematologic remissions in relapsed acute myeloid leukaemia. *J Clin Oncol* 1992; **10**: 364–70.

45 Ball ED, Rybka WB. Autologous bone marrow transplantation for adult acute leukaemia. *Haematol/Oncol Clin N Am* 1993; **7**: 201–31.

46 Applebaum FR, Clift RA, Buckner CD *et al.* Allogeneic marrow transplantation for acute nonlymphoblastic leukemia after relapse. *Blood* 1983; **61**: 949–53.

47 Peterson FB, Lynch MHE, Clift RA *et al.* Autologous marrow transplantation for patients with acute myeloid leukemia in untreated first relapse or in second complete remission. *J Clin Oncol* 1993; **11**: 1353–60.

48 Clift RA, Buckner CD, Applebaum FR *et al.* Allogeneic marrow transplantation during untreated first relapse of acute myeloid leukaemia. *J Clin Oncol* 1992; **10**: 1723–9.

49 Warrell RP Jr, Frankel SR, Miller WH Jr *et al.* Differentiation therapy of acute promyelocytic leukemia with tretionon (all-trans retinoic acid) *N Engl J Med* 1991; **324**: 385–1393.

50 Adamson PC, Balis FM, Smith MA *et al.* Dose dependent pharmacokinetics of all-trans retinoic acid. *J Natl Cancer Inst* 1992; **84**: 1332–5.

51 Koller E, Kriegen O, Kasparu H, Lutz D. Resoration of all-trans retinoic acid sensitivity by interferon in acute promyelocytic leukaemia [Letter] *Lancet* 1991; **338**: 1154–5.

52 Bergman L, Mitrou P.S., Hoelzer D. Interleukin-2 in the treatment of acute myelocytic leukemia: in vitro data and presentation of clinical concept. In *Acute Leukemias (Haematol and Blood Transfusion)* Hiddeman W, Büchner T, Schellong G., eds, 1992: 601–7.

53 Foa R, Fierro MT, Cesano A *et al.* Defective lymphokine-activated killer cell generation and activity in acute leukaemia patients with active disease. *Blood* 1991; **78**: 1041–6.

54 Foa R, Meloni G, Tosti S *et al.* Treatment of acute myeloid leukaemia patients with

recombinant IL-2; a pilot study. *Br J Haematol* 1991; 77: 491–6.

55 Arienti F, Gambacorti-Passerini C, Borin L *et al.* Increased susceptibility to lymphokine activated killer (LAK) lysis of replasing vs newly diagnosed acute leukaemic cells without changes in drug resistance or in the expression of adhesion molecules: *Ann Oncol* 1992; 3: 155–62.

56 Cesano A, Lista P, Belloni G *et al.* Effect of human interleukin 3 on the susceptibility of fresh leukaemic cells to interleukin-2 induced lymphokine activated killing activity. *Leukemia* 1992; 6: 567–73.

57 Uhr JW. Immunotoxins: an overview. *Semin Cell Biol* 1991; 2: 1–6.

58 Wade JC. Management of infection in patients with acute leukaemia. *Haematol Oncol Clin N Am* 1993; 7: 293–315.

59 Oksanen K, Elonen E. Impact of leucocyte-depleted blood components on the haematological recovery and prognosis of patients with acute myeloid leukaemia. *Br J Haematol* 1993; 84: 639–47.

60 Williamson LM, Wimperis JZ, Williamson P *et al.* Bedside filtration of blood products in the prevention of HLA immunisation—a prospective randomised study. *Blood* 1994; 83: 3028–35.

61 Sivakumaran M, Norfolk DR, Tan L *et al.* Evaluation of the "Handling Capacity" of Pall RC100 leucocyte removal filters and the effect of air introduction on its performance. *Br J Haematol* 1994 86(Suppl 1): Abstr P209.

62 Green RHA, Palmer JB, Parker AC *et al.* The clinical efficacy of platelet transfusions. *Br J Haematol* 1994; 86: Abstr 113.

63 Metcalf D. Thrombopoietin—at last. *Nature* 1994; 369: 519–20.

64 Morris-Jones PH, Craft AW. Childhood cancer: cure at what cost? *Archiv Dis Child* 1990; 65: 638–40.

65 Steinherz LJ, Sternherz PG, Tan CTC *et al.* Cardiac toxicity 4 to 20 years after completing anthracycline therapy. *JAMA* 1991; 266: 1672–77.

66 Hann IM, Stevens RF, Burnett AK *et al.* Randomised comparison of DAT versus ADE as induction chemotherapy in children and younger adults with acute myeloid leukaemia. Results of the Medical Research Council's 10th AML Trial (MRC AML 10). Submitted for publication.

67 Childhood Cancer, anthracyclines and the heart. *Lancet* (Editorial) 1992; 339: 1388–9.

68 Dorr RT. Chemoprotectants for cancer chemotherapy. *Semin Oncol* 1991; 18(Suppl 2); 48–58.

69 Halliwell B, Bomford A. ICRF-187 and doxorubicin-induced cardiac toxicity. *Lancet* (Letter) 1989; 320: 339–40.

70 Green MD, Alderton P, Gross J *et al.* Evidence of the selective alteration of anthracycline activity due to modulation by ICRF 189 (ADR-529) *Pharmac Ther* 1990; 48: 61–9.

71 Herman EH, Ferrans VJ. Examination of the potential long-lasting protective effect of ICRF-187 against anthracycline-induced chronic cardiomyopathy. *Canc Treat Rev* 1990; 17: 155–60.

72 Ozsahin M, Belkacemi Y, Pene F *et al.* Total body irradiation and cataract incidence: Results in a series of 495 patients. *Bone Marrow Transpl* 1994; (EMBT Suppl): Abstr 519.

73 Tichelli A, Gratwohl A, Schonenberger A *et al.* Cataract formation after bone marrow transplantation (BMT). *Bone Marrow Transpl* 1994; (EMBT Suppl): Abstr 520.

74 Tichelli A, Duell T, Weiss M *et al.* The keratoconjunctivitis sicca syndrome after bone marrow transplantation. *Bone Marrow Transpl* 1994; (EMBT Suppl); Abstr 388.

75 Ropponen P, Siimes MA, Rautonen J, Aalberg V. Psychosexual problems in male childhood malignancy survivors. *Acta Psychiatr Scand* 1992; 85: 143–6.

76 Baruch J, Benjamin S, Treleaven J *et al.* Male sexual function following bone marrow transplantation. *Bone Marrow Trans.* 1991; 7 (Suppl 2): 52.

77 Aaronson NK, Ahmedzai S, Bergman B *et al.* The European Organisation for Research and treatment of Cancer QLQ - C30: a quality of life instrument for use in international clinical trials in incology. *J Natl Cancer Inst* 1993 85: 365–76.

14: Acute lymphoblastic leukaemia

SALLY E KINSEY

Acute lymphoblastic leukaemia (ALL) is the most common childhood malignancy and one of the most common in the adolescent age group.[1] The peak age of presentation with ALL in the UK is between the ages of 1 and 7 years with a trend from 50 years of age to increase in incidence with increasing age. The incidence in later life does not, however, reach the same as that in early childhood.[2] The recent advances in understanding the biology and management of ALL in childhood have been reviewed[3] and it remains a major problem. Over the last 20 years there has been an undoubted improvement in remission rates, event-free survival, and overall survival in children treated for acute lymphoblastic leukaemia (ALL). The majority will achieve long-term remission and may be considered cured.[4-7]

Improvement in response to induction and continuing treatment has been seen across the whole spectrum of paediatric patients from young children to adolescents. However, infants and older children continue to have a worse prognosis.[8] Remission rates and event-free survival in adults presenting with ALL have also improved over the same time period but those improvements have not been as great as those seen in children.[9]

Despite improvement in both remission rates and event-free survival with more intensive treatment, older children (>10 years) still fare less well than children between the ages of 1 and 10 years.[8 10-12] There are important features which distinguish childhood and adult ALL and also contribute to a worse overall prognosis; these include higher leucocyte count at presentation, bulky disease, poor risk immunophenotype, and cytogenetic abnormalities.[13 14]

The clinical features of patients with ALL change progressively with age. Young children (1–10 years) tend to have features which imply a better prognosis; the older child (>10 years) is more likely to present with poor risk "adult" features. The accumulation of poor risk features increases with age, suggesting the need for continued attempts at understanding clinical and biological features at presentation, their implication with respect to intensification of treatment, and their contributions to relapse. In the UK Medical Research Council (MRC) ALL trials, treatment has not been stratified for age or immunophenotype except for those with B-cell disease. These have traditionally been treated with lymphoma protocols. Some centres have chosen to treat T-cell ALL on an intensive chemotherapy protocol coordinated by United Kingdom Children's Cancer Study Group (UKCCSG).[15]

This chapter will briefly review our knowledge of ALL and will consider further specific risk factors associated with this disease in the adolescent and the approach to management of high risk disease. Because of the prolonged duration of therapy for ALL, chemotherapy management presents some difficulties and compliance in the adolescent age group cannot always be guaranteed. This problem will also be addressed.

Aetiology

The cause of ALL in childhood and adolescence is still unknown. Greaves[16] has put forward the hypothesis that most cases of childhood ALL are the consequences of an abnormal response to common infections occurring in early life. Early, perhaps in utero, mutational events may contribute to this. Recent reports of an increasing incidence of ALL presumably reflect a change in exposure to environmental agents although statistical variation may also be a factor in this observation.[17] Constitutional genetic defects can predispose to acute leukaemias (trisomy 21, Fanconi's anaemia, and germ cell p53 mutations, for example) although the specific link to the lymphoblastic subtype is not always clear. In children with Down's syndrome the position is complex. Children of less than 3 years tend to develop AML whereas ALL is the characteristic leukaemia of older children and adolescents with Down's syndrome.[18 19] The potential importance of exposure to ionising radiation has been discussed elsewhere in this book.

Haematopathology

In leukaemogenesis, lymphoid progenitor cells are blocked at a particular stage of differentiation and accumulate as a result of a failure to regulate clonal expansion. The process can result in a number of different immunologically and genetically defined malignant processes.[3 20] Morphological subdivision of ALL has been attempted using the French/American/British Classification (FAB) which divides ALL into subtypes L1, L2, and L3 (see below). These distinctions are sometimes difficult to make under light microscopy and not all haematologists are happy that the distinction between the small L1 lymphoblasts and the larger more pleomorphic L2 lymphoblasts is always consistent and a reproducible observation between different laboratories. Granular ALL is recognised by some authorities[21] but is not included in the FAB system.

Major improvements in the understanding of the clinical biology of ALL have come from the process of immunophenotyping leukaemic cells to identify antigens which are associated with specific developmental and immunological characteristics. ALL can be broadly classified as having either a T lymphocyte or a B lymphocyte origin and the B lineage ALLs can be further sub-divided into early pre-B ALL, pre-B ALL and B ALL. The fourth subtype of a transitional B-cell ALL has been recently described to be associated with an improved prognosis.[22] Subdividing T-cell ALLs according to the stage of thymocyte differentiation has not so far achieved the same significance as that of B-cell leukaemias.[22-24] There may also be prognostic significance of surface antigen expression such as CD34 which may be studied even though it does not directly relate to T cell or B cell differentiation.

Pui[3] has reported the subdivisions and frequency of ALL in 600 consecutive cases of newly diagnosed ALL seen at St Jude Children's Research Hospital from 1984 to 1992 and including all of those cases up to 18 years of age (Table 14.1). In this series numerically early pre-B cell ALL and pseudodiploid karyotype were the commonest.

A mixture of expression of lymphoid and myeloid lineage specific antigens is described in acute leukaemias without any consistency in the literature about the proportion of cases which show this.[21 25 26] This mixture of lineage antigens may be associated with a poor prognosis.[27 28] The biology underlying this lack of lineage specificity is not understood.

Molecular genetics and cytogenetics

Studies of the karyotype of leukaemic cells have been very informative. More than 80% of cases reveal clonal chromosomal abnormalities. ALL can be classified by the number of chromosomes or DNA content and it is useful, as described below, to divide cases into hyperdiploid (>50 chromosomes/cell) and hypodiploid (<45 chromosomes). Chromosomal

Table 14.1   Classification of ALL (Data from Pui[3])

	Frequency
Immunophenotype	
Early pre-B cell (cCD22+, cCD79a+, CD19+, CS22+, clgμ-, and slg-	57%
Pre-B cell (clgμ+)	25%
Transitional pre-B cell (clgμ+, slg+, slg$_\kappa$ −, slg$_\lambda$ −)	1%
B cell (slg+, slg$_\kappa$+ slg$_\lambda$+)	2%
T cell (cCD3+ and CD7+ plus CD5+ or CD2+)	15%
	100%
Ploidy	
Hypodiploid	7%
Diploid	8%
Hyperdiploid	42%
47–50 chromosomes	27%
>50 chromosomes	15%
Triploid or tetraploid	1%
	100%

214

Table 14.2   Common non-random chromosomal translocations in ALL (Data from Pui[3])

Chromosomal translocation	Frequency (%)	Genetic alteration
t(1;19) (q23;p13.3)	5–6	*E2A-PBX1* fusion
t(9;22) (q34;q11)	3–5	*BCR-ABL* fusion
t(4;11)(q21;q23)	2	*MLL-AF4* fusion
t(8;14)(q24;q32.3)	1–2	*MYC-IGH* fusion
t(11;14)(p13;q11)	1	*TTG2-TCRD* fusion
dic(9;12)(p11-p12;?p12)	1	?

translocations are described in ALL. Table 14.2 shows the common identified translocations. There are important lessons to be learned from the cytogenetic analysis of ALL. The first is a significant association between specific translocations and the phenotype of the cells. The second is the association between the translocation, the molecular changes which it brings about, and the changes in the control of cell proliferation and differentiation which result in the leukaemic process. For instance, the t(8;14) translocation is associated with B cell ALL occurring predominantly in boys who often have bulky extramedullary disease. This translocation brings together the *MYC* oncogene from chromosome 8 under the control of regulatory sequences which normally influence the regulation of immunoglobulin genes on chromosome 14. The dysregulation of *MYC* and its subsequent interaction with another cellular protein known as MAX brings about a change in nuclear regulatory processes which influence transcription and a whole series of changes in gene expression.

The t(9;22) translocation which is characteristic of chronic myeloid leukaemia (CML) is also found in a small proportion of ALL cases and these tend to be of B-cell phenotype. The fusion gene resulting from this translocation in ALL is distinct from that usually found in adult CML. A smaller fusion protein of molecular weight 185 kDa is produced. This fusion protein is a tyrosine kinase, with the same biological effect as the fusion protein produced in CML, but it does appear to have more potent transforming activity.[29] All of the BCR-ABL fusion proteins seem to be associated with blast cells which are very resistant to chemotherapy.[30][31]

Other links between specific translocations, the phenotype of leukaemic cells, and the molecular biology of leukaemogenesis are being clarified. This field presents one of the most exciting links between molecular biology and cancer medicine. The links between aetiological factors, such as environmental agents, and the molecular genetic abnormalities seen in ALL remain elusive. However, it is not unreasonable to expect that in the next decade a clearer understanding at a molecular level of the sequence of events from exposure to environmental leukaemogens, through changes in gene expression, to the cellular changes responsible for the phenotype of the leukaemia and its clinical features will be obtained. It is to be hoped that this detailed knowledge will result in a clearer understanding of the value of different approaches to treatment and better outcomes for patients.

Minimal residual disease

When young people with ALL are in complete remission their total body burden of leukaemic cells may still be in excess of 10^9. Significant progress has been made in identifying this minimal residual disease. Immunological stains can help to identify cells in bone marrow or cerebrospinal fluid.[3] These are particularly helpful in T-cell ALL but are also useful in other subtypes. Fluorescence in situ hybridisation relies on chromosome specific DNA probes to identify specific chromosomes including those that may be abnormal in ALL. Major advances have come from the use of the polymerase chain reaction (PCR) which is a means of amplifying very small quantities of RNA or DNA. This can focus either on the fusion gene transcripts described above which result from specific translocations or, of particular value in ALL, the junctional regions generated by immunoglobulin or T-cell receptor gene rearrangements.[32] Using all of these approaches PCR has a potential to detect minimal residual leukaemia in 90% or more of ALL,[33 34] although false negatives can occur. The value in assessing the completeness of remission and suitability for intensive treatments of these approaches is only beginning to be fully evaluated.

Clinical and biological features

Male sex, increased age, presenting leucocyte count, and immunophenotype are the poor prognostic features mentioned above. They influence response to treatment and survival.

A change is seen in ALL immunophenotypes with increasing age. The immunophenotype with the worst influence on prognosis, null-ALL seen in older adult patients, is seen with increasing frequency with increasing age during adolescence. There is a peak incidence of T-cell ALL in adolescence and young adults (10–29 years) with the incidence in males being greater than in females in the ratio of 2:1.[2] A greater proportion of individuals presenting with ALL in the adolescent age group will have T-cell immunophenotypic characteristics than at any other age.

Information regarding identification of patients who will fare less well with a high probability of treatment failure is increasing. This is largely due to improved analysis of features at the time of diagnosis which includes presenting leucocyte count, age, bulky disease, sex, immunophenotype, cytogenetic characteristics, leukaemic cell ploidy (DNA index), and blast cell morphology. In addition, mediastinal disease, time taken to achieve disease remission, presence of CNS disease at diagnosis, blast PAS positivity, and even immunoglobulin levels are also of prognostic importance. The morphological characteristics of acute lymphoblastic leukaemia cell are classified according to the FAB group[35] and has been shown by several groups to be of prognostic importance.[36] Features seen by light microscopy of Romanowsky stained peripheral blood and bone marrow smears subclassify ALL into three groups, L1, L2, and L3. L3 phenotype are invariably B-cell ALL and are characteristically large cells with deeply basophilic cytoplasm often with prominent cytoplasmic vacuolation. Lymphoblasts are classified as L1 or L2 in appearance by virtue of cell size, nuclear indentations, prominence of nucleoli, abundance of cytoplasm.[37] The L1 phenotype is of better prognosis than the L2 phenotype. In addition the periodic acid Schiff (PAS) reaction in lymphoblasts has some prognostic bearing in relation to other morphological and immunophenotype features.[38] Haemoglobin level at diagnosis may also be of prognostic importance particularly in children over 13 years with T-cell disease.[39]

Analysis of cellular DNA content by flow cytometry determines the DNA ploidy of cells. By comparison of DNA content of the constitutional cell line with that of the abnormal clone a DNA index may be calculated, ie a DNA index of 1·0 infers diploidy (indistinguishable from the normal cell line), 1·01–1·5 hyperdiploidy <53 chromosomes, >1·16 increasing hyperdiploidy >53 chromosomes. A DNA index of 2·0 implies tetraploidy ($4n$).

In a retrospective analysis of adolescents, defined in this study as individuals older than 11 years, Crist et al.[13] found that adolescents were more likely to be males ($p=0·02$), have bulky disease (mediastinal mass, $p=0·0001$), marked lymphadenopathy ($p=0·0001$) with higher white cell count and to have lower serum immunoglobulins ($p=0·0001$) compared with children younger than 11 years. Of patients older than 11 years 24% had T-cell phenotypic disease compared with 13% under the age of 11 years. Santana and colleagues[14] have similarly reported more adverse features in the adolescent age group (10–21 years), including T-cell phenotype, L2 morphology, higher white cell count, and increased lactate dehydrogenase (LDH) activity.

Individuals presenting with ALL in later childhood (older than 10 years) and adolescents are also more likely to express cytogenetic abnormalities associated with poor prognosis and with increasing similarity to those cytogenetic abnormalities seen in the adult age group. In particular there is increasing likelihood of Philadelphia chromosome positivity (Ph[1]) (translocation t(9;22)). Interestingly, in childhood Ph[1] positive ALL the majority have the M-bcr breakpoint (72%) compared with equal frequency of M-bcr and m-bcr in adult ALL.[40]

Other chromosomal translocations and a lower incidence of hyperdiploidy with the associated DNA index >1·16 are likely to be seen.[12] Both structural and numerical chromosomal abnormality are of prognostic significance. The St Jude Children's Research Hospital data[12 41] and the Group Français de Cytogenetique Hematologique[42] identify that prolonged continuous complete remission was most likely to be seen in those with hyperdiploidy >50 chromosomes. Those with pseudodiploidy or hypodiploidy in the malignant clone had the poorest outcome, with those demonstrating diploidy being intermediate. The French group identified a poor subgroup within the hyperdiploid group as those with additional structural chromosomal abnormalities as previously identified by Pui et al.[41] particularly isochrome 17q.

Other cytogenetic data in childhood ALL[43] suggested that there were some cytogenetic abnormalities present which were not prognostically important and that with increasingly intensive treatment differences with respect to outcome due only to cytogenetics were nullified. In addition Fletcher's group suggested that there was an increasing incidence in the proportion of children with demonstrable cytogenetic abnormalities. This has attributed to a better approach to cytogenetic investigation and improved and quicker handling of specimens, direct or short-term culture techniques and improved chromosome preparations and banding. With increased efficiency more frequent recognition of subtle cytogenetic changes have been allowed and this may account for a decrease in numbers of diploid ALL and concurrent increase in pseudodiploid cases.[41] Look et al.[44] defined a "favourable" ALL group as those with DNS index >1.16, corresponding to >53 chromosomes. These patients had a significantly longer continued complete remission than those with DNA index <1.16 ($p = 0.002$).

An improved overall and event-free survival has been seen in all patients with ALL over the last 20 years. However, despite improvements in MRC studies in the United Kingdom, boys consistently have a less good survival than girls.[8] This has been confirmed in other published studies.[45 46] However, recent results of protocols from the United States and Germany[47 48] showed no difference in outcome between the sexes. Despite the fact that 10% of boys will relapse in the testis (girls do not have an equivalent extramedullary site) there is also an excess of bone marrow relapse in boys compared with girls. Testicular irradiation did not afford improvement in overall survival in boys when used prophylactically.[49] UKALL VIII identified a difference in response between boys and girls, being worse in boys ($p < 0.005$ for event-free survival and remission rates), and this was independent of any other factors. This feature became more marked after two years' treatment, suggesting that therapy during the later stages of continuing treatment was failing to keep the disease under control or that there was a sex difference in handling of therapeutic agents or compliance with them.[8] UKALL X continued to show a poorer outlook for boys. There is emerging evidence which suggests that continuing treatment may be less effective in boys than girls[50] due to different handling of 6-mercaptopurine. This may be due to sex variation in intracellular enzymes important for metabolism of thiopurines.[51 52]

Treatment

The mainstay of treatment of ALL in American, European, and British protocol trials is induction, intensification, central nervous system directed treatment, and continuing chemotherapy for 2–3 years. Steroids, vincristine, and asparaginase will induce remission in more than 95% of children with ALL[53] and this comprises standard induction treatment. The addition of a fourth drug (usually an anthracycline) may contribute to better relapse-free survival.[5 54] However, it may also contribute to increased mortality during induction from infection. The German Berlin–Frankfurt–Münster (BFM)[55] United Kingdom,[7] and St Jude[47] groups have shown that intensification treatment given within the first six months of therapy is beneficial for all risk groups with childhood ALL. Survival is now expected in 60–65% of children. It is unclear whether further intensification will improve event-free survival and the attendant problems of long term toxicity with additional chemotherapy must be recognised.

Continuing (maintenance) therapy for ALL is important. Continuing treatment with mercaptopurine and methotrexate for two years from diagnosis is beneficial. Earlier trials discontinuing treatment 12–15 months from diagnosis were associated with a high relapse rate.[56] The addition of intermittent vincristine and prednisolone to 6-mercaptopurine and methotrexate may decrease relapses.[57]

Treatment outcome may be influenced during the maintenance phase by a genetic variation in 6-mercaptopurine metabolism,[52] the degree of myelosuppression achieved[51] and compliance of both patients and clinicians to treatment.[58] Smith et al.[59] have attempted to measure non-compliance with oral anti-cancer treatment in children by measuring urinary steroid metabolites.

CNS directed therapy is an essential component of the management of ALL in children and adolescents. Without it, the majority of children relapse in the CNS resulting in the necessity for aggressive treatment and a reduction in long term survival.[60 61] The most frequently used modalities are regular intrathecal methotrexate (with or without additional intrathecal drugs), intravenous methotrexate (with folinic acid rescue at very high doses), and cranial irradiation.

At present in the United Kingdom the treatment of most adolescents with ALL is within an MRC trial (UKALL XI) into which children with ALL older than 1 year and up to 16 years at presentation may be entered. Based upon the best arm from UKALL X, all patients receive induction chemotherapy (vincristine, prednisolone, asparaginase, and intrathecal methotrexate) followed by two intensification blocks at 5 and 20 weeks (cytosine, daunorubicin, etoposide, thioguanine). Children are randomised to receive, or not, a third intensification block at week 35 which is outpatient based and spans eight weeks. The first 4 weeks comprise vincristine weekly, asparaginase, and dexamethasone, the second 4 weeks comprise cyclophosphamide, cytarabine and thioguanine. In addition, CNS directed therapy is randomised depending upon white cell count at presentation. For white cell count $<50 \times 10^9$/l children are randomised to either continuing weekly intrathecal methotrexate or three cycles of high dose methotrexate with folinic acid rescue with additional intrathecal methotrexate. Patients with a high white cell count at presentation ($>50 \times 10^9$/l) are randomised in the same way to receive cranial irradiation (18 Gy) or high dose methotrexate and folinic acid rescue with intrathecal methotrexate as for the lower count patients. This trial will assess if additional benefit (i.e. reduction in bone marrow relapse) may be achieved by high dose methotrexate in those with low leucocyte counts ($<50 \times 10^9/l$) and if it may be used in those with high leucocyte counts ($>50 \times 10^9/l$) as a substitute for cranial irradiation.

Continuing therapy comprises daily 6-mercaptopurine with dose modifications to maximise the dose by inducing leucopaenia but not neutropaenia, with weekly oral methotrexate, monthly pulsed courses of intravenous vincristine, and oral prednisolone. In addition, lumbar puncture with intrathecal methotrexate instillation continues at three-monthly intervals. This trial also incorporates a prospective evaluation of long-term effects of therapy.

"Intensification" or alternative treatment strategies

Adolescents fare less well on conventional therapy for ALL due largely to the increased likelihood of poor prognostic features with increasing age. It is logical to consider intensifying treatment for those in whom the long-term prognosis is likely to be poor. What differences in management are available to these individuals and how may they be identified?

Several groups (MRC,[8] Rome,[62] St Jude[12]) have described risk or "hazard" scores. The MRC hazard score for childhood ALL is related to age, gender and leucocyte count and is as follows:

$$0\cdot8 = 0\cdot22 \times \log_e (WBC + 1\cdot0) + 0\cdot0043 \times age^2 - 0\cdot39 \times sex$$
$$sex: male = 1, female = 2$$

When applied to UKALL X patients and their features, patients with standard risk hazard score $<0\cdot8$ had an event-free survival of 66% at five years compared with 39% for the worse risk group hazard score $>0\cdot8$.[8]

The Rome group[62] classified patients as standard risk if they were aged between 1 and 9 years and with white count $<50 \times 10^9/l$. The same UKALL X data analysed by this process results in a five year event-free survival of 51% in high risk patients and 68% in standard risk patients. However, taking as high risk anyone with a presenting white count $>100 \times 10^9/l$, event-free survival for high risk would be 48% at five years and for standard risk 65% at five years. Therefore it becomes clear that the MRC UKALL X hazard score is a useful discriminant and may potentially be used to modify therapy to prevent overtreatment of those at lower risk and for maximising early intensive treatment for those who fall into the high risk category.

The St Jude Group[12] have presented a calculated "hazard ratio" for adolescents estimating the proportional increase in risk of failure for those having "worse" compared with "better" prognostic factors for several variables; (common ALL antigen expression, age immunophenotype, ploidy, leucocyte count). Thus far no details from this group have suggested any modification of therapy by virtue of hazard ratio, but this would be the logical next step.

Intensify with what therapy?

The options for intensification treatment are limited. Treatment protocols (CCG, MRC, BFM) are already very intensive and use a wide range of agents administered in several ways in order to achieve maximal cytotoxic/cytostatic effect. Increasingly the importance of prognostic factors is changing. All prognostic risk groups have benefited from more intensive therapy and it is apparent that prognostic features should be interpreted in the context of therapy received; it is not valid to directly extrapolate prognostic factors from one therapy protocol to another.

Bone marrow transplantation in first remission has to be considered for those deemed to be at very high risk, for whom, despite the procedure related mortality and morbidity, it offers a greater chance of event-free survival or cure. Morbidity and mortality varies depending on selection of donor for bone marrow transplantation (sibling or other related versus unrelated donor). In ALL, the selection of patients for bone marrow transplantation in first complete remission remains difficult. Those in whom it seems most appropriate are failures to respond to initial therapy,[63] for example no remission at day 28 in the current UKALL XI MRC trial; or particular cytogenetic abnormalities, such as Philadelphia chromosome or near haploidy. The frequency of cytogenetic abnormalities is greater in the adolescent age group than in younger children (as previously discussed). However, the number of patients falling into these very high risk groups is small.

From the MRC UKALL X trial[8] a group of children comprising approximately 11% of the total with a five year survival of <40% can be identified when the hazard score is applied, which is based on clinical features (age, sex, white count). Adding together those with high risk cytogenetic abnormalities and high risk features based on clinical criteria, the numbers for whom bone marrow transplant seems an appropriate choice of management remains very small (about 3%). In the adolescent age group who are more likely to be at high risk by virtue of laboratory and clinical criteria, a greater proportion are more likely to be selected for bone marrow transplant procedures, compared with a younger age group.

Late effects of the treatment of ALL

The late effects of the treatment of childhood cancers are discussed elsewhere in the book. These are particularly important for the management of ALL. Second malignancies have been a significant concern and in a recent study of 9720 children treated for ALL, Neglia et al.[64] found a seven-fold increase in secondary malignancies. In particular the excess of CNS tumours was 22-fold. Cranial irradiation of young children appeared to be an important risk factor. Patients treated for ALL with genotoxic drugs which include epipodophyllotoxins are at risk of a secondary acute myeloid leukaemia. Young children or those who receive high doses of anthracyclines are at risk of cardiomyopathy, and cranial irradiation has been implicated in neuropsychological and endocrine dysfunctions.

Conclusion

A satisfactory explanation for the poorer outcome of adolescents with ALL has not been found. Many studies have suggested that the increasing likelihood of poor prognosis features (as covered above) may contribute to poorer response and survival following chemotherapy. In addition, differential pharmacokinetic handling of some chemotherapeutic agents (especially thiopurines) may result in inadvertent undertreatment of a group of patients who need continued aggressive management. Another important contributing factor is patient and parent non-compliance with prescribed medication. This probably plays a significant role in the overall outcome in a minority of patients.

The role of intensified treatment in adolescents at particularly high risk needs to be examined. The options available are not great in number but must include bone marrow transplantation (with appropriate conditioning therapy) or further intensification of "standard" therapy introducing for instance chemotherapy conventionally considered for acute myeloid leukaemia.

In the approach to the management of adolescents, ALL therefore represents not only the challenge of managing children and adolescents when they present but also the problems of managing the late effects of treatment in childhood which are seen in adolescents. Long-term follow up, multidisciplinary care and a clear awareness of the risk of late effects of the management of ALL in young people is becoming crucially important.

1 Stiller CA, Bunch KJ. Trends in survival for childhood cancer in Britain diagnosed 1971–85. *Br J Cancer* 1990; **62**: 806–15.
2 McKinney PA, Alexander FE, Cartwright RA *et al*. Acute lymphoblastic leukaemia incidence in the UK by immunophenotype. *Leukaemia* 1993; 7: 1630–4.
3 Pui C-H. Medical progress: childhood leukaemias. *N Engl J Med* 1995; **332**: 1618–30.
4 Medical Research Council UKALL Trials 1972–84. Improvements in treatment for children with acute lymphoblastic leukaemia. *Lancet* 1986; i: 408–11.
5 Eden OB, Lilleyman JS, Richards S *et al*. Results of MRC trial UKALL VIII. *Br J Haematol* 1991; **78**: 187–96.
6 Chessells JM, Bailey CC, Richards S. MRC UKALL X. The UK protocol for childhood ALL: 1985–1990. The MRC Working Party on Childhood Leukaemia. *Leukaemia* 6 1992; suppl. 2: 157–61.
7 Chessells JM, Bailey C, Richards SM. Intensification of treatment and survival in all children with lymphoblastic leukaemia: results of UK MRC trial UKALL X. *Lancet* 1995; **345**: 143–8.
8 Chessells JM, Richards SM, Bailey CC *et al*. Gender and treatment outcome in childhood lymphoblastic leukaemia: report from the MRC UKALL trials. *Br J Haematol* 1995; **89**: 364–72.
9 Hoelzer D. Therapy and prognostic factors in adult acute lymphoblastic leukaemia. *Bailliere's Clin Haem* 1994; 7: 299–320.
10 Sather HN. Age at diagnosis in childhood acute lymphoblastic leukaemia. *Med Pediatr Oncol* 1986; **14**: 166–72.
11 Pullen DJ, Boyett JM, Crist WM *et al*. Pediatric oncology group utilization of immunologic

markers in the designation of acute lymphoblastic leukaemia subgroups. Influence on treatment response. *Ann NY Acad Sci* 1984; **428**: 26.

12 Rivera GK, Pui C-H, Santana VM *et al*. Progress in the treatment of adolescents with acute lymphoblastic leukaemia. *Cancer* 1993; **71**: 3400–5.

13 Crist W, Pullen J, Boyett J *et al*. Acute lymphoid leukaemia in adolescents; clinical and biologic features predict a poor prognosis—a pediatric oncology group study. *J Clin Oncol* 1988; **6**: 34–43.

14 Santana VM, Dodge RK, Crist WM. Presenting features and treatment outcome of adolescents with acute lymphoblastic leukaemia. *Leukaemia* 1990; **4**: 87–90.

15 Mott MG, Chessells JM, Willoughby MLN *et al*. Adjuvant low dose radiation in childhood T cell leukaemia/lymphoma. *Br J Cancer* 1984; **50**: 457–62.

16 Greaves MA. A natural history for pediatric acute leukaemia. *Blood* 1993; **82**: 1043–51.

17 Ries LAG, Hankey BF, Miller BA *et al*. (eds). *Cancer Statistics Review 1973–88*. NIH publication no 91–2789. Bethseda MD; National Cancer Institute.

18 Kojima S, Matsuyama T, Samo T *et al*. Down's syndrome and acute leukaemia in children: an analysis of phenotype by use of monoclonal antibodies and electron microscopic platelet peroxidase reaction. *Blood* 1990; **76**: 2348–53.

19 Pui C-H, Raimondi SC, Borowitz MJ *et al*. Immunophenotypes and karyotypes of leukaemic cells in children with Down's syndrome and acute lymphoblastic leukaemia. *J Clin Oncol* 1993; **11**: 1361–7.

20 Pui C-H, Crist WM, Look AT. Biology and clinical significance of cytogenetic abnormalities in childhood acute lymphoblastic leukaemia. *Blood* 1990; **76**: 1449–63.

21 Cerezo L, Shuster JJ, Pullen DJ *et al*. Laboratory correlates and prognostic significance of granular acute lymphoblastic leukaemia in children: a Pediatric Oncology Group study. *Am J Clin Path* 1991; **95**: 526–31.

22 Koehler M, Behm FG, Shuster J *et al*. Transitional pre-B cell acute lymphoblastic leukaemia of childhood is associated with favourable prognostic clinical features and an excellent outcome: a Pediatric Oncology Group study. *Leukaemia* 1993; **7**: 2064–8.

23 Pui C-H, Behm FG, Crist WM. Clinical and biological relevance of immunologic marker studies in childhood acute lymphoblastic leukaemia. *Blood* 1993; **82**: 343–62.

24 Campana D, van Dongen JJM, Mehta A *et al*. Stage of T cell receptor protein expression in T cell acute lymphoblastic leukaemia. *Blood* 1991; **77**: 1546–54.

25 Pui C-H, Behm FG, Singh B *et al*. Myeloid associated antigen expression lacks prognostic value in childhood acute lymphoblastic leukaemia treated with intensive multi-agent chemotherapy. *Blood* 1990; **75**: 198–202.

26 Pui C-H, Raimondi SC, Head DR *et al*. Characterisation of childhood acute leukaemia with multiple myeloid and lymphoid markers at diagnosis and at relapse. *Blood* 1991; **78**: 1327–37.

27 Wiersma SR, Ortega J, Sobel E *et al*. Clinical importance of myeloid antigen expression in acute lymphoblastic leukaemia of childhood. *N Engl J Med* 1991; **324**: 800–8.

28 Fink F-M, Koller U, Mayer H *et al*. Prognostic signficance of myeloid associated antigen expression on blast cells in children with acute lymphoblastic leukaemia. *Med Pediatr Oncol* 1993; **21**: 240–6.

29 Lugo TG, Pendergast A-M, Muller AJ *et al*. Tyrosine kinase activity and transformation potency of BCR-ABL oncogene products. *Science* 1990; **247**: 1079–82.

30 Marin T, Butturini A, Kantarjian H *et al*. Survival of children with chronic myeloid leukaemia. *Am J Pediatr Hematol Oncol* 1992; **14**: 229–32.

31 Fletcher JA, Tu N, Tantravahi R, Sallam SE. Extremely poor prognosis of pediatric acute lymphoblastic leukaemia with translocation (9;22): updated experience. *Leuk Lymphoma* 1992; **8**: 75–9.

32 Potter MN, Cross NCP, van Dongen JJM *et al*. Molecule evidence of minimal residual disease after treatment for leukaemia and lymphoma: an updated meeting report and review. *Leukaemia* 1993; **7**: 1302–14.

33 Brisco MJ, Condon J, Hughes E *et al*. Outcome prediction in childhood acute lymphoblastic leukaemia by molecular quantification of residual disease at the end of induction. *Lancet* 1994; **343**: 196–200.

34 Steward CG, Goulden NJ, Katz F *et al*. A polymerase chain reaction study of the stability of lg heavy chain and T cell receptor–gene rearrangements between presentation and relapse of childhood B lineage acute lymphoblastic leukaemia. *Blood* 1994; **83**: 1355–62.

35 Bennett JM, Catovsky D, Daniel MT *et al*. French-American-British (FAB) Co-operative group proposal for the classification of acute leukaemias. *Br J Haematol* 1976; **33**: 451–8.

36 Miller DR, Krailo M, Bleyer WA *et al.* Prognostic importance of blast cell morphology in childhood acute lymphoblastic leukaemia: A report from the Children's Cancer Study Group. *Cancer Treat Rep.* 1989; **69**: 1211–21.

37 Bennett JM, Catovsky D, Daniel MT *et al.* The morphological classification of acute lymphoblastic leukaemia; concordance among observers and clinical correlations. *Br J Haematol* 1981; **47**: 553–61.

38 Lilleyman JS, Britton JA, Anderson LM *et al.* Periodic acid Schiff reaction in childhood lymphoblastic leukaemia. *J Clin Pathol* 1994; **47**: 689–92.

39 Hann IM, Scarffe JH, Palmer MK *et al.* Haemoglobin and prognosis in childhood acute lymphoblastic leukaemia. *Arch Dis Child* 1981; **56**: 684–6.

40 Secker-Walker LM, Craig JM. Prognostic implications of break point and lineage heterogeneity in Philadelphia-positive acute lymphoblastic leukaemia: a review. *Leukaemia* 1993; **7**:147–51.

41 Pui C-H, Raimondi SC, Dodge RK *et al.* Prognostic importance of structural chromosomal abnormalities in children with hyperdiploid (>50 chromosomes) acute lymphoblastic leukaemia. *Blood* 1989; **73**: 1963–7.

42 Group Français de Cytogenetique Hematologique. Collaborative study of karyotypes in childhood acute lymphoblastic leukaemias. *Leukaemia* 1993; **7**: 10–19.

43 Fletcher JA, Kimball VM, Lynch E *et al.* Prognostic implications of cytogenetic studies in an intensively treated group of children with acute lymphoblastic leukaemia. *Blood* 1989; **74**: 2130–5.

44 Look AT, Roberson PK, Williams DL *et al.* Prognostic importance of blast cell DNA content in childhood acute lymphoblastic leukaemia. *Blood* 1985; **65**: 1079–86.

45 Sather H, Miller D, Nesbit M *et al.* Differences in prognosis for boys and girls with acute lymphoblastic leukaemia. *Lancet* 1981; **i**: 741–3.

46 Lanning M, Garwicz S, Hertz H *et al.* Superior treatment results in females with high-risk acute lymphoblastic leukaemia in childhood. *Acta Paed Scand* 1992; **81**: 66–8.

47 Rivera GK, Raimondi SC, Hancock ML *et al.* Improved outlook in childhood ALL with reinforced early treatment and rotational combination chemotherapy. *Lancet* 1991; **337**: 61–6.

48 Niemeyer CM, Reiter A, Riehm H *et al.* Comparative results of two intensive treatment programmes for childhood acute lymphoblastic leukaemia: the Berlin-Frankfurt-Münster and Dana-Farber Cancer Institute protocols. *Ann Oncol* 1991; **2**: 745–9.

49 Eden OB, Lilleyman JS, Richards S. Testicular irradiation in childhood lymphoblastic leukaemia. *Br J Haematol* 1990; **75**: 496–8.

50 Hale JP, Lilleyman JS. Importance of 6-mercaptopurine dose in lymphoblastic leukaemia. *Arch Dis Child* 1991; **66**: 462–6.

51 Lennard L, Lilleyman JS. Variable mercaptopurine metabolism and treatment outcome in childhood lymphoblastic leukaemia. *J Clin Oncol* 1989; **7**: 1816–23.

52 Lennard L, Lileyman JS, van Loor J *et al.* Genetic variation in response to 6-mercaptopurine for childhood acute lymphoblastic leukaemia. *Lancet* 1990; **336**: 225–9.

53 Ortega JA, Nesbit ME, Donaldson MH *et al.* L-asparaginase, vincristine and prednisolone for induction of first remission in acute lymphocystic leukaemia. *Cancer Res* 1977; **37**: 535–40.

54 Van der Does-van der Berg A, van Wering ER, Sucin S *et al.* Effectiveness of rubidomycin in induction therapy with vinc, pred and L-asp for std risk childhood ALL; Results of a Dutch Phase III study (ALL V). *Am J Pediatr Hematol Oncol* 1989; **11**: 125–33.

55 Riehm H, Feickert JH, Schrappe M *et al.* Treatment results in five ALL-BFM studies since 1970: Implication of risk factors for prognosis. *Haematol Blood Trans* 1987; **30**: 139–46.

56 Gale RP, Butturini A. Maintenance chemotherapy and cure of childhood acute lymphoblastic leukaemia. *Lancet* 1991; **338**: 1315–18.

57 Bleyer WA, Sather HN, Nickerson HJ *et al.* Monthly pulses of vincristine and prednisolone prevent bone marrow and testicular relapse in low-risk childhood acute lymphoblastic leukaemia: A report of the CCG-161 study by the CCSG. *J Clin Oncol* 1991; **9**: 1012–21.

58 Peeters M, Koren G, Jakubovicz D *et al.* Physician compliance and relapse rates of acute lymphoblastic leukaemia in children. *Clin Pharmacol Therapeut* 1988; **43**: 228–32.

59 Smith SD, Rosen D, Trueworthy RC, Lowman JT. A reliable method for evaluating drug compliance in children with cancer. *Cancer* 1979; **43**: 169–73.

60 Chessels JM. Treatment of childhood acute lymphoblastic leukaemia: present issues and future prospects. *Blood Rev* 1992; **6**: 193–203.

61 Chessels JM. Central nervous system directed therapy in acute lymphoblastic leukaemia.

Ballieres Clin Haematol 1994; 7: 349–63.

62 Mastrangelo R, Poplack DG, Bleyer WA *et al.* Report and recommendations of the Rome workshop concerning poor-prognosis acute lymphoblastic leukaemia in children: biologic bases for staging, stratification and treatment. *Med Pediatr Oncol* 1986; 14: 191–4.

63 Forman SJ, Schmidt GM, Nademanec AP *et al.* Allogeneic bone marrow transplantation as therapy for primary induction failure for patients with acute leukaemia. *J Clin Oncol* 1991; 9: 1570–4.

64 Neglia JP, Meadows AT, Robinson LL *et al.* Second neoplasms after acute lymphoblastic leukaemia in childhood. *N Engl J Med* 1992; 325: 1330–6.

15: Late effects of treatment on paediatric oncology

GEORGE KISSEN

Introduction

It would be inappropriate to start any description of the late effects of treatment of childhood cancers without first pointing out that we are able to recognise these late effects only because there are now significant numbers of long-term survivors. The improvement in survival of victims of cancer in childhood is a major success story. An illustration of that improvement is given by the data for long-term survival in acute lymphoblastic leukaemia (ALL) from the Manchester Children's Tumour Registry which have improved from around 2% for those diagnosed between 1954 and 1963, through 10% for the 1964–73 cohort, to 40% for the 1974–83 cohort.[1] Subsequent data from United Kingdom Acute Lymphoblastic Leukaemia (UKALL) trials show a continuing improvement likely to result in long term survival for at least 70% of those diagnosed currently.

Although this degree of success has not been repeated for all cancers, the overall survival has improved dramatically and for children treated in centres affiliated to the United Kingdom Children's Cancer Study Group the overall survival now exceeds 60%. The reasons for this include advances in therapeutic regimens and centralisation of treatment.[2 3] This has resulted in an ever increasing number of long term survivors, now totalling over 14 000 in Britain who are aged 18 or over (M Hawkins, personal communication). A graph representing the 10 000 survivors over the age of 18 years whose diagnosis was registered since 1970 and the rate of increase in that population is shown in Figure 15.1 (C Stiller, personal communication). The age distribution of these survivors is of course biased to be very largely in their third decade or early fourth decade of life. The result of this is that 1/1000 of young people aged 20–29 will soon be a survivor of cancer.

An accurate figure of the numbers of teenage long term survivors is not

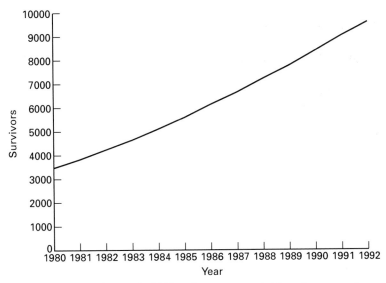

Fig 15.1 Known survivors of childhood cancer aged 18 and over at the end of successive calendar years, representing those registered with the Children's Cancer Research Group since 1970 (courtesy of C Stiller)

available but could be based on the following estimations (C Stiller, personal communication). In the United Kingdom each year there are approaching 700 new cases of cancer in people aged 13–19 years, and, if the children who are now teenagers but who were diagnosed aged 12 or less is added, the total number of teenagers who are either long term or as yet short term survivors of cancer will be approaching 3000. This correlates with the fact that the total number of survivors aged 18 or over is increasing at a rate of around 500 per year. This is now a relatively stable number and will increase only in proportion to any increase in incidence or survival.

These numbers are of considerable significance when it comes to planning for the provision of long term follow up. A centre which has around 100 new cases per year will already have a cohort of survivors aged over 18 numbering in excess of 1000 and a cohort of teenaged patients (survivors) of approaching 250. Centres which were involved in the treatment of childhood cancer from the start may have substantially more.

Why should this group be a cause for concern? What is the risk and what are these late effects?

Late effects can be either those effects of treatment which are apparent during therapy but persist long after therapy has finished or effects which only become manifest at a later date. Such effects have now been recognised affecting almost every body system. The catalogue of these effects is continuing to expand both with our increasing awareness of these effects and increasingly intensive treatment regimes.

The risk of late effects is to a large extent dependent on the treatment a patient has received for their cancer rather than the diagnostic group. This

---

Late effects

Psychosocial	Cataracts
Neuropsychological	Breast
Renal	Bladder
Cardiac	Dental
Respiratory	Hearing
Hepatic	Gastrointestinal
Skin	Thyroid
Skeletal	Uterine
Hypothalamic–pituitary	Gonadal
Second neoplasms	

---

is not only because treatment has changed and progressed over the years but also because, with stratification of treatment dependent on prognostic factors or following relapse, the treatment that two patients with the same diagnosis may receive can be substantially different.

To illustrate this, a long term survivor treated for ALL in 1963 is now aged 32. He received only vincristine, corticosteroids, mercaptopurine, and methotrexate, with no central nervous system (CNS) directed therapy and no radiotherapy. A patient with the same diagnosis who is cured after relapse with current therapy would in addition to the previously mentioned drugs also have received high dose methotrexate, intrathecal methotrexate, daunorubicin, epirubicin, asparaginase, etoposide, cyclophosphamide, cytarabine, thioguanine, and possibly whole body irradiation and an allogeneic bone marrow transplant. The risk of late effects is very different for these two patients. Each modality of treatment—surgery, chemotherapy, radiotherapy—carries potential risks, and these risks may interact.

ALL 1963	Cured after relapse 1993
Vincristine	Vincristine
Corticosteroids	Corticosteroids
Mercaptopurine	Mercaptopurine
Methotrexate	Methotrexate
No CNS therapy	oral
No RT	high dose
	intrathecal
	Daunorubicin
	Epirubicin
	Asparaginase
	Ectoposide
	Cyclophosphamide
	Cytarabine
	Thioguanine
	TBI
	BMT

Endocrine and growth effects

Perhaps the best described of these effects are those on the endocrine system and those affecting growth. Infertility is an important late effect and is the subject of a separate chapter.[30] It will not therefore be discussed further here.

The hypothalamic–pituitary axis is sensitive to the effects of radiation, and the extent of dysfunction is dose dependent. Growth hormone related problems appear at lower doses and panhypopituitarism at higher doses. The speed of onset of pituitary hormone deficiency is also dose dependent, but the first to appear is growth hormone deficiency.[4] Work in adults suggests that the other hormone deficiencies may occur after a long latent period extending many years after therapy.[5] Both the pituitary and the hypothalamus can be affected by radiotherapy, but the hypothalamus is more radiosensitive and is the more important at lower doses of radiation. The effect at lower doses of radiation may be a subtle disturbance of the periodicity of growth hormone secretion pulses and a quantitative reduction in growth hormone secretion which may be restricted to puberty.[6 7] The timing of puberty may also be affected by radiotherapy and these children are at risk of an early or precocious puberty.[8 9]

The combination of growth hormone deficiency or an attenuated pubertal growth spurt together with an early onset of puberty is of considerable clinical importance. The clinical implication is that if it is unrecognised it can result in loss of final height, and even if it is recognised it shortens the available time for treatment with growth hormone. It is essential that this combination is recognised early. Monitoring by charting of both growth and puberty must be performed at least six monthly for all patients at potential risk until a normal pattern of pubertal growth spurt is established (Figure 15.2). This growth chart illustrates the effect in a female patient of the onset, and treatment, of ALL with loss of growth velocity initially. The subsequent acceleration of growth is due not only to catch-up growth but the early onset of puberty and a suboptimal pubertal growth spurt which may go unrecognised until the onset of menstruation (M in Figure 15.2). It is deviation from an appropriate rate of growth, for an appropriate pubertal stage, at an appropriate age, that should alert the observer to a potential problem. It is this loss of harmony between the

---

Dose of radiation to hypothalamic–pituitary axis:

Less than 24 Gy	*More than 24 Gy*
At risk of:	At risk of:
early puberty	early puberty
attenuated pubertal	growth hormone deficiency
growth spurt	
	multiple pituitary
	hormone deficiency

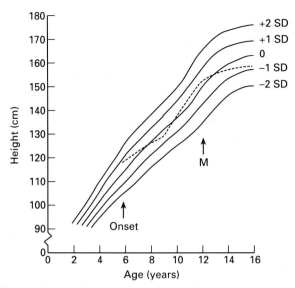

Fig 15.2 Growth chart of female patient with ALL showing the effect on growth of treatment and subsequently early onset of puberty

variables that is the critical factor in recognising the patient at risk. Recognition can then allow appropriate endocrine assessment to be performed to allow consideration of the use of growth hormone. It may also be combined with a luteinizing hormone releasing hormone analogue to arrest puberty and allow lengthening of the time available for growth hormone therapy.

It is of course important to take into account the other factors which can influence growth, in particular the effects of radiation therapy. For example, spinal irradiation will result in severe restriction of spinal growth at puberty and resulting disproportion. Also if the gonads have received a sufficient insult to affect their secretion of sex hormones this will result in an incomplete or absent pubertal response. Normal thyroid function is necessary for normal growth.[10] The thyroid is sensitive to the effects of radiotherapy. Patients who have received radiotherapy to any field with possible involvement or scatter to the thyroid require regular monitoring of thyroid function for life and regular palpation of the gland due to the

Factors affecting growth

- Growth hormone
- Sex hormones
- Thyroxine
- Skeletal radiotherapy
- Parental height
- The illness

increased risk of thyroid tumours.[11] The onset of either complication may be very late. Biochemical monitoring is essential because of the difficulty in recognising thyroid dysfunction clinically and also the implications of an isolated raised thyroid stimulating hormone. Those with low thyroxine and raised thyroid stimulating hormone clearly need replacement therapy but those with isolated raised thyroid stimulating hormone and normal thyroxine should receive replacement therapy sufficient to suppress the raised level. There is concern that an increased thyroid stimulating hormone level increases the already elevated risk of thyroid tumours in the irradiated gland. It is also important in the case of an already short child to ensure normal thyroid function before starting any other therapy.

Recently interest has turned to the effect of pubertal disturbance and growth hormone on bone density. Bone mass in later life is dependent on the peak reached at the end of puberty[12] and if this is reduced there may be an increased risk of osteoporosis. Since girls may be at risk of early menopause this is of particular significance to their long-term risk of developing osteoporosis.

Before leaving the subject of growth and radiotherapy it is worth remembering the effect on other parts of the skeleton. Any area of bone treated in early childhood will demonstrate poor growth. The extent of this may not become apparent until well on in puberty and the subsequent development of deformity can be a distressing problem. This is particularly true when it affects the facial bones and is an obvious cosmetic problem, but can also be an embarrassment when it affects the spine or thorax and may result in self-imposed restriction of activity.

Cardiotoxicity

Cardiac function can be affected by both chemotherapy and radiotherapy. Radiotherapy has been associated with the development of coronary artery disease in young adults[13] although this has been at doses to a field including the heart which is uncommon in radiotherapy practice in this country.

The greatest concern at present is in respect of anthracycline drugs, adriamycin, and daunorubicin. It has been known for some time that these drugs could produce an acute cardiotoxicity, and total dose limitation was recommended.[14] It has become apparent that cardiac function can be affected even many years later with development of cardiomyopathy.[15] Radiotherapy to any field which includes the possibility of scatter to the heart increase the risk of developing anthracycline cardiomyopathy. This can be progressive, severe, and ultimately fatal. There are now a number of patients who, having survived their childhood cancer, are now surviving their cardiac transplant.[16 17] The mechanism of this effect is a loss of myocytes occurring at the time of treatment with subsequent fibrosis and ultimate thinning of the myocardium. These changes are recognisable on endomyocardial biopsy specimens.[18]

More worryingly, it is clear that if sophisticated techniques are used abnormalities can be identified in currently asymptomatic individuals and at very much lower doses.[19] It is not clear which of those in whom an abnormality can be recognised will go on to develop clinically significant problems. Heart failure has developed suddenly in patients undertaking physically stressful activities. Initially this was reported in association with pregnancy and labour[20] but also now with weightlifting programmes and other strenuous activity. This has considerable implications for the advice we might give these patients and their management during pregnancy and labour. This group of drugs has been of importance in improving survival, so the risk of this late effect must be seen in the appropriate context. Strategies are also being used to reduce toxicity such as administration over longer periods[21] and the development of cardioprotective agents.[22] There is, however, a sizable cohort of survivors already exposed to these drugs for whom this is and will continue to be a very important issue. Guidelines have been produced for the use of echocardiography in surveillance of this group[23] and are also included in the guidelines for long term follow up produced by the author and Dr WHB Wallace on behalf of the late effects group of the United Kingdom Children's Cancer Study Group.

Cyclophosphamide has been implicated as being potentially cardiotoxic. This does not result in a significant clinical problem at present, but introduction of new techniques to allow dose escalation may change that and result in different patterns of late effects.

Pulmonary effects

The lung can be affected by certain chemotherapy, radiotherapy, and surgery.[24] It is also susceptible to the consequences of infection and the effects of smoking (both active and passive). Asthma is common and is more easily recognised when awareness of respiratory symptoms is raised. This can make it difficult to assess the exact reason for a given patient's respiratory symptoms, and indeed they are often multifactorial.

The more important chemotherapeutic agents which can affect the lung are carmustine (BCNU), lomustine (CCNU), busulphan, cyclophosphamide, and bleomycin. Bleomycin is of importance to the long term survivor because of the risk of hypersensitivity to oxygen with general anaesthesia. Patients who have received this drug should carry a warning of this risk.

Carmustine is an agent which may be toxic after a long latent period. In 1978 a death from lung fibrosis was reported in a patient treated for medulloblastoma at the age of 2 years. She died within six months of treatment, having received 1550 mg/m^2.[25] A recent series of 31 patients who had received carmustine between 1972 and 1976 has reported the outcome of the 17 survivors of the initial tumour. Of these 17, 6 died of pulmonary fibrosis 1–13 years after completion of treatment and of the remaining 11, 8 were available for study. Six of these patients had abnormal radiographs and all had evidence of lung fibrosis. Since that report two further patients have died of pulmonary fibrosis. The median age at treatment of those who died was 2·5 years. The nine long term survivors had a median age of 10 years. All five patients treated below the age of 5 years died of lung fibrosis.[26]

Research conducted in Manchester on long term survivors of ALL and Wilm's tumour has suggested that, in addition to the previously mentioned factors, the anthracycline drugs may also have an effect on lung function. These effects may be asymptomatic but identifiable on testing pulmonary function. Research is continuing to establish if this is a static or progressive effect (M Jenney, personal communication).

The late effects of radiotherapy on the lung are the result of fibrosis and a restriction of growth. The effects are dependent on the volume of lung irradiated, the dose, and the fractionation of the dose.

The previously mentioned research in Manchester confirms the clinical impression that some survivors of childhood cancer have reduced exercise capacity when measured objectively. However, it is also true that they participate in less habitual exercise than their peers but whether this "couch potato syndrome" is the cause, or an effect, is not clear.

Renal effects

Renal and bladder function can be affected by both chemotherapy and radiotherapy. Patients who have had a nephrectomy and even minimal chemotherapy for Wilm's tumour are at a small but recognisable risk of late renal decompensation.

Glomerular function may be affected by the platinum drugs but this is an effect that will be present from the time of treatment from when it may either improve or worsen. If glomerular function is normal at the end of treatment it has not been reported to worsen later.

Renal tubular function may be affected by therapy with ifosfamide. In the same way it is likely that any effect will be apparent at the time of treatment, but it too may improve or deteriorate and survivors have gone on to develop renal rickets and tubular acidosis. They also show a tendency for glomerular filtration rate to fall.

Other drugs including the nitrosoureas, melphalan, and very high dose methotrexate have been implicated in renal dysfunction and this has implications for developing megatherapy and rescue therapy.

Radiotherapy to a field involving the kidney may result in arterial or arteriolar constriction with resulting renal impairment. This is recognised by the associated development of raised blood pressure which occurs. The bladder can be affected by fibrosis and reduced capacity or more severe impairment of this function.

Skin

Many patients treated with chemotherapy develop multiple pigmented naevi.[27 28] This does not appear to be restricted to any individual drug or combination. The appearance of these naevi is often quite atypical, which can lead to concern about malignancy. Malignant melanoma has been described as a second malignancy in association with retinoblastoma. The presence of large numbers of naevi is one of the known risk factors for malignancy in the general population. Patients need to be given advice on reduction of the other risk factors for malignant melanoma. The aetiology probably relates to immunosuppression as increased naevi have also been seen following renal transplant and treatment with cyclosporin.[29]

Radiotherapy may affect the skin, and hair growth may be poor or absent. Basal cell naevi may occur and in the case of Gorlin's syndrome where there is a genetic predisposition the effect may be dramatic. One such patient received craniospinal irradiation for medulloblastoma and the radiotherapy field became demarcated by multiple basal cell carcinoma.

Genetic predisposition

The fact that some cancers could be familial has been long recognised, for example retinoblastoma. So has the association between malignancy and other familial syndromes such as neurofibromatosis.[30] The recognition of other cancer families and in particular the Li–Fraumini syndrome and the association with the p53 gene has been more recent.[31]

These syndromes are of importance to a small group of long term survivors for two reasons. Firstly, their cancer may be the first to be recognised as indicating a familial factor which will have implications for the rest of the family and secondly, this will have implications for their own risks of further malignancy as well as the risk to any offspring they may have.

This is in contrast to the risk of cancer in the offspring of the whole cohort of long term survivors which has not, as yet, shown any excess over the general population.[32]

Second neoplasms

The development of a second neoplasm indicates an increased likelihood of the presence of a genetic predisposition. This does not account for all second neoplasms, and all survivors of childhood cancer are at increased risk of other second malignancies. Apart from the specific genetic factors previously mentioned the additional risk factors include radiotherapy, treatment with alkylating agents, and treatment with epipodophylotoxins.[33]

The incidence following ALL is around 2% and following Hodgkin's disease around 8% representing an increased risk of four- and 10-fold respectively. By contrast, following genetic retinoblastoma the risk is 30-fold increased.[34]

The commonest second tumour is bone or soft tissue sarcoma but others include basal cell carcinoma, other carcinoma, glioma, meningioma, and acute leukaemia.[35 36] These second tumours may take many years to appear

234

and it is not yet known if the risk eventually tails off. While radiotherapy is certainly a very important etiological factor, it may simply accelerate the onset of a malignancy which would have occurred later. In those who have not received radiotherapy we may have longer to wait to see the full picture.

The epipodophylotoxins are associated with an increased risk of acute myeloid leukaemia occurring relatively early, within about three years of completing therapy. Radiotherapy is an associated factor increasing the risk, as may therapy with alkylating agents.[37]

The experience of seeing patients with second malignancy is certain to become more common with more survivors and increasing time from completion of treatment.

Neuropsychological effects

Treatment directed at the CNS can affect cognitive function. The experience of being treated for childhood cancer almost inevitably disrupts the other normal experiences of childhood, including schooling, thus increasing the problems for these survivors. Both radiotherapy and chemotherapy have been implicated in their effect on cognitive function. The effects of radiotherapy are directly related to dose and inversely to the age when treated. The presence of intracranial calcification on computed tomography has been associated with an increased risk of learning difficulty. Survivors of brain tumours may therefore have experienced quite severe problems[38] which may have required special schooling and significantly influence their prospects for employment.

Survivors of ALL will generally have received lower doses of CNS irradiation, but they too have been shown to experience learning difficulties. These may be specific, affecting particular skills most, for example concentration, short term memory, and number skills.[39 40] However, it has also been estimated that the mean loss of intelligence quotient scores for children treated before 4 years of age is 17 points compared with 7 points for those treated over this age.[41] The full effect of this loss may not develop until some time after treatment. This raises the question of remedial help at school or statement of special educational need, and for how long that help may be required.

The most recent acute lymphoblastic leukaemia trial in the UK (UKALL XI) of course omits cranial irradiation in favour of chemotherapy directed at the CNS in an attempt to reduce sequelae. However, learning difficulties have been reported without radiotherapy[42 43] and psychological assessments are being performed on the survivors as part of that trial. Intracranial calcification has been seen in association with parenteral methotrexate and no CNS directed therapy at all. Impairment of memory, both immediate and delayed, has been shown to be related to the presence of cerebral atrophy and intracranial calcification on computed tomography.

Perhaps the surprising thing is that achievements of these survivors at school leaving age seem to compare quite well with the general population.[44 45] This probably reflects the specific nature of some of these effects which allows the individual to focus on those areas of least problem. This naturally leads in the direction of a career for which they are best equipped and least disadvantaged. In this respect they are no different from their peers.

Psychosocial effects

It is important to realise that the psychosocial effects of treatment for childhood cancer are to be found not only in the survivor but also in their siblings, parents, carers, and society in general.

The psychosocial outcome for a survivor of childhood cancer must be the result of not only their experience of being treated but also their own personality, family setting, schooling, and peer group. The experience of other late effects will also influence the outcome. The worry of possible relapse or of possible late effects can continue to hang over them. This has been called the Damocles syndrome. The studies which have been done so far point to a good outcome for the majority of patients, apart from those treated for brain tumours where the effects on cognitive function will affect social development.[46]

The impression gained in the long term follow up clinic is that while the majority do have a good outcome, some do not. Those treated so young that they have little or no recollection of their therapy or life before it seem to do well, but those treated in later childhood or adolescence may have a tendency to do less well. Figure 15.3 is the work of a patient treated for Hodgkin's disease at 13 years of age. He accepted his treatment stoically and gave the impression of being a quiet, shy person. Seven years later he finally spoke of his feelings both at the time of his treatment and subsequently. He found it difficult to verbalise his experience, but described loss of his previous outgoing personality and subsequent social isolation. This developed into a desire for solitude, which resulted in him choosing a career as a gamekeeper. He also experienced a feeling of having been damaged by his treatment (he is infertile) while recognising the fact that it had cured him. The following year when he returned he brought this picture with him. He feels it illustrates those feelings. The next year he was rather dismissive of his own work, stating that perhaps he had overstated its significance. It would be consistent to see this as part of his own capacity to work through his emotions and then be able to move on. It should also be said that other patients describe a very positive outcome from their experience of childhood cancer and feel they have gained as a result.

Further research is under way to improve our knowledge and understanding of the factors which result in different outcomes and how they may interact.[47]

Attention has lately been directed at systems of health status assessment which could be used as an object measure of outcome.[48] One system, described by Feeny *et al.*[49] has already been incorporated into a current United Kingdom Children's Cancer Study Group trial. These instruments are still being refined and developed and it is likely they will be more widely used in the future.[50]

Long-term follow-up

In the emotional tension that exists when a child is treated for cancer, there is the moment when it is possible to inform the patient and the parent that it is now highly likely that their cancer is cured. It is not always easy to be prepared to temper that moment with the reality of potential late effects. However, there is a responsibility to provide long-term follow-up for the survivors and that follow-up should be lifelong.[51][52] It is important to discuss the possibility of late effects from an early stage. The necessity and reasons for long-term follow-up should be discussed at appropriate times during treatment and prior to completion of therapy as well as in the long-term follow-up clinic.

Concern has been expressed that continuing to recall patients who are thought to be cured may perpetuate illness behaviour and therefore may itself be harmful. This needs to be balanced with the harm we can do by failing to recognise late effects. There is potential for harm both for the

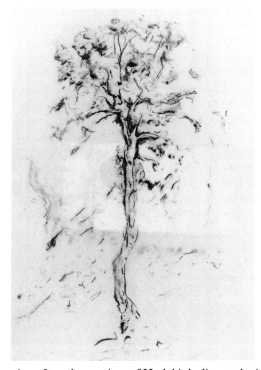

Fig 15.3 Drawing of tree by survivor of Hodgkin's disease depicting his feelings

Recommendations for follow-up

- All survivors should be followed up annually by tertiary care providers for life
- Providers of follow-up should be aware of potential harm including insurability, employability, and the completeness of cure
- Follow-up should be tailored to the patient, taking into account type of cancer, therapy, and psychosocial need
- A team approach, including paediatric oncologist and an internist trained in late effects, together with nurse practitioner, psychologist, social worker, and others as needed
- Follow-up should initially be in a paediatric setting but after a period of overlap should make the transition to the adult care environment
- Primary care providers should be educated as to their patients' risks and incorporated into the process
- Research must be conducted into outcomes
- A registry of survivors and adverse sequelae and outcomes should be established

individual and for subsequent generations of survivors. That care needs to include provision of information about their risks, appropriate surveillance for late effects, treatment and health promotion, and should be done in a way that changes as the patient matures. It is important that continuity exists and as patients may only return annually this is not a task for staff on short term contracts. The statistics provided earlier indicate the extent of the need and how it will grow in the future.

At the Royal Manchester Children's Hospital long term follow up is provided in a separate clinic for adolescent and adult survivors. This is a joint clinic with an endocrinologist, a hospital practitioner, a senior registrar, and a clinic nurse who has a longstanding knowledge of the patients. Contacts have been established with other specialists, both paediatric and adult, to share the care of particular problems. Occasional evening clinics are provided in order to minimise disruption for those who do not wish to take time off work. A consultation without the presence of the parents is actively encouraged from an age that is variable but dependent on the maturity of the individual. The parent is also allowed a consultation, but it is made clear the patient's consultation is confidential. The patients and their parents will have been used to an open, honest approach during treatment, and this is continued by informing them of likely or possible late effects. In respect of risks of infertility, for example, this can be done in a way that allows the patient to mature in the knowledge of the possible problems and decide when it is appropriate from their perspective to clarify the position by further investigation. In this way the patient is able to take at least some of the responsibility for their care and retain a degree of control. The intention has been to make it a positive rather than a negative experience for both patients and clinic staff.

The American Cancer Society Workgroup on Long-term Care and Lifetime Follow-up have produced a set of recommendations (see box).[53] There is now a need to debate the appropriateness of these recommendations to the situation in the United Kingdom. If care is to be transferred into an adult care environment, who is going to take it on? Is it necessary to do so, or can care be provided by those involved in the follow-up of children and adolescents in a way that meets the needs of adult survivors? What will constitute the appropriate background and training for the late effects specialist? How can best use be made of the skills of nurses in these clinics? How can the outcome be monitored for those who decline to attend for follow-up?

Whatever the answers to these questions, those involved in the treatment of childhood cancer have been privileged to be part of a remarkable success story. That success has left a duty to those survivors. The increasing knowledge of late effects and the enlarging cohort of survivors presents a problem, but until late effects can be prevented it is a problem we should be pleased to have. Late effects will be common but rarely fatal. To have a late effect you need to be a survivor of a previously fatal disease. Most survivors are well, employable, and indistinguishable from their peers.

1 Birch JM, Marsden HB, Morris Jones PH et al. Improvements in survival from childhood cancer: results of a population based survey over 30 years. Br Med J 1988; 296: 1372–6.
2 Stiller C. Centralisation of treatment and survival rates for cancer. Arch Dis Child 1988; 63: 23–30.
3 Pediatric Oncology Group. Progress against childhood cancer: the pediatric oncology group experience. Pediatrics 1992; 89: 597–600.
4 Shalet SM. Growth and hormonal status of children treated for brain tumours. Child's Brain 1982; 9: 284–93.
5 Shalet SM, Clayton PE, Price DA. Growth and pituitary function in children treated for brain tumours or acute lymphoblastic leukaemia. Horm Res 1988; 30: 53–61.
6 Crowne EC, Wallace WHB, Moore C et al. A novel variant of growth hormone (GH) insufficiency following low dose cranial irradiation. Clin Endocrinol 1992; 36: 59–68.
7 Moell C, Garwicz S, Westgren U et al. Blunted pubertal growth after leukaemia: A new pattern of growth hormone insufficiency. Horm Res 1988; 30: 68–71.
8 Leiper A, Stanhope R, Preece MA et al. Precocious or early puberty and growth failure in girls treated for acute lymphoblastic leukaemia. Horm Res 1988; 30: 72–6.
9 Winter RJ, Green OC. Irradiation-induced growth hormone deficiency: Blunted growth response and accelerated skeletal maturation to growth hormone therapy. J Pediatr 1985; 106: 609–12.
10 Shalet SM. Endocrine consequences of treatment of malignant disease. Arch Dis Child 1989; 64: 1635–41.
11 Shalet SM, Rosenstock JD, Beardwell CG et al. Thyroid dysfunction following external irradiation to the neck for Hodgkin's disease in childhood. Clin Radiol 1977; 28: 511–15.
12 Cooper C, Eastell R. Bone gain and loss in premenopausal women. Br Med J 1993; 206: 1357–8.
13 Green DM, D'Angio GJ. Cardiac toxicity and cardiomyopathy after cancer therapy. New York: Wiley, 1993.
14 Borrow KM, Henderson IC, Neuman A et al. Assessment of left ventricular contractility in patients receiving doxorubicin. Ann Int Med 1983; 99: 750–6.
15 Steinhertz LJ, Steinhertz PG, Tan CTC et al. Cardiac toxicity 4 to 20 years after completing anthracycline therapy. JAMA 1991; 266(12): 1672–7.
16 Edwards BS, Hunt SA, Fowler MB et al. Cardiac transplantation in patients with preexisting neoplastic diseases. Am J Cardiol 1990; 65: 501–4.

17 Arico M, Pedroni E, Nespoli L *et al.* Long term survival after heart transplant for doxorubicin induced cardiomyopathy. *Arch Dis Child* 1991; **66**: 985–6.

18 Billingham ME, Mason JW, Bristow MR, Daniels JR. Anthracycline cardiotoxicity monitored by morphologic changes. *Cancer Treat Rep* 1978; **62**(6): 865–72.

19 Lipshultz SE, Colan SD, Gelbur RD *et al.* Late cardiac effects of doxorubicin therapy for acute lymphoblastic leukaemia in childhood. *N Engl J Med* 1991; **324**: 808–15.

20 Davis LE, Brown CE. Peripartum heart failure in a patient treated previously with doxorubicin. *Obstet Gynecol* 1988; **71**: 506–8.

21 Shapira J, Gotfried M, Lishner M, Ravid M. Reduced cardiotoxicity of doxorubicin by a 6-hour infusion regimen: a prospective randomized evaluation. *Cancer* 1990; **65**: 870–3.

22 Bu'Lock FA, Gabriel HM, Oakhill A *et al.* Cardioprotection by ICRF187 against high dose anthracycline toxicity in children with malignant disease. *Br Heart J* 1993; **70**: 185–8.

23 Steinhertz LJ, Graham T, Hurwitz R *et al.* Guidelines for cardiac monitoring of children during and after anthracycline therapy: report of the cardiology committee of the childrens cancer study group. *Pediatrics* 1992; **89**: 942–9.

24 Makipernaa A, Heino M, Laitinen L, Siimes M. Lung function following treatment of malignant tumors with surgery, radiotherapy or cyclophosphamide in childhood: a follow-up study after 11 to 27 years. *Cancer* 1989; **63**: 625–30.

25 Bailey CC, Marsden HB, Jones PH. Fatal pulmonary fibrosis following 1,3-bis(2-chloroethyl)-1-nitrosorea (BCNU) therapy. *Cancer* 1978; **42**: 74–6.

26 O'Driscoll BR, Haselton PS, Taylor PM *et al.* Active lung fibrosis up to 17 years after chemotherapy with carmustine (BCNU) in childhood. *N Engl J Med* 1990; **323**: 378–82.

27 Hughes B, Bailey CC. Excess benign melanocytic naevi. *Br Med J* 1989; **299**: 854–5.

28 Baird EA, McHenry PM, MacKie RM. Effect of maintenance chemotherapy in childhood on numbers of melanocytic naevi. *Br Med J* 1992; **305**: 799–801.

29 McGregor JM, Barker JN, MacDonald DM. The development of excess numbers of melanocytic naevi in an immunosuppressed identical twin. *Clin Exp Dermatol* 1991; **16**(2): 131–2.

30 Draper GJ, Heaf MM, Kinnear Wilson LM. Occurrence of childhood cancers among sibs and estimation of familial risks. *J Med Genetics* 1977; **14**: 81–90.

31 Li FP, Fraumeni JF, Mulvihill JJ. A cancer family syndrome in twenty-four kindreds. *Cancer Res* 1988; **48**: 5358–62.

32 Hawkins MM, Draper GJ, Smith RA. Cancer among 1,348 offspring of survivors of childhood cancer. *Int J Cancer* 1989; **43**: 975–8.

33 Meadows AT, Hobbie WL. The medical consequences of cure. *Cancer* 1986; **58**: 524–8.

34 Hawkins HM, Draper GJ, Kingston JE. Incidence of second primary tumours among childhood cancer survivors. *Br J Cancer* 1987; **56**: 339–47.

35 Soffer D, Pittaluga S, Feiner M, Beller AJ. Intracranial meningiomas following low-dose irradiation to the head. *J Neurosurg* 1983; **59**: 1048–53.

36 Meadows AT, Baum E, Fossati-Bellani F *et al.* Second malignant neoplasms in children: an update from the late effects group. *J Clin Oncol* 1985; **3**: 532–8.

37 Hawkins MM, Kinnier Wilson LM, Stovall MA *et al.* Epipodophyllotoxins, alkylating agents, and radiation and risk of secondary leukaemia after childhood cancer. *Br Med J* 1992; **304**: 951–8.

38 Bamford FN, Morris Jones PM, Pearson D *et al.* Residual disabilities in children treated for intracranial space-occupying lesions. *Cancer* 1976; **37**: 1149–51.

39 Moore IM, Kramer JH, Wara W *et al.* Cognitive function in children with leukaemia: effect of radiation dose and time since irradiation. *Cancer* 1991; **68**: 1913–17.

40 Eiser C. Cognitive deficits in children treated for leukaemia. *Arch Dis Child* 1991; **66**: 164–8.

41 Cousens P, Waters B, Said J, Stevens M. Cognitive effects of cranial irradiation in leukaemia: a survey and meta-analysis. *J Child Psychol Psychiatry* 1988; **29**: 839–52.

42 Mulhern RK, Fairclough D, Ochs J. A prospective comparison of neuropsychological performance of children surviving leukaemia who received 18 Gy, 24 Gy or no cranial irradiation. *J Clin Oncol* **9**: 1348–56.

43 Ochs J, Mulhern RK. In: *Late effects of treatment of childhood cancer.* Green DM, D'Angio GJ eds. New York: Wiley Liss, 1992.

44 Hays DM, Landsverk J, Sallan SE *et al.* Educational, occupational, and insurance status of childhood cancer survivors in their fourth and fifth decades of life. *J Clin Oncol* 1992; **10**: 1397–1406.

45 Meadows AT, McKee L, Kazak AE. Psychosocial status of young adult survivors of childhood cancer: a survey. *Med Pediatr Oncol* 1989; **17**: 466–70.
46 Eiser C, Havermans T. Long term social adjustment after treatment for childhood cancer. *Arch Dis Child* 1994; **70**: 66–70.
47 Green DM, Zevon MA, Hall B. Achievement of life goals by adult survivors of modern treatment for childhood cancer. *Cancer* 1991; **67**: 206–13.
48 Billson AL, Walker DA. Assessment of health status in survivors of cancer. *Arch Dis Child* 1994; **70**: 200–4.
49 Feeny D, Leiper A, Barr RD *et al.* The comprehensive assessment of health status in survivors of childhood cancer: application to high-risk acute lymphoblastic leukaemia. *Br J Cancer* 1993; **67**: 1047–52.
50 How can one assess damage caused by treatment of childhood cancer? *Lancet* (Editorial) 1992; **340**: 758–9.
51 D'Angio GJ. Cure has its tomorrows. *Int J Radiation Oncol Biol Phys* 1976; **1**: 373–4.
52 Meadows AT, Krejmas NL, Belasco JB. The medical costs of cure: sequelae in survivors of childhood cancer. In *Status of the curability of childhood cancers.* van Eys J, Sullivan MP editors. New York: Raven Press, 1980.
53 Bleyer WA, Smith RA, Green DM *et al.* Workgroup #1: long-term care and lifetime follow-up. *Cancer* 1993; **71**: 2413–25.

16: Where should patients be treated?

ANN BARRETT

Oncologists have become increasingly aware of the need for special facilities for patients who present with cancer during adolescence. All patients with cancer need help to understand the disease and its treatment, to learn to cope with side effects and to develop psychosocial strategies by which they can reach and maintain a reasonable level of adjustment to what is always a personal disaster. Adolescents in particular need open and honest communication at an appropriate level and a way of continuing their threatened normal development. They need support from their peers and at the same time both independence and increased help from their parents.

Paediatricians have shown a particular interest in the development of special adolescent units, but many of these patients are still treated in adult units.[1] Data from the Scottish Cancer Registration Scheme has been used to determine the pattern of adolescent cancer in Scotland to try to identify how appropriate care could be provided. Patients have been arbitrarily divided into groups: age 13–16 representing early adolescence, 16–19 mid adolescence, and 20–25 late adolescence or early adulthood. The needs of patients in these age groups are obviously different, but a survey in our own centre has indicated that even the younger adolescents would be quite happy to be cared for with adults up to the age of 25. In the 12 year period 1980–91 there was a total of 2628 patients with cancer in these age groups from a total population in Scotland of 5 million. There were 248 males and 210 females diagnosed between the ages of 13 and 16, 289 males and 23 females aged 16–19, and 850 males and 792 females aged 20–25. The male to female ratio is about 1·1:1 in each group. There are twice as many patients presenting over the age of 21 as in the two groups up to age 19.

There has been no obvious change in the number of incident cases by age group, sex or year of diagnosis, as shown in Figure 16.1. The graph shows minor fluctuations from year to year, but no significant variations. The range of numbers of registrations per year varies between a minimum of 124 in 1990 and a maximum of 149 in 1981.

Data are collected from 15 health boards in Scotland. There are paediatric oncology centres in Lothian, Greater Glasgow, and Grampian,

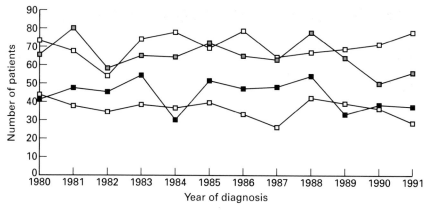

Fig 16.1 Numbers of diagnoses by age group, year of diagnosis, and sex. ■, male 13–19; □, female 13–19; □, male 20–25; □, female 20–25

and additional adult oncology centres in Tayside and Highland. Table 16.1 shows the number of patients by age group coming from each health board. Figure 16.2 shows the wide geographical distribution of these patients and underlies the difficulties that may arise because of the need to travel to large centres for treatment. An additional factor to be taken into account is that independent hospital trusts have been set up recently in each of these health boards and this is already changing referral patterns.

Although the total number of registrations has remained constant over the study period, there has been an apparent fall in the mortality rate by year of diagnosis in all age groups (Figure 16.3). Although the apparent improvement in the later years may be due in part to shorter time of follow up, it is also likely to reflect improvements in treatment as reported by the

Table 16.1   Number of patients by age group coming from each Scottish health board

Health board	13–19 years	20–25 years
Argyll and Clyde	72	127
Ayrshire and Arran	66	109
Borders	17	31
Dumfries and Galloway	28	55
Fife	64	117
Forth Valley	62	75
Grampian	96	203
Greater Glasgow	187	291
Highland	37	66
Lanarkshire	109	162
Lothian	161	294
Orkney	3	1
Shetland	3	9
Tayside	73	102
Western Isles	2	5
Total	980	1647

243

United Kingdom Children's Cancer Study Group. Recent data from Scotland clearly indicate improvement in survival for those tumours amenable to treatment.[2]

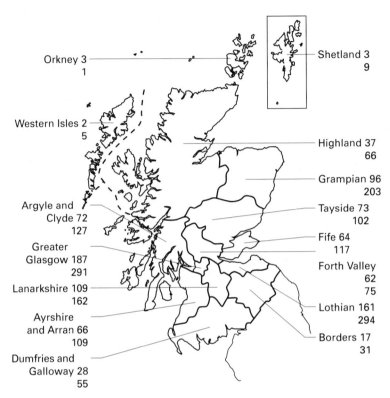

Fig 16.2 Number of patients in each region. The first figure indicates number of patients treated at ages 13–19, the second figure those treated at ages 20–25

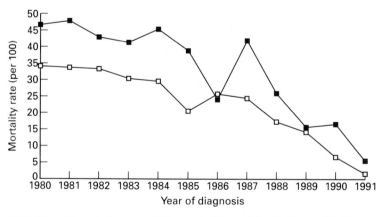

Fig 16.3 Mortality rate by year of diagnosis. ■, age 13–19; □, age 20–25

It is important to appreciate the different spectrum of disease that is seen in this age group, compared with children or older adults (Figure 16.4). Tumours of the genitourinary system constitute the largest proportion, accounting for about 24% of patients. In the 13–19 age group, testicular tumours occurred in 67 patients and ovarian tumours in 26. Tumours of the bladder and kidney were rare (6 and 7 respectively). In the 20–25 year age group, testicular tumours accounted for 251 patients, carcinoma of the cervix 96, and ovarian cancer 49. Twenty-nine patients had bladder cancer and 10 tumours of the kidney. Approximately one quarter of the patients had lymphoma. Out of the total of 232 patients under the age 19, 73 had non-Hodgkin's lymphoma, 158 Hodgkin's disease, and 1 multiple myeloma. In the 20–25 age group, 273 had Hodgkin's disease, 93 non-Hodgkin's lymphoma, and 1 myeloma. Thirteen per cent of patients in both groups had skin tumours: more of these were malignant melanoma than non-melanoma skin cancers. The incidence of central nervous system tumours, bone and soft tissue sarcomas, and leukaemia was equal at 9·1%. Other tumours such as carcinoma of the thyroid, gastrointestinal tract, and head and neck region were much less common than in older patients.

In the 11 year period studied, 9 hospitals treated more than 25 patients aged 13–19; this represented 51% of the whole population. In the 20–25 age group, 20 hospitals were involved in treating more than 25 patients and these represented 76% of the total patient numbers. The remaining cases were treated in 69 other hospitals throughout Scotland.

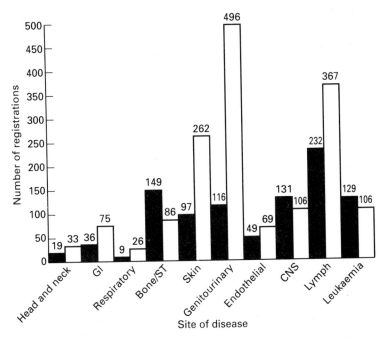

Fig 16.4 Number of registrations by site of disease. Black bars, age 13–19; white bars, age 20–25

Analysis of this registration data leads to the following conclusions:

- The cancer incidence in males and females is similar, but it is twice as common in the age group 20–25 as in the 13–19 year olds. This slightly older group of patients share some of the specific problems of adolescents with cancer and also benefit from separate facilities.
- The number of patients presenting with cancer has not changed over the last 10 years. The patients, however, are scattered very widely and likely to be treated in a large number of different hospitals. At the same time there is a probable improvement of the outcome of treatment, which other studies in Scotland have indicated may, in part, be due to increased centralisation of care.[3]

With current treatments, most patients will require management by specialists in a number of different disciplines. The study of this data highlights potential conflicts of interest in providing optimum care for adolescents with cancer. There is evidence of improved outcome for patients with rare tumours when they are treated by multimodality teams of specialists in a centralised treatment facility. However, most patients prefer to be treated near to home and this is particularly a problem where there may be other young family members requiring the attention of parents as well as the adolescent patient. An individual patient is likely to prefer to have all his care delivered by familiar team of experts and to prefer admission to the same place, whenever necessary. A special adolescent unit is ideal from this point of view, but centralisation of facilities may cause problems for staff.

Nursing staff will need to be specially selected for work on adolescent units, but even then it is well recognised that they may suffer considerable stress, particularly at times when the outcome of treatment is unsuccessful. The death of an angry questioning teenager may be much more harrowing to someone of a similar age than the death of an older person, considered to be near the end of their natural life.

Some of the major problems arise, however, from the small number of patients in this age group. The costs of running a very small unit may be too high for efficiency and such units may not have high priority in the new NHS market system. One way of overcoming the small numbers is to create mixed units where patients with, for example, diseases such as diabetes and cystic fibrosis are cared for together with those with cancer. This is sometimes not considered convenient by medical staff and in some cases there may be a risk of cross-infection or other problems, which staff would prefer to avoid.

I believe some of the desirable features specified for adolescent units are in fact basic requirements for the treatment of all patients with cancer and differ quantitatively rather than qualitatively.

Adolescents or young adults have a great need for privacy and a way of maintaining modesty and self esteem, when they are very aware of their body image and often fearful of being thought different. They need both psychological and physical space in which to continue their normal development and in this they need to be supported by those of their own age. It is particularly important for contact to be maintained with their friends at school and at home as this will make it much easier for them to re-integrate into their normal society. However, since they often experience some rejection, which is presumably based on fear in people whose health remains normal, it may be beneficial to have the opportunity to meet others in the same situation who will provide support and encouragement.

It is important for the family to be recognised as a unit and proper provision made for parents and siblings to visit and stay as appropriate. Flexible and specialised staff are needed who have a genuine interest in adolescents — people who are not frightened of frank discussion, who don't mind criticism (sometimes personal), who are not rigid in their ways of doing things, and who are prepared to consider all sorts of options to make treatment acceptable to their patients. One of my hardest decisions was deciding whether a 16-year old with Ewing's sarcoma undergoing treatment was safe to take part in a stunt motorbike jumping competition, at the nadir of his blood count after chemotherapy. He obviously expected it to be approved or he would not have mentioned it until afterwards.

Various models for nursing care exist, and it is beyond my competence to discuss the appropriateness of these. However, in practice it seems as if those trained in paediatric oncology nursing cope more naturally with the demands of adolescents than those experienced in other nursing practices. Nursing opinion tends to be fairly divided between those nurses who particularly enjoy these patients and those who are frightened, find them threatening, or feel inadequate to cope with their demands.

In the oncology centres in Glasgow at present there are no specific facilities for adolescents. The current policy is that patients over the age of 16 are either treated by the consultant to whom they were originally referred or, if initially seen by a speciality team, will be treated in the adult cancer centre, with or without time in the appropriate surgical unit. Children under the age of 13 or presenting before puberty will usually be treated in the children's hospital except for any necessary radiotherapy. There may be exceptions in patients referred for surgical procedures to individual consultants. For patients between the ages of 13 and 17, a wide variety of practices exists. If such patients are referred to an oncologist initially, the decision as to whether they would be more appropriately treated in the children's or adult unit is made after parents and patients have seen the two units. Within the oncology units, accommodation is either in single-bedded units or in units of 4–6 beds. In the adult wards, adolescents will be allocated side wards as a priority. One or other parent, usually the mother, is present for much of the day, but overnight accommodation is available for emergencies only. It is rarely requested, but this may be because there is no expectation for such provision. In the children's wards, the needs of immunosuppressed patients for isolation facilities will be paramount.

247

My clinical commitment is equally divided between the paediatric and adult oncology unit and my special interest in paediatric cancer, sarcomas, and lymphomas means that the majority of my patients fall into the age groups under discussion. In the absence of specific facilities, it has been possible to compare to a certain extent the responses of adolescents to care in the different units. There is obviously a tendency for the younger patients to be treated in the children's hospital, but considerable flexibility is maintained in mid adolescence. Adolescents nursed in the adult ward are allocated private rooms wherever possible, but we have observed that, whether they have a room of their own or are in the open ward, they make little effort to talk to other patients or interact with them socially. This is true even when there are patients of the same age in the ward at the same time. In general they do not undertake much specific activity during their hospital admissions, which are usually short and during which they may be restricted by sedation given to counteract effects of chemotherapy or by intravenous antibiotic therapy for intercurrent infections. They watch television and the boys occasionally play pool, but many patients become relatively reclusive.

Since the majority of patients in the oncology centre are adults, the investigative facilities outside the department are obviously adult orientated and there may be an unreasonable expectation of cooperation of these young patients. For example, there may not be such free use of lignocaine cream before intravenous procedures as in the children's ward and less explanation and preparation may be given for procedures such as computed tomography and magnetic resonance imaging.

There is no formal provision for education or occupational therapy for these patients. The educational service based in the children's hospital willingly assist when resources permit, but these patients usually make individual arrangements with their school for home tuition. We find the parents to be relatively undemanding, being content with on average twice-weekly discussions with the consultant in charge. Social work support is provided as to other patients, but there are none of the special arrangements such as the Malcolm Sargent social workers with access to specific help, which are so helpful in the children's hospital.

Within the paediatric setting, there is a much more supportive environment for the patients, which makes it easier to cope if they regress. There is access to all the appropriate educational, social and financial support needed and more appropriate preparation for possibly painful procedures. Parents benefit from support from one another, although there is sometimes confusion as parents compare and contrast diagnoses and treatments. We have noted that there is a tendency for adolescents to make friends with younger patients rather than their peers, even when they are in hospital at the same time. It may be that providing help and encouragement to younger patients helps to maintain their self esteem and reduces their feelings of depression and self pity. The parents are noticeably more overtly anxious and demanding. Because of a different pattern of working in the paediatric unit, they expect more frequent interaction with the consultant and a greater depth of detailed information about their child's condition. It is sometimes more difficult to establish an individual rapport with the child under these circumstances than when he is forced into greater independence on an adult ward.

It is difficult to evaluate directly which of these patterns of care is best, since there is some patient selection already in determining where patients are treated and it is not always easy to separate the distress associated with the disease and its treatment from that produced by unsatisfactory and remediable external circumstances.

The current concern with adolescents needs to be expanded to take account of the many adolescents who are at present treated outside paediatric units and for whom it is unrealistic to expect referral to a specialised unit in the immediate future. While we are waiting the development of more adolescent units, (if these prove to be viable numerically and economically), what is needed is adequate supportive care for adolescents wherever they are treated at present. This needs to take account of social, educational, and financial factors as well as the needs of parents and the direct medical and psychological needs of the patients. This immediate improvement can probably only be achieved by staff education and training. Specific teaching about the care of adolescents should be incorporated into all existing oncology training courses and particularly into the education of surgical trainees. It seems likely that the development of any new units will need to continue to be supported by charities such as the Teenage Cancer Trust, who have worked so well to provide the existing facilities. It is unlikely to be cost effective for any individual trust to give this area priority in the current environment. It may be that for large regional centres, consideration should be given to the development of more than one small specialised nursing area for this patient group until the general education of the profession has reached the stage of overcoming professional pride and need for ownership and lack of interdisciplinary cooperation. No amount of effort to improve services can be too much for these patients who have diseases that threaten both their quantity and quality of life. However, the toll on staff undertaking this work must be recognised and provision made for adequate variety of work and support in what can be a very taxing and emotionally draining area. We must also guard against guilt at our lack of achievement, which seems to be a result of increasingly high patient expectation.

In summary, therefore, we need a programme of education to supplement the present sporadic provision of care for adolescents to ensure a general improvement. I have no doubt that if one is faced with a stark choice, these patients benefit from all the additional support which is normally available in a department of paediatric oncology. It would, however, be appropriate for adult departments to incorporate many of these assets into their own practice.

I finish with a quotation from a patient of mine treated at age 15 for an osteosarcoma and then subsequently with relapse of her disease at the age of 20.

> At 15 you think you are grown up and then you discover suddenly that you can't cope. I was the first person I knew who had cancer as young as me. I felt really sorry for myself, all the people in the ward with me were really old, they had already lived, no one was trying to cure them like they were me. If I had been in a ward with younger children rather than the same age, I would have had a better sense of perspective. You think there can't be anyone worse off than you, until you see the really young children with cancer. It would definitely be best though to be in a teenage unit with Mega-drives, decent music, videos, and SKY.

1 Stiller CA. Centralisation of treatment and survival rates for cancer. *Arch Dis Child* 1988; **63**: 23–30.
2 Black RJ, Sharp L, Kendrick SW. *Trends in cancer survival in Scotland 1968–1990.* National Health Service in Scotland, Directorate of Information Services, Information and Statistics Division. 1993.
3 Harding PJ, Paul J, Gillis CR, Kaye SB. Management of malignant teratoma: does referral to specialist unit matter? *Lancet* 1993; **341**: 999–1002.

17: Interacting with teenagers with cancer

MARGARET EVANS

Introduction

> "Our youth love luxury; they have bad manners, contempt for authority, they show disrespect for elders and love chatter in place of exercise. Children are now tyrants, not the servants of their households. They no longer rise when elders enter the room. They contradict their parents, chatter before company, gobble up their food, and tyrannize their teachers." (Plato, quoting from Socrates in the 5th century BC).[1]

It seems that very little has changed over the years, and teenagers are still considered by society to be a problematic group. However, although they are not adults, they do become less problematic when they are treated like adults and when an attempt is made to understand their specific needs.

Teenagers with cancer not only struggle with challenging developmental tasks but also struggle with coming to terms with a life-threatening illness —and yet we have been slow to recognise this in the hospital setting, paying very little attention to their unique needs and often caring for them in an inappropriate environment. We do not allow them to express their views and often treat them like children.

This chapter addresses some of the problems associated with interacting with this age group and considers ways of alleviating them.

The normal teenager

The teenager years are a unique and turbulent period of life when young people experience many physical and emotional changes. Attempts by society to categorise teenagers are confusing, especially as they are often expected to be adults one minute and children the next. In reality, they are teenagers whether they like it or not.

The developmental age of teenagers is difficult to define of maturity differs in individuals, but it does span roughly of 12 and 20. In its wisdom, society grants permission for become adults at the age of 16 and allows them to marry w consent, have sex (although homosexuals must wait until t school, find a job, smoke, sign their own consent, and ride a moped. At 17, they are allowed to drive a car but not a heavy goods vehicle until they are 21. At 18 they can vote, drink, own a credit card, and leave home. At 20 they are no longer teenagers.

Kuykendall[2] comments on the arbitrary nature of this categorisation and suggests that a developmental approach is much more viable. Erikson[3] has defined a developmental approach in relation to identity versus role confusion.

The teenage years are a time when young people reorganise their personality structure, and it is a time for existential confrontation. A new identity, new roles, and new exploratory relationships with both sexes allows teenagers to forge ahead into the future, developing autonomy and a personal value system. At the same time, they are experiencing a confusing sense of loss by attaining emancipation from their parents and the security of a home.

Teenagers need to live in the present and gradually orient themselves towards the future to allow their confidence to grow. They are trying to take responsibility for their own behaviour in terms of financial and social independence and competence, but this is sometimes imposed on them or questioned because they seem out of control—at least according to socially acceptable norms which do not always take account of the fact that protest, searching, and disorganisation are part of the process of development.

Developing to sexual maturity with an associated change in body image can be embarrassing and confusing for this age group. Body image is related to how a person feels about himself or herself and it may be a conscious or unconscious attitude. It certainly contributes to a positive self esteem and self confidence. Body ideal is the way a person wants to look, and, with teenagers, may undermine their own body image which may be influenced by significant others, the environment, and the maturation of the central nervous system.

Teenagers' peer groups are the most influential significant others in their lives, and conformity to peer group norms in appearance and behaviour is evident. Peer group pressure is powerful, and exclusion from a gang can be potentially destructive for teenagers.

During this time of transition, teenagers develop cognitive skills and the ability to think in abstract terms. Previously held perceptions are re-examined, analysed and changed—thus it is a time of great conflict, not only with others, but also within themselves, and this accounts for much of the misunderstanding experienced by this age group. Conflicts such as separation versus reunion, independence versus dependence, or closeness versus distance result in an ambivalence between childhood and adulthood as the ego is redefined and confidence is built. At the same time, teenagers are developing the ability to control and take responsibility for their own behaviour in accordance with the values of society.

If teenagers complete their development successfully, they will emerge into adulthood with a positive self esteem, a comfortable body image, an established identity, emotional independence, and a realistic view of the future.

Teenagers with cancer

In the United Kingdom 1 in 800 teenagers develop cancer: although the number is small, their needs are great, because they are experiencing a crucial stage in their lives.

The complex nature of cancer treatments, coupled with teenage developmental tasks, challenge coping strategies and exacerbate the natural ambivalence between childhood and adulthood which has already been discussed. In addition, at a time when they need autonomy from parents, the hospital experience is likely to contribute to lack of independence, regression, and confusion as to responsibilities—parents quite naturally become overprotective and want to take over, which often causes conflict. Changes in social relationships are common, especially if long absences from school or college create distancing from peers and other significant people in their lives.

A diagnosis of cancer, then, is enormously threatening and places young people at risk of psychosocial disturbance, since the developmental tasks of this age group focus on identity and independence. Major changes in daily living must be faced as they endeavour to adjust to the shock of debilitating disease and treatment.

Teenagers want to be treated as adults and feel that they should be able to cope with their fears, but at the same time they long for the comfort and the security of childhood. This inherent dichotomy only serves to intensify their distress.

Interacting with teenagers

The professionals who come into contact with teenagers need to have developed a clear understanding of the developmental tasks which they are confronting and in order to manage this age group, appreciate that at times they may be rebellious, moody, self centred, paranoid, or antagonistic. Teenagers are particularly susceptible to loss of control and, clearly, this is intensified during a period of serious illness, when control may shift from the teenager to the hospital and it may feel as if dependence and regression are being reinforced. It is well known that loss of control is a major stressor in life and is often associated with a feeling of being unable to cope. The teenager needs to regain control and it is important to identify what is adaptive and what is maladaptive for this age group, when so many issues are being confronted.

It is therefore fundamental to the care of teenagers that their independence is restored and that those who are interacting with them are able to gain their trust.

How can this be achieved?

253

Involving teenagers in decision making

There are two issues which need to be addressed in relation to decision making; the first is interactions with parents, and the second is the ability to make choices.

Interacting with parents

Many parents have great difficulty coping with the increasing mood swings of their offspring and have a tendency to encourage childlike behaviour in their efforts to diminish the pain of the cancer experience. In addition, parents may be suffering from the loss of their children during the teenage years and will naturally grasp any opportunity to retrieve them. Teenagers, may, however, see their parents as having double standards, because they have been encouraged to conform to adult behaviour prior to their illness and, in their confusion, will tend to vacillate between dependence and independence.

Parents often cause much unnecessary antagonism by being over-protective and families may need help to encourage mutual understanding during this stressful and difficult time.

Ability to make choices

"The key to respecting teenagers' rights is the belief that they can be trusted to make informed and wise decisions when they are given enough information, support, and respect" (Tipping et al.).[4]

It is fundamental to the care of teenagers to maintain open lines of communication and to treat them as equals in an environment of mutual trust and honesty. This means including them in all decision making and discussions. Teenagers need to be involved and to understand the implications of what is happening to them. They need to be given enough responsibility to be able to take control. They also need to know what options are available to them so that they can make choices and seek information when they require it. Knowledge is power for teenagers, and helps to restore independence which is so vital to their coping strategies.

Jamison et al.,[5] in a study of the psychosocial impact of cancer on adolescents, found that knowledge of cancer was positively related to self image and suggested that increased knowledge may help with adjustment.

Parents often try to take control, assuming that teenagers are too unwell to be given autonomy, but undermining their freedom of choice will only cause antagonism and resentment and teenage patients are then likely to cease to comply and respond and may even opt out of treatment.

Teenagers do need to maintain the support and understanding of their parents but at the same time want to avoid regression to childlike behaviour and dependence on others. Allowing them to make their own decisions will help to facilitate this and will return some control to them when they badly need to feel that their feelings and values are respected.

Control can also be facilitated by negotiating with teenagers to become

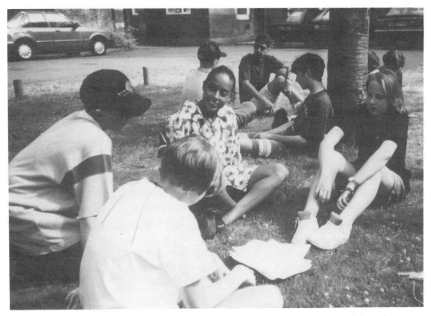

Fig 17.1 Group holidays help teenagers keep their freedom and independence.

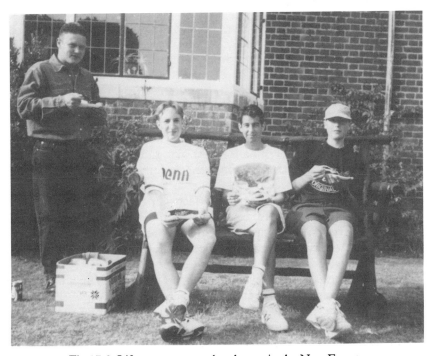

Fig 17.2 Life goes on: a weekend away in the New Forest.

active participants in their own care which, again, will give them a sense of responsibility and help to minimise their concerns.

Threat to body image and peer support

Sometimes teenagers will give vent to anger, frustration and sadness—especially when they are confronted with so many insults to their body image, in terms of delayed sexual maturity, alopecia, debilitation, weight changes, or lack of energy. It is particularly difficult for girls to lose their hair because it is a very visible sign of sexual attractiveness and loss of hair sets them apart from their peers. Weight gain or loss may be very alarming, and although teenagers are encouraged to resume normal activity, sustaining that activity may be difficult, if energy levels are low.

Sadly, some teenagers must endure the indignity of limb amputation, when not only do they grieve over the loss of a limb but also grieve over a loss of freedom and function and find themselves dependent on others—their independence, peer relationships, and future plans may all be compromised.

The reality of the damage caused by cancer may be difficult to accept because a physical disability needs to be adapted to and a value system changed, so that they are able to accommodate a new perception of the "self" and a change of status within the peer group. Clearly, their opportunity to socialise may be severely limited.

Peer group approval and the need to conform may actually force teenagers to hide their feelings and emotions—unless peers are educated to help with this adjustment, teenagers may find themselves increasingly isolated and once again their self image is distorted and their self esteem is damaged. A great deal of constructive support is required to make so many adjustments.

Older teenagers may be involved in a relationship and may feel unable to continue with it or, worse still, their partner may leave. At this stage they may feel the need to rejoin the family even though it may feel like a substantial blow to their pride.

Hospitalisation inevitably limits socialisation and contact with peers, and teenagers who have experienced treatment for cancer will argue strongly in favour of a return to school or college to restore a sense of mastery, independence, normality, and social contact.

It is difficult to appreciate this, however, during the treatment phase when energy levels are low, physical activity is limited, and frequent absence is unavoidable. It is difficult to overcome a distorted self image and a natural self consciousness.

It is important that liaison with schools or colleges is facilitated so that other pupils are receptive to them and studies are compromised as little as possible. It is also helpful if oncology units are flexible with treatment protocols, to allow teenagers to resume as normal a lifestyle as possible. Tutorial assistance may be helpful, but it is still necessary to encourage socialisation in school or college, if at all possible.

Denial

Teenagers may use denial as a means of reinforcing their perception of their own indestructibility, and it appears that for teenagers with cancer, denial is a part of the process of adjustment to their diagnosis. If it is used as a coping mechanism then it is important that nurses respect this and allow them to progress at their own pace.

Chesler *et al*[6] have commented that denial of bad feelings and bad outcome is a common and relatively healthy coping mechanism for teenagers with cancer. They also suggest that these patients may hide their distress from doctors and parents to protect themselves from intrusive procedures and their parents from further pain and burden.

Hinds[7] discusses the concept of adaptive denial which may be healthy—but it is also important to be aware when denial is maladaptive, because professionals could fall into the trap of ignoring cues. It may be necessary to assess the nature of denial in each person, and to work with it, according to individual needs.

Provision of own space

Socialisation is a crucial developmental task for teenagers, and during their time in hospital they should be provided with their own space wherever they are looked after. This will allow them to pursue normal teenage activity or non-activity if they so wish. It may also provide the opportunity to socialise with other people with similar problems. It is helpful to this age group if they are able to participate in group activities like a weekend away or a support group.

The Macline

Teenagers need help to regain a degree of equilibrium and control in their lives, and it was with this in mind that Cancer Relief Macmillan Fund launched a new helpline for teenagers with cancer.

A questionnaire circulated to 25 teenagers with cancer indicated that they welcomed this initiative, and the helpline was launched in 1993. CancerLink, a charity associated to Cancer Relief, took up the challenge and their experienced counsellors are now operating the line. It is a free and confidential service open to all teenagers with cancer and their relatives.

This type of initiative will contribute to teenagers feeling that society believes their needs to be worthy of consideration, as would more interest in the setting up of teenage units.

Adolescent units

Recognition of the very specific needs of teenagers with cancer is fundamental to their care and to their future quality of life and the question arises as to whether teenagers should be nursed on a teenage unit where the environment is tailored to their individual requirements. Based on the fact that teenagers fall between childhood and adulthood, it would be easier to meet their needs on a purpose-built unit where appropriate facilities and resources are provided; and where they have the chance to interact with people of their own age. Many people have made recommendations to this effect.

In 1959 the Platt report[8] recommended separate accommodation for teenagers, but this was largely ignored. In 1985 the British Paediatric Association[9] made detailed recommendations regarding accommodation and highlighted some problems inherent in nursing adolescents with either adults or children. It was suggested that a ward for teenagers would benefit them because their developmental needs should assume more importance than their clinical disorders. They also identified the need for privacy, education, and recreation. They stated that teenagers would be frustrated with the noise and lack of privacy on a children's ward and would feel like misfits on an adult ward. It was suggested that transfer to adult services should take account of level of maturity rather than age.

This can be a particularly difficult time for teenagers because it is hard to leave the safety of familiar staff and a familiar environment and they require comprehensive preparation and explanation. It is also important to consider transferring this age group to an adult service before events like relapse occur.

In 1986 the World Health Organization[10] contributed to the debate by stating that teenagers would find adult wards unaware of their needs and children's wards would be an unacceptable setting.

The 1991 report of NAWCH (now named Action for Sick Children)[11] made clear recommendations for the hospitalised care of adolescents and these were supported by the UK Department of Health in 1991.[12]

In the wake of the Allitt inquiry in 1994 the Royal College of Nursing[13] have reviewed guidelines for the care of sick children and state that although adolescents deserve special attention, services for them are particularly poor.

It could be argued that symptom distress would be reduced if adolescents were nursed in an appropriate environment. Gillies and Parry Jones[14] suggest that by nursing teenagers in an appropriate environment their anxiety would be reduced, and it would be easier to relieve their symptoms—outcome would be improved and discharge could be earlier.

Blunden[15] looked at where adolescents would choose to be nursed. She questioned 85 healthy adolescents. The 11 + age group opted for a children's ward; the 12 + and 13 + age group opted for an adolescent ward. When asked to choose between a children's and an adult ward, the 11 + chose a children's ward, more of the 12 + chose a children's ward, and the 13 + group were almost equally divided between the two. It was interesting to note that when she asked if they felt that young people should have a voice in decisions about care in hospital, 100% answered in the affirmative.

Teenagers do speak a different language at times, and staff need to be able to communicate with them and know how to set limits on unacceptable behaviour. Blunden[15] looked at the syllabus for nurse training and found that those with a mental health training were best qualified to understand this age group. The children's nurses covered teenagers in less depth and the general trained nurses, hardly at all. This research indicates that nurses require more comprehensive training if they are to fulfil the needs of teenagers. They also require strong and mature leadership to supervise their interactions, as most nurses will be of a similar age and need to be aware of boundaries of involvement. In 1976 the Court report[16] recommended that staff caring for adolescents should receive additional training to help meet their specific needs, and yet it is clear that very little has been done about it.

There appear to be a number of reasons why all these recommendations have not been implemented. Staff who care for this age group may not be trained well enough to be aware of their needs. The internal market system in the NHS has created a change in patterns of care delivery and increased the emphasis on cost effectiveness. Adolescents are considered to be a small group, and the financial implications make the creation of specialist accommodation with specialist staff unattractive to providers of health care.

The Teenage Cancer Trust has made a substantial and welcome contribution to the provision of units for this age group, but it cannot be expected to pick up running costs which should be the responsibility of the provider unit. Research is needed to demonstrate that meeting the social and emotional requirements of adolescents will improve their long term outlook, and more importantly, in the eyes of the providers, will reduce costs, although this will be difficult to prove.

Teenagers and death

Many nurses caring for teenagers may feel able to identify with them because they have not long since left this stage of life behind. They may find it difficult to confront their own mortality, and experience great difficulty in dealing with the death of this age group. Sensitive support from senior members of staff may well be needed.

Zeltzer et al.[17] have observed that teenagers see themselves as immortal and view death as something possible only in the distant unforeseeable future. Teenagers certainly have a compulsive need to prove that they are alive and that they are invincible—hence their need to defy death by driving fast cars or motorbikes. Thus, although they are mature enough to consider death in concrete terms, if fears about it surface they will have great difficulty in confronting it.

Adolescence is, of course, a time of life when many losses are experienced which are related to leaving childhood behind and progressing into adulthood. The death of teenagers, therefore, is particularly poignant because they are on the threshold of adult life and have a strong orientation towards the future. Their sense of loss encompasses both the loss of the past and the loss of the future. Questions such as 'Why me?' 'What did I do?' 'Why can't I be? . . .' can be bitter and painful and have no answers.[18] Elizabeth Kubler-Ross[19] said, "Everyone has a right to know that they are dying but not everyone needs to know". It does seem, that for young people in particular, there is a conflict between what is known intellectually and what is known emotionally. They understand that they are going to die, but at the same time, in order to remain in touch with life and make the most of it, they deny it at some level.

Although it can be helpful to use denial as a means of compartmentalising death, it may contribute to mutual pretence when teenagers and parents, in an effort to protect each other, find that they are unable to communicate. This only adds to the teenagers' loneliness and fear, and causes unnecessary emotional pain. They may then find that they are unable to confide in anyone before they die because there is no one they feel able to trust.

Parents may require support and help to be honest, because their fear may heighten their need to protect their children from painful knowledge. If they are able to be honest they will be able to maintain or regain trust, which is so necessary for interactions with this age group.

It may be that teenagers are not ready to give vent to their feelings or discuss their many anxieties, but it is important that they know that they have permission to do so and that they can feel safe. At this time, probably more than at any other, teenagers need to feel in control.

Teenagers are likely to be uncertain about an afterlife and may need to discuss this area. They must also be given the opportunity to ask questions about issues related to symptom control, and be able to express fears about the time of death. They should be given the opportunity to talk about their anger and frustration, and, most important of all, they need the chance to say goodbye. It is for this last reason that home care is so vital for this age group if at all possible. They are then able to set their affairs in order and make the most of the time they have left. It seems that teenagers are particularly mature in this respect and often become a source of support and strength to their family.

Late effects

The cure rate for children and young adults treated for cancer has improved dramatically over the last 20 years. By the year 2000 approximately 1 in 1000 young adults will be a survivor of childhood cancer.[20] This success has been due to the use of increasingly toxic treatment regimes and better supportive care — but a price has had to be paid in terms of toxic side effects, for example short stature, intellectual deficits, and infertility. As more and more children survive childhood cancer, the long term effects of treatments are becoming evident.

For teenagers, by far the most worrying effect is infertility because of its impact on their role as sexual partners and parents. Sensitive guidance and support are required and alternative suggestions made such as adoption or in vitro fertilisation. If possible, boys should be offered the facility of sperm banking. Muscle wasting, compromised growth, and impaired endocrine and intellectual functioning are all particularly problematic for teenagers, but improvements in techniques and more rigorous follow up is helping to counteract these problems.

Some late effects have only recently come to our attention, in particular with regard to the psychosocial consequences of disease and treatment, which could compromise long term adjustment.

The way that the future is viewed depends upon the developmental stage of the person and the essence of their past experience and for teenagers part of growing up involves an orientation towards the future in terms of career, relationships, and a way of life. They need to be able to set realistic goals and have a sense of purpose to provide direction and a sense of fulfilment. Adolescents may be concerned that the effects of disease and treatment may limit their future possibilities. The threat of recurrence and second malignancy, therefore, are particularly problematic for this age group, and help may be required to re-establish direction and motivation and a positive self esteem.

Achieving a positive self esteem is challenging for everyone in life and it is debatable whether the cancer experience causes difficulties with adult adjustment or whether it allows teenagers to grow into stronger people. Greenberg et al.[21] and Koocher and O'Malley[22] found that survivors of childhood cancer had a poorer self concept and greater adjustment problems than a similar group of well children, and these problems could therefore be attributed to the sequelae of the cancer experience. Kellerman et al.[23] on the other hand, found that the consequences of childhood cancer are incorrectly seen as lowering the person's self esteem. Chesler[24] felt that self esteem issues are a major worry for adolescent cancer survivors and second only to physical health worries. Overbaugh et al.[25] have commented on the fact that parents' attitudes and concerns will influence teenagers' attitudes to themselves and their future orientation.

Teenagers embarking on a career may find it difficult to obtain insurance cover or indeed employment, and they may be discriminated against if they are trying for military service or the police force, because there is still much ignorance about the cure rate for childhood cancer.

Fortunately, clinicians have recognised the importance of long term follow up for survivors of childhood cancer, and clinics are being set up for this specific purpose. Efforts are, however, often concentrated on monitoring the physical sequelae of treatment and more time needs to be given to psychosocial screening and education regarding a healthy lifestyle. The reality of the damage caused by cancer may be difficult for teenagers to accept, and they may need help to realise that life is back to normal and that they have left their cancer behind. Responsibility for progress in survival can only be justified if there is quality to that survival.

261

Conclusion

We make too many assumptions about teenagers based on the rather negative attitudes of society, and yet in the face of cancer they are capable of demonstrating a special kind of courage and wisdom.

Teenagers are experiencing a stage of rapid learning both cognitively and emotionally, and their self esteem is easily bruised, especially when they are faced with a life-threatening illness. They are old enough to be aware of the dangers of cancer and yet they are young enough to feel cheated out of life.

Recognition of the needs of this age group is fundamental to their future development and subsequently to their quality of life. Professionals need to develop the skills to be able to recognise problems which are specific to this age group and aim to care for them in the context of their unique world helping them to restore positive expectations about the future.

The challenge of looking after teenagers with cancer is unique. They need boundaries and they need freedom to keep their independence intact. As one young man said: "Just treat us like regular human beings".

1 Elder SL. Impact of major life transitions on adolescent development. In: Morgan JD ed. *The dying and the bereaved teenager*. Philadelphia: The Charles Press, 1990.
2 Kuykendall J. Adolescence. Teenage trauma. *Nurs Times* 1989; 5 July; **85**(27): 26–8.
3 Erikson EH. *Identity, youth and crisis*. New York: Norton, 1968.
4 Tipping G, Schwartz C, Chapman R. Teenagers in hospital. *Cascade* 1993; July: 4–5.
5 Jamison RN, Lewis S, Burish TG. Psychological impact of cancer on adolescents: Self-image, locus of control, perception of illness and knowledge of cancer. *J Chron Dis* 1986; **39**: 609–17.
6 Chesler MA, Weigers M, Lawther T. How am I different? Perspectives of childhood cancer survivors on change and growth. In Green DM, D'Angio GJ ed. *Late effect of treatment for childhood cancer*. Bognor Regis: Wiley-Liss, 1992, 151–8.
7 Hinds PS. Quality of life in children and adolescents with cancer. *Seminars in Onc Nurs* 1990; **6**(4): 285–92.
8 Platt H. *Report of the committee on the welfare of children in hospital*. London: HMSO, 1959.
9 British Paediatric Association. *Report of the working party on the needs and care of adolescents*. London: BPA, 1985.
10 World Health Organisation. *Young people's health—a challenge for society*. Geneva: WHO, 1986.
11 National Association for the Welfare of Children in Hospital. *Setting standards for adolescent in hospital*. Quality Review Series. London: NAWCH, 1990.
12 Department of Health. *Welfare of children and young people in hospital*. London: HMSO, 1991.
13 Gillies M, Parry-Jones WLI. Adolescents in a children's hospital. A report of a prospective study. *Arch Dis Child* 1992; **67**: 1506–9.
14 Royal College of Nursing. *The care of sick children—a review of the guidelines in the wake of the Allitt Inquiry*. London: RCN, 1994.
15 Blunden R. An artificial state. *J Paediatr Nurs* 1989; **1**: 12–13.
16 Court S. *Fit for the future: the report of the committee on child health services*. London: HMSO, 1976.
17 Zeltzer LK. The adolescent with cancer. In Kellerman J, ed., *Psychological aspects of childhood cancer*. Springfield Ill: Charles C. Thomas, 1980.
18 Hodson D. The special needs of children and adolescents. In Penson J. ed., *Bereavement: A guide for nurses*. London: Harper & Row, 1990, 151.
19 Kubler-Ross E. *On death and dying*. London: Tavistock, 1971.
20 Meadows AT, Hobbie WL. The medical consequences of cure. *Cancer* 1986; **58**: 524–8.

21 Greenberg HSX, Kazaak AE, Meadows AT. Psychologic functioning in 8 to 16 year old cancer survivors and their parents. *J Pediatr* 1989; **114**: 488–93.

22 Koocher GP, O'Malley JE. *The Damocles syndrome. Psychosocial consequences of surviving childhood cancer.* New York: McGraw-Hill, 1981.

23 Kellerman J, Zeltzer L, Elleberg L *et al.* Psychological effects of illness in adolescence. 1. Anxiety, self-esteem, and perception of control. *J Pediatr* 1980; **97**: 126–31.

24 Chesler MA. Surviving childhood cancer: The struggle goes on. *J Pediatr Oncol Nurs* 1989; **7**: 57–9.

25 Overbaugh KA, Sawin K. Future life expectations and self-esteem of the adolescent survivor of childhood cancer. *J Pediatr Oncol Nurs* 1992; **9**(1): 8–16.

263

18: The impact of treatment: adolescents' views

CHRISTINE EISER

A diagnosis of cancer is likely to have devastating effects whenever it occurs, but is especially damaging during adolescence. Unlike younger children, adolescents are well enough informed to realise that something is seriously wrong. However, they may not be as able as older adults to deal with the knowledge. First, information is complex and difficult to understand. Second, adolescents may be less able to deal with the uncertainties. Third, compared with older people, adolescents with cancer have little peer and social support. They are becoming independent of the nuclear family, but may not yet have formed close interpersonal relationships on their own. Fourth, a diagnosis of a life-threatening disease during adolescence is out of time. Thus, there is a far greater and more negative disruption of normal activities and impact on self esteem. More than at any other time of life, therefore, adolescents may find that the experience of cancer is a crisis that has to be managed alone.

We have not previously treated adolescents as a distinct group, but rather assumed that their experiences and needs can be inferred from a knowledge of the impact of cancer during childhood more generally. This failure to recognise the uniqueness of adolescence means that we are forced to make assumptions about the effects of cancer based on studies involving children across a wide age span. This practice stems from the limited survival times which characterised many child cancers until recently. It remains very much a numbers problem. Few centres have large populations of adolescents, and certainly not populations at a similar stage of illness. We must look toward the development of multicentre collaborative projects in order to recruit samples of sufficient size that relevant findings are statistically likely to emerge.

It is also important that work develops more systematically from established theories of adolescent development. Many of our findings are based on anecdotal reports or small scale clinical projects which use measures of convenience rather than those which might be hypothesised to be important during this particular phase of the life cycle. Adolescents with cancer live in two worlds; that of the hospital patient and that of the healthy. However, everyday difficulties and daily hassles—completing homework on time, resolving disagreements with parents, making employment decisions—which affect all adolescents can appear magnified when these are combined with the demands of treatment. The point has been made previously by van Eys:[1]

> It must be considered normal to have cancer. Life, the business of the child, must be on-going, not in spite of the cancer, but with the cancer.

Thus, it is important that understanding of the impact of cancer on adolescents parallels and reflects issues which affect all adolescents.

Healthy development during adolescence

Adolescence is often a difficult time for young people and their parents. Although it is no longer recognised to be universally a period of "storm and stress",[2] it is undoubtedly a potentially difficult time. It is characterised by transitions, changes, and decisions.[3] Transitions are made from school to work, and from the nuclear family to independent relationships. There are many changes, most notably with respect to physical appearance. Decisions must be made with respect to career choice, marriage, where and how life is lived.

Certainly many parents point to the time when their child was adolescent as one of the most stressful. Pasley and Gecas[4] reported that 62% of mothers and 64% of fathers said it was the most difficult part of bringing up a child. Parents reported difficulties in that they had less control over what the adolescent did, so that they became increasingly concerned about individual safety. They were also annoyed by adolescent behaviour. Adolescents like their music too loud, they dress scruffily, and they leave things lying around. Experimentation with alcohol, drugs, and sexuality create concerns among parents and conflicts within the family as acceptable limits of behaviour are negotiated between parent and child. These conflicts are very much part of our culture. A few years ago, when we were just entering the world of being parents to an adolescent, I can remember suggesting to my son that he was being a bit hard to live with lately. He snapped back: "I'm an adolescent; it's my job to be difficult . . .".

The hallmark of adolescent development is the ability to "think about thinking".[5] This preoccupation is not without its costs. The assumption that everyone else thinks about the same things as the adolescent, coupled with a concern about their own appearance and behaviour, results in a logical error so that adolescents are convinced that they are the centre of everyone's attention. Hence, the belief that no one, or no previous generation, has ever experienced emotions so intensely, or lived life so fully, as themselves.

This egocentric confusion has two consequences. First, there is the creation of an *imaginary audience*. Adolescents believe that everyone else is looking at them and they are therefore overly concerned with their own appearance. The audience is imaginary, in that others are rarely as fascinated by their behaviour as adolescents believe. Nevertheless, the result can be a painful embarrassment and self consciousness. The belief in the imaginary audience declines in late adolescence, but a second confusion, the *personal fable*, lasts much longer. Adolescents believe their own thoughts and actions are original and special, unique and intense. The belief in a personal fable may cloud judgements and result in a belief in personal invulnerability. A diagnosis of a life-threatening disease is incompatible with such a belief.

The challenge of adolescence is to achieve independence and autonomy, while at the same time maintaining close and supportive ties with the nuclear family.[6] This may be specially difficult for adolescents with cancer to achieve, in that increased dependence on parents is inevitable. Emotional bonds may be deepened through awareness of the potentially life-threatening nature of the condition. There are practical ties too resulting from parents' involvement in home-based treatments.[7]

For the adolescent with cancer, some of the normative decisions are even more complex. In addition, there may be other complications. Some careers may simply not be available.[8] Life insurance and a driving licence may be difficult to obtain.[9] The break from the nuclear family may be more difficult. The child with cancer is dependent on parents in many ways. Dependence is increased because parents may be responsible for some aspects of home care; they will certainly have acted as advocates for their child in interactions with medical staff. The crisis of treatment for a life-threatening disease may very much influence the relationship. For some, the result is increased closeness and empathy; for others, the occurrence of illness is more divisive. While it can be more difficult for the adolescent to break free of the family, it may also prove hard to establish new relationships. At what point do adolescents decide to tell a new friend that they are being, or have been, treated for cancer? Adolescents who do disclose may experience rejection. However, keeping the information secret may cause problems and in fact jeopardize the establishment of new relationships, as friends sense that something is being hidden. In most relationships, there comes a time when it is necessary to reveal information about the illness. Adolescents must balance the need to be honest with friends against the risk of rejection and loss of self image.

Methodological issues

Given current methodologies, it is difficult to discuss the impact of treatment specifically from the perspective of the adolescent, since most contemporary research includes clinic populations covering wide age ranges. These studies indicate concerns generally, but do not give insight as to the unique experience during adolescence. Much of what follows, therefore, is based on a selective review of the literature to include work which involves samples of older children and adolescents. Issues which are most clearly of relevance for preschool children[10] are not included.

Knowledge and beliefs about the illness

Given the complexity of information about cancer, it is not surprising that adolescents often seem poorly informed about basic aspects of their illness. Levenson et al.[11] asked 55 cancer patients (aged 11–20 years) and their parents to complete written questionnaires to determine disparities in knowledge of cancer-related tests and treatments, relative importance of disease-related information, responses evoked by information, and need for additional information. They reported significant differences in three of the four areas, the exception being responses evoked by information. Parents were more concerned about self-help efforts, the effects of patient behaviour on health, and sociopersonal factors, and wanted more information compared with their children. Discrepancies between parents and children were not related to demographic variables. The authors concluded that some family conflict may be the result of differences in knowledge between parents and their children. Some conflict may be resolved by ensuring a degree of consensus within the family, especially with regard to information about the severity of the disease, rationale for treatment and impact of general health behaviour (especially drinking and smoking) on the effectiveness of therapy.

Other work suggests that many adolescents have little clear idea about their illness. Everhart[12] used a questionnaire to determine knowledge in children over 12 years of age. She concluded that knowledge was often characteristic of much younger children. For example, one 12-year-old survivor of Wilm's tumour explained that "they took out my kidney and gave me another stomach. So now I have two stomachs. That's why I eat so much". While it is to be expected that knowledge in some survivors will be inadequate, small scale studies of this type need to be interpreted carefully. On the one hand, it is perhaps surprising that the child's natural curiosity had not led her to determine something about her medical history. On the other hand, she had first been treated when she was 2 years old, and appears to have since been well; perhaps there is little point in discussing history, unless it has some implications for current health.

Communication and compliance

Knowledge has also been considered important for its implications for parent–child communication and compliance with treatment. Tebbi et al.[13] studied 16 parent–child pairs. Children had cancer and were under 17 years. There was much similarity in response in terms of knowledge about illness, medication, treatment, and compliance. Parent–child correlations increased with age. It was concluded that good parent–child communication is important for compliance.

Cohen et al.[14] focused on quantity and quality of parent–child communication. A correlational analysis was used to indicate agreement between parents and child about the amount of communication about the disease. Frequency of communication increased with the number of side effects experienced by the child.

These studies suggest considerable consistency between parents and children. If there is disagreement, it tends to be in terms of estimates of the impact of the disease, with mothers reporting greater impact than their children. It is unlikely that such a discrepancy would be detrimental in terms of adolescent's compliance with treatment, though it might account for reports of overprotectiveness by parents. Again, we have the example of how normal parent–child conflict during adolescence can be magnified by cancer. There has been a tendency to assume that any differences between parents and children will be negative. In fact, the nature of the discrepancies may be important. Reports of parental restrictions may follow from disagreements about the impact of the disease. Disagreements about responsibility for self care may be more likely to have a direct effect on compliance and physical health.

What does a diagnosis of cancer mean to adolescents?

Some years ago, it was considered wise to protect children and adolescents from the knowledge that they had a life-threatening condition.[15] This decision was usually justified in the light of the very poor prognosis which inevitably followed the diagnosis of cancer. A number of factors have contributed to the more open approaches generally favoured today. Prognosis has improved significantly; the fact that cancer is no longer an absolute death threat means that information does not need to be thoroughly negative and pessimistic. Modern therapies increasingly involve a degree of self care; therefore it is necessary to involve the adolescent and offer some explanation as to why compliance with treatment advice is essential. Secondly, there was evidence that adolescents were curious about their condition; if they were not given a satisfactory explanation, they set about finding out for themselves.[16] The consequences of inadequate knowledge appeared significant. Spinetta and Spinetta[17] showed that terminally ill children who did not have the opportunity to discuss their concerns were withdrawn and distressed. In contrast, Slavin et al.[18] showed that children were better adjusted to the condition where they were informed either on diagnosis, or within one year if they were initially less than 6 years old. Most recently, Claflin and Barbarin[19] concluded that the effect of withholding information was to make children feel lonely and isolated; "If the goal of limited disclosure was to spare young children from emotional arousal, the goal was not achieved in the long-term".

Increasingly, it is seen necessary not only to inform children about their condition, but also to make efforts to involve them actively in decision making about treatment. Ellis and Leventhal[20] administered questionnaires to 50 children (aged 8–17 years) and 60 accompanying parents about their informational needs and decision making preferences. The study points only to population differences between parents and their children in the sort of information they would like. Children wanted information about all aspects of the disease. Although 76% of children specifically wanted information about prognosis, only 38% of parents felt this was appropriate for their children. Otherwise the study only hints at disagreements. Children accepted that decisions about initial treatment should be made by others, but wanted more say in decisions about palliative therapy. Ten percent of children and 44% of parents felt that the child made personal decisions about treatment. However, 39% of patients and 16% of parents felt that they had little or no say in treatment decisions. Such decisions were seen to be made almost exclusively by physicians. Other potential conflicts might be anticipated from the finding that only 37% of children considered their condition to be serious, in contrast to 75% of parents. Such a discrepancy may reflect lack of knowledge in the adolescent, or be part of the general feeling of personal invulnerability typical of adolescence. However, as adolescents demand more say in their treatment, it seems imperative that we consider more systematically their understanding of the disease, in that this will form the basis on which they are likely to make decisions about continuing or terminating therapy.

Adolescents' concerns: some interviews

Our awareness of how cancer affects adolescents is therefore based on a handful of studies which have adopted a limited number of methods. These have included formal questionnaires, especially to assess knowledge or beliefs about the condition and its prognosis, or more informal semi-structured interviews. The fact that work tends to be based on small samples in specialist clinics means that it is not possible to infer how the majority of children and adolescents experience and understand the illness. What does cancer mean to an adolescent? Much of what we know is based on parents' reports. Yet parents are not always reliable informants for their children.[21]

In considering what adolescents think about cancer, we are therefore forced to rely on a number of separate studies, often based on small samples and clinical anecdote. It is easy to criticise these studies from methodological perspectives. Yet in the absence of any formal assessment tool, there is little choice. In the remainder of this chapter, I would like to consider some of the key elements which should be included in any comprehensive assessment of adolescents' concerns.[22] I would like then to present some preliminary findings in which we have attempted to develop a more formal instrument to assess adolescents' experiences of cancer.

I am drawing on literature which describes views of parents, children and teachers about the impact of cancer and will consider the findings in relation to eight "themes". These include physical appearance, activity, restrictions, integration in school, effects on the family, manipulation, disclosure, preoccupation with the illness, and impact of treatment.

First, adolescents express concern about changes in their physical appearance as a result of cancer. The problem is particularly acute for newly diagnosed patients who must endure very visible changes in their appearance. Loss of hair has frequently been cited as a major cause of concern in young people.[23][24]

Second, there is a reduction in activity[25] partly through sickness or tiredness, partly through rejection.[26][27] Ross and Ross[28] reported that children with leukaemia cite being teased on return to school because of hair loss or visible changes in weight as worse than the physical pain from the disease or diagnostic procedures. Children with cancer have been reported to be isolated and have difficulties with peer relationships.[29] This peer rejection has implications for integration in school. Children "must be prepared to handle teasing, questions, and comments from peers, in addition to allaying their own concerns about feeling different and unattractive".[30] Although hospital policy is generally to encourage children to return to school as soon as possible after diagnosis, many experience some difficulties. Absences[31][32] and in extreme cases, school phobia, have been reported.[33] Teachers report that they are uncertain about how to handle sick children, especially in setting limits to their behaviour. There is some suggestion that children use the illness to their advantage; they become adept at manipulation.[34] This has consequences for the family.[35] The literature has long suggested that parents overprotect sick children. For the children the result is limited activities which in turn can become a source of conflict.[36] Conflict can also be created through lack of communication. In particular, the very early literature suggested that children and adolescents were aware of the seriousness of their disease and deliberately did not discuss their fears in order not to distress their parents further.[37] In their study of a Dutch population, Veldhuizen and Last[23] reported that one quarter of children interviewed did not want to ask their parents questions about the illness in attempts to protect them; there was a lack of disclosure. The threat of recurrence can result in a preoccupation with illness.[38] Given the extended follow ups and need for care and treatment beyond the initial treatment phase, it is not surprising that many parents report continual anxiety about the child. Finally, for those on treatment, there are mood swings, concerns about infection resulting in restricted activities, and general uncertainties which mean that the period on treatment is traumatic.[39]

In a preliminary study, we attempted to confirm how far adolescents themselves identified these areas to be problematic. We conducted informal interviews with 13 adolescents who had been diagnosed with a range of cancers. At the time of interview, all were well and in remission. Adolescents were told that we wanted to hear from them about their experiences so that we would be better able to help others in the future. To help them remember, it was suggested that they tried to recall their stories historically, i.e. beginning from when they realised something was wrong, through the diagnosis, immediate hospitalisation and therapy, through to the period on maintenance therapy and return to school. Here are a few of their comments.

Physical appearance

My hair fell out, that was one of the worst parts actually because when you are at school and I just thought I am a real man now, cos I had some hair growing under my arms. Yeah, real man and then it all fell out. My eyebrows that was the worst, cos you look in the mirror, fair enough you are bald on top, cos everyone knows your hair falls out there, but no one realises about your eyebrows and all your hair on your arms and you are just completely bald and that was what I didn't like much. They said I could wear wigs but I didn't want that; if I was bald, I was bald.

Activity

I can't walk very fast and I worry about falling over. It's difficult to go out unless someone gives me a lift. I worry about crossing the road as if there's a bump I might fall over.

Rejection

At school, they just talk about their girlfriends and boyfriends. I don't know half the people they are talking about and they just exclude me.

I used to think that if I saw someone talking to somebody else it was about me. At 15, that's the way you think.

It's not the time away from school that matters but that all your friends have moved on. When I went back it was leading up to choosing options. Lots of others had no idea what they wanted to do but I went by the marks I got. Go for subjects that you really like and teachers I liked. Lots of people just took options that looked easy. I wasn't interested in that. They were all at the age of just being interested in going into town and getting legless; I wasn't interested in that.

Integration in school

They can put you on a pedestal; Matthew must go for lunch first, Matthew can leave early today, Matthew doesn't need to worry about finishing that painting . . . They are like that if you are bald.

Sometimes you feel a bit tired and stuff but because I never liked school I used to get bored. One thing I really hate is I could do something wrong and the teacher would just say "don't do that" but if my mate was to do something exactly the same, he had to go out and I reckon they should have treated me the same. Just because I had leukaemia, they decided to be a bit soft. I just wanted to be treated as normal, like before, like I was the same as everyone else. Afterwards they treated me completely different, like no one likes being told off and kicked out of the class, but near the end I did go a bit far and they said he is not a special boy any more and then I got expelled for one day and I thought yes this is like back to normal.

I just rebelled, I don't want people to feel sorry for me. I just wanted to get into trouble cause my mates used to tease me, they never meant harm. They used to say you won't get into trouble, you can do anything and that is half the reason I done it.

Manipulation

I used to have pains in my leg and my dad would put cream on but that didn't work, and my mum and dad said are you going to the doctor? and I said yes, and my mum said I hope you're not doing this for school and I said no and I went to the doctor.

271

Family

> Dad wraps me up in cotton wool and treats me like a little girl and wonders if I'll manage to do a lot of things.

Disclosure

> People are always asking me "what's it like having cancer? Why did your hair fall out? Why do you go to the hospital so much?" I get really annoyed, as I don't want to talk about it.

> I wanted to know the chances, but I didn't want to ask in front of my parents; I didn't want them to know. We were trying to protect each other. It would have been good if I could have spoken to the consultant on my own.

Preoccupation with illness

> I have cataracts in both eyes . . . I wonder if it will ever stop.

> I was very anxious. When you are on treatment it's like a support, because you know the cells are being killed off. Then you're let out and there's nothing stopping these cells. I was very worried it would come back. I felt safer on the drugs. I am always checking to see if I look pale. I don't think I could stand to do it again if I relapsed, because you know what it is.

Treatment

> I had aching in my legs. The doctors tested me for TB. They thought it was an infection on the bone and gave me antibiotics. Then they took me off painkillers to see if I was faking. One consultant knew about cancer but the tests were cancelled because they thought I was putting it on . . . The nurse still thought I was putting it on. They said if you're really in pain you'll have to stop crying or they won't be able to tell the doctors. So I would stop crying and then they said see it's not so bad.

> The treatment is horrid, be careful the line doesn't get jammed. I hated that. Don't get ratty and don't feel sorry for yourself, don't winge and don't get spoiled. It was boring. I got tired and fed up and in the end moody.

Interviews are often lengthy and time consuming. Some adolescents feel uncomfortable answering detailed interviews, and can resent personal questions.[40] For those circumstances in which interviews are less appropriate we put together a questionnaire which reflected some of the main themes coming through the interviews.[41] A preliminary sample of 70 items were put together, including 8 which were specifically concerned with the effects of treatment. These statements were presented as a series of ideas that other children had had about how their illness had affected their lives. Adolescents were asked to rate how much they agreed or disagreed with each one. Ratings were made on five point scales, with higher scores indicating greater awareness or perceived impact.

The questionnaires were administered to 41 young people with cancer attending the Royal Victoria Infirmary, Newcastle. A parallel version of the scale was completed by 35 of their patients (the remaining 6 patients attended clinic by themselves).

From discussions with the adolescents and preliminary statistical analyses, we were able to put together a briefer and more focused questionnaire, but one which included the themes we identified through the literature. Some examples which make up the subscales include the following:

- Physical appearance (I feel my illness has made me look different; I feel embarrassed about the way I look)
- Family (My parents use my illness to stop me doing things)
- Manipulation (I use my illness to get out of things I don't want to do).

In addition, there was a separate subscale to measure

- Impact of treatment (My treatment makes me very moody).

All subscales consisted of four items apart from physical appearance which included just two. Thus the total scale includes 38 items. Preliminary work on the scale suggests good internal reliability for the separate subscales described, as well as a combined score based on responses to all items. Significant correlations were also found between ratings made by patients and their parents on all subscales apart from disclosure and impact of treatment.

Conclusions

It is sometimes difficult to see the "adolescent" separately from the "adolescent with cancer". We have become increasingly aware of the need to provide interventions to help the child or adolescent with cancer cope with painful treatments.[42] There have been more limited attempts to tackle the extent to which they may also need help in dealing with everyday difficulties, such as being teased at school, or explaining to potential employers about the illness.[43]

The need for multicentre projects

Progress can only be made through intensive studies focusing on a specific age group and this requires collaboration across centres. Much can also be learned through the study of long term survivors, necessarily involving adolescents and young adults.[44]

The need for a developmental theory to understand the impact of cancer during adolescence

The fact that little work focuses exclusively on the adolescent as opposed to children in general is a limiting factor in our ability to understand the impact of cancer during different stages of development. It is clear from the work reviewed that research is not guided by contemporary theories of adolescence. Instead, research is guided by hunches about how cancer might be expected to influence any individual. Methodologies do not take into account the specific issues which are unique to adolescence and most likely to be adversely affected. Adolescents with cancer are ordinary people coping with exceptional circumstances. Assessments need to recognise this. General scales which focus on negative behaviours, or were developed for

273

psychiatric or learning-disabled children, are not appropriate. Our measure hopefully represents a first attempt to draw together some of the concerns as they uniquely affect adolescents with cancer. Assessments need to include issues relating to family dynamics and adolescent–parent relationships, the initiation of new social and peer relationships, self presentation, integration in the workforce and career, and other life decisions. Too much emphasis on interviews can be limited, in that adolescents may often be reluctant to discuss their feelings openly with a stranger. The need to present a positive self image may lead to a real underestimation of the extent to which cancer affects daily routines and functioning.

Although I have identified some themes which are important for adolescents with cancer, these are not substantially different from the issues which affect adolescence generally. All adolescents agonize over their looks, they are concerned with their own feelings and how they seem to others and they hate to be singled out and made to appear different or special in any way. Only by seeing adolescents with cancer *as adolescents* will we ultimately be acceptable as sources of support.

Acknowledgements

The author is funded by the Cancer Research Campaign, London (CP1019/0101). I would like to thank Joy Berrenberg and Dick Eiser for comments on an earlier version of this paper, Trudy Havermans for help in the collection of data and Professor A Craft, Dr J Kernahan, Dr A McNinch and Dr T Parkyn for allowing me to work in their clinics.

1 van Eys J. The truly cured child? *Pediatrician* 1977; **18**: 90–95.
2 Hall GS. Adolescence. In: *Psychology and its relations to physiology, anthropology, sociology, sex, crime, religion and education.* New York: 1904. Appleton.
3 Montemayor R, Adams GR, Gullotta TP (eds). (1990). *From childhood to adolescence: a transitional period?* London: Sage Publications.
4 Pasley K and Gecas V. Stresses and satisfaction of the parental role. *Person Guidance J* 1984; **2**: 400–4.
5 Elkind D. Egocentrism in adolescence. *Child Dev* 1967; **38**: 1025–34.
6 Erikson EH. Identity and the life-cycle. *Psych Issues* 1959; **1**: 18–164.
7 Zeltzer LK. The adolescent with cancer. In J Kellerman (ed.), *Psychological aspects of childhood cancer.* Springfield, Il: Thomas Publishers, 1980, 70–99.
8 Green DM, Zevon MA, Hall B. Achievement of life-goals by adult survivors of modern treatment for childhood cancer. *Cancer* 1991; **67**: 206–13.
9 Hays DM, Landsverk J, Sallan SE *et al.* Educational, occupational and insurance status of childhood cancer survivors in their fourth and fifth decades of life. *Psycho-Oncol* 1992; **10**: 1397–1406.
10 Horwitz WA, Kazak A. Family adaptation to childhood cancer: Sibling and family system variables. *J Clin Child Psychol* 1990; **19**: 221–8.
11 Levenson PM, Copeland DR, Morrow JR *et al.* Disparities in disease-related perceptions of adolescent cancer patients and their parents. *J Ped Psychiatr* 1983; **8**: 34–45.
12 Everhart C. Overcoming childhood cancer misconceptions among long-term survivors. *J Ped Oncol Nursing* 1991; **8**: 46–8.
13 Tebbi CK, Richards ME, Cummings M *et al.* The role of parent adolescent concordance in compliance with cancer chemotherapy. *Adolescence* 1988; **91**: 599–611.
14 Cohen S, Friedrich WN, Pendergrass TW. Instruments to measure parent-child communication regarding pediatric cancer. *Child Health Care* 1989; **18**: 142–5.

15 Share L. Family communication in the crisis of a child's fatal illness; a literature review and analysis. *Omega* 1972; **3**: 187–201.

16 Kendrick C, Culling J, Oakhill A, Mott M. Children's understanding of their illness and its treatment within a paediatric oncology unit. *ACPP (newsletter)* 1986; **8**: 16–20.

17 Spinetta JJ, Spinetta D eds. *Living with childhood cancer.* St Louis: Mosby, 1981.

18 Slavin LA, O'Malley JE, Koocher G, Foster DJ. Communication of the cancer diagnosis to pediatric patients: Impact on long-term adjustment. *Am J Psychiatr* 1982; **139**: 179–83.

19 Claflin CJ, Barbarin OA. Does telling less protect more? Relationships among age, information disclosure, and what children with cancer see and feel. *J Pediatr Psychol* 1991; **16**: 169–92.

20 Ellis R, Leventhal B. Information needs and decision-making preferences of children with cancer. *Psycho-Oncol* 1993; **2**: 277–84.

21 Mulhern RK, Crisco JJ, Camitta BM. Patterns of communication among pediatric patients with leukaemia, parents and physicians; prognostic disagreements and misunderstandings. *J Pediatr* 1989; **83**: 480–3.

22 Noll RB, Bukowski WM, Davies WH *et al.* Adjustment in the peer system of adolescents with cancer: A two-year study. *J Pediatr Psychol* 1993; **18**: 351–64.

23 van Veldhuizen AM, Last BF. *Children with cancer: communication and emotions.* Amsterdam: Swets & Zeitlinger.

24 Varni JW, Setoguchi Y. Correlates of perceived physical appearance in children with congenital/acquired limb deficiencies. *J Develop Behav Pediatr* 1991; **12**: 171–6.

25 Tebbi C. The role of social support systems in adolescent cancer amputees. *Cancer* 1985; **56**: 965–71.

26 Spirito A, DeLawyer DD, Stark LJ. Peer relations and social adjustment of chronically ill children and adolescents. *Clin Psychol Rev* 1991; **11**: 539–64.

27 Noll RB, LeRoy S, Bukowski WM *et al.* Relationships and adjustment in children with cancer. *J Pediatr Psychol* 1991; **16**: 307–26.

28 Ross DM, Ross SA. Childhood pain: the school-aged child's viewpoint. *Pain* 1984; **20**: 179–91.

30 La Greca AM. Social consequences of pediatric conditions: fertile area for future investigation and intervention. *J Pediatr Psychol* 1990; **15**: 285–307.

31 Eiser C. How leukaemia affects a child's schooling. *Brit J Soc Clin Psychol* 1980; **19**: 365–8.

32 Charleton A, Larcombe IJ, Meller ST *et al.* Absence from school related to cancer and other chronic conditions. *Arch Dis Child* 1991; **66**: 1217–22.

33 Lansky SB, Lowman JT, Vats T, Guylay JE. School phobia in children with malignant neoplasms. *Am J Dis Child* 1975; **129**: 42–6.

34 Eiser C, Town C. Teachers' concerns about chronically sick children. Implications for pediatricians. *Dev Med Child Neurol* 1987; **29**: 56–63.

35 Kupst MJ. Long-term family coping with acute lymphoblastic leukaemia in childhood. In: LaGreca AM, Siegel LJ, Wallander JL, Walker CE (eds), *Stress and coping in child health.* New York: Guilford Press, 1992, 242–61.

36 Cappelli M, McGrawth PJ, MacDonald NE *et al.* Parental care and overprotection of children with cystic fibrosis. *Br J Med Psychol* 1989; **62**: 281–9.

37 Binger CM. Childhood leukaemia: emotional impact on patient and family. *N Engl J Med* 1969; **280**: 414–18.

38 Chesler MA. The child with cancer and the family. Paper given at the First International meeting in Psychosocial Oncology for Social Workers, University of York, UK.

39 Harris JC, Carel CA, Rosenberg LA *et al.* Intermittent high dose corticosteroid treatment in childhood cancer: Behavioural and emotional consequences. *J Am Acad Child Psychiatr* 1986; **25**: 120–4.

40 Dindia K, Allen M. Sex differences in self-disclosure: a meta-analysis. *Psych Bul* 1992; **112**: 106–24.

41 Eiser C, Havermans T, Craft A, Kernahan J. Development of a measure to assess the perceived illness experience after treatment for cancer. *Arch Dis Child* 1995; **72**: 302–7.

42 Dahlquist LM, Gil KM, Armstrong D *et al.* Behavioral management of children's distress during chemotherapy. *J Behav Exper Psychiatr* 1985; **16**: 325–9.

43 Varni JW, Katz ER, Colegrove R, Dolgin M. The impact of social skills training on the adjustment of children with newly diagnosed cancer. *J Pediatr Psychol* 1993; **18**: 751–68.

44 Eiser C, Havermans T. Treatment for childhood cancer and implications for long-term social adjustment: A review. *Arch Dis Child* 1994; **70**: 66–70.

275

19: Benefits and problems of an adolescent oncology unit

RL SOUHAMI, J WHELAN, JF MCCARTHY,
and A KILBY

In the United Kingdom about 600 cases of cancer will occur each year in the age group 13–20. In this age group leukaemias, lymphomas, brain tumours, and sarcomas are the most frequent tumours. The overall cure rate of cancer in adolescence is now about 60%, and the two major problems which concern oncologists are how to limit treatment side effects in those patients who are currently cured, and how to increase the cure rate in the remaining patients.

After the establishment of the London Bone Tumour Service in 1987 the referral of increasing numbers of adolescents led us to consider whether special provision for the care of the patients was necessary. After three years of planning, a 10-bed adolescent unit was opened in 1990. This paper discusses the way in which we manage the unit and the successes and difficulties which go with it. Other units have been, and are being, developed in the United Kingdom and elsewhere and we hope that our experiences may prove of value.

What are the special needs in the care of adolescents with cancer that made us consider that such a unit was necessary? Patients aged 13–20 fall uneasily between paediatric and adult care. For patients with cancer, where the diagnosis is life threatening and treatment may be extremely difficult, the reactions to the illness at this age are not the same as those of an infant or an adult. Teenagers often have an adult understanding of the disease and its possible prognosis, but may not always have the emotional resources to cope. The diagnosis has come at a time of life which, for healthy teenagers, has its own problems. The pressures caused by school work and examinations, growing apart from family, and discovering yourself, are at an intensity which is different from that which younger children experience and which becomes somewhat less in the twenties. The parents of a patient of any age with a life-threatening illness suffer dreadfully, but such an illness in a healthy teenager produces exceptional stress. Parents need to feel not

Table 19.1   Number of new cases per year

Type of cancer	1992	1993		Total
Osteosarcoma	14	10	9	33
Ewing's	3	4	7	14
Other sarcoma	0	0	6	6
Lymphoma	1	1	1	3
Teratoma	3	0	1	4
Total	21	15	24	60

only that the best is being done for their child but that they too can receive the help they need. These considerations and the wish to concentrate technical expertise led us to establish the unit.

The ward has 10 beds with three cubicled rooms and a seven-bed open plan area. The patients have their own dayroom, bathroom, and kitchen. There is a small room where parents or friends can stay overnight and where we can have quiet conversations. We now think we should have had a larger room for resident visitors and at least one other room for conversation with parents or patients, or for discussions between staff. A seminar room for teaching and larger meetings is adjacent to the unit.

Admissions policy

The number of new cases seen in the period June 1992–December 1993 is shown in Table 19.1. The number of admissions and bed days occupied for 1993 is shown in Figure 19.1 in relation to age. The unit admits

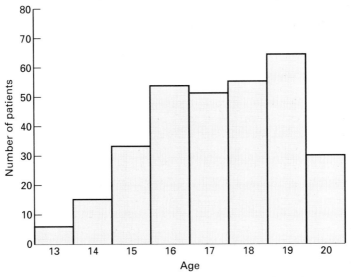

Fig 19.1 Admissions to adolescent unit by age, 1993–4. The total number of admissions was 308.

approximately 40 new patients a year, aged between 13 and 20. The bed occupancy of 1400 bed days per year means that, excluding weekends and national holidays when the occupancy is deliberately reduced, about 7 of the 10 beds are occupied by this age group. The admissions policy of the unit is decided by the nursing and medical team. If the unit is going through a period of relatively low occupancy we have agreed that the upper age limit can be extended. On other occasions the unit is too busy to allow this. Prolonged periods of both over- and under-activity are bad for morale. We estimate that for patients in the diagnostic categories which we are treating at present (Table 19.1) a unit of 10 beds could cope with 60 new cases per year aged 13–20. A unit which treated a larger number of patients with acute leukaemia might need more beds. As treatments become more complex, for example with very high dose chemotherapy regimens, the number of beds needed will increase. If the age limit is extended to 28 years, the additional number of potential cases will be almost double the total in the age range 13–20. The diagnoses will also be different, with more carcinomas and melanomas. Admissions policy is therefore an important medical, social, and economic issue in the management of these units when resources are limited.

It is essential that the admissions policy is formulated and discussed by all members of the medical team, and agreed with other members of hospital staff who might be affected by the policy (such as staff on other wards and services, administrative staff). All hospital units develop their own territorial boundaries. In the case of an adolescent cancer unit we have found it important to define this policy carefully since it greatly influences working practice.

Specialisation of medical practice

For rare cancers, best results are obtained in specialised centres familiar with the diseases. This is well illustrated by the success of paediatric oncology units where cure rates are either higher than on general paediatric wards, or equivalent results are achieved with lower toxicity. We do not yet know if this will be true for adolescent units, but there is every reason to believe that specialisation will be beneficial. While children aged 13–16 are expertly treated on paediatric oncology wards, older patients may be admitted to adult wards without great experience of the tumours concerned.

The technical problems are well illustrated by the management of osteosarcoma and Ewing's sarcoma. The interlinking of complex specialised surgery with intensive combination chemotherapy is perhaps the most difficult challenge. Local control of the tumour may require radical surgery especially at sites such as the pelvis or vertebral column. The cure rate with current chemotherapy regimens is 55–60%. Increasing the cure rate will require still more intensive treatment. In patients at low risk it may be possible to reduce short term and long term chemotherapy toxicity.

Current problems in osteosarcoma management

- Good prognosis cases
  To limit treatment complications
- Bad prognosis cases
  Metastases
  Large volume tumours
  Surgically challenging tumours

New developments in treatment of osteosarcoma

- Good prognosis cases
  Skilful reconstructive surgery
  Careful use of chemotherapy
  Analysis of risk
- Bad prognosis cases
  More intensive chemotherapy
  More radical surgery
  Increasing use of thoracotomy
  Introduction of new agents
- Close daily collaboration between medical and surgical teams

---

Similar technical problems are found in developing strategies to increase the cure rate in Ewing's sarcoma. In this tumour the outlook is still poor for those patients who have metastases at presentation, or who have large volume tumours. Intensification of treatments are being investigated, including the use of chemotherapy at high dose with autologous bone marrow as haematological support, or by using peripheral blood stem cells.

These examples, which are typical of the problems of cancer therapy in this age range, require experience of the tumours and of the treatments. Concentration of experience and expertise is essential. A major aim of the adolescent unit has been to provide a multidisciplinary medical team able to judge the necessary steps in treatment.

Staff training and support

When our unit opened, our experience in the care of adolescents with cancer was derived from care of these patients either on adult wards, or in a ward with paediatric oncology beds. In planning the staff structure we based our working practice largely on that of a paediatric oncology unit but recognised that there would need to be special provision for the adolescent age group.

279

Problems in management of Ewing's tumour

- Good risk cases
  Limit chemotherapy toxicity
  Limit radiation sequelae
- Poor risk cases
  Very intensive chemotherapy
  Increasing use of surgery
  Increasing interest in combined radiotherapy and chemotherapy

---

Medical teams on the adolescent unit

- Medical oncology
- Paediatric oncology
- Radiotherapy
- Haematology

Medical staff

The medical teams working on the unit all have extensive clinical commitments apart from the adolescent unit, although the unit constitutes a considerable proportion of the work of the medical oncology team. Most of the responsibility for the initial reception of the patient and the family lies with the senior medical staff, both consultant and senior registrar grade. The establishment of a warm and open relationship with senior team members is an important first step in allaying some of the anxiety about the initial diagnosis and proposed management. Discussions of treatment choices, especially those involving radical surgery or amputation, and the role of alternatives such as radiation, can only take place with senior, experienced staff, ready and able to respond to detailed questioning. We consider it very important for a member of the nursing team (usually the "key nurse") to be present and for details of these conversations also to be passed on to junior medical staff and colleagues in counselling, social work, and education. Senior staff also take the responsibility of discussing important results, changes in treatment policy and, especially, the significance of relapse if this occurs. This is a time consuming and tiring role for the staff concerned.

Junior medical staff will usually have had little experience in the management of cancer in this age group. The more junior members of the team may also have had no previous training in cancer medicine. Some, but usually a minority, may have had paediatric training. It is hardly surprising that they find the unit a considerable challenge, especially when they first arrive. It is, however, important not to exaggerate the stresses. Most of those who have worked in the unit have found it hard work, but enjoyable and rewarding, and have been able to form happy and comfortable relationships with the patients. Nevertheless there are moments of difficulty. Perhaps the most important source of disquiet is when the unit, and other work outside, becomes so busy that the staff feel they have too little time to spend with their patients. Fiscal and administrative efficiency can be the enemy of good working practice. Junior staff need to take time to get to know their patients and to learn what is expected of them. Secondly, all cancer units go through periods in which everything seems to be going wrong: tumour recurrence in several patients at once, unexpected or extreme toxicities, tension between staff members. At these times junior medical staff may need extra support and encouragement. The most junior among them may not see patients away from the ward and only meet patients during treatment or on relapse when the patients' morale may be low. The third source of stress comes from a serious setback in a patient to whom one of the team is particularly close. On its own this is sad but usually not a serious problem. Combined with long working hours, or an external event such an unsuccessful job interview or examination, the stress can be greater and longer lasting.

Support and training comes first of all from a recognition of these problems and encouragement of open discussion with senior staff. This goes a long way to preventing individual unhappiness and, so far, we have not identified a need for more detailed counselling for medical staff members. There are two aspects to training. The technical aspects of cancer medicine and of management of specific tumours are taught in exactly the same way as in any other branch of medicine: by experience, teaching on rounds, and in department pathology and radiology meetings, by reading and discussion of individual cases. Training in the psychological aspects of cancer medicine in this age group presents a more difficult problem. Junior staff are not greatly different in age from the patients and, although this is often a help in the relationship, it can be difficult for parents to regard the younger doctors as having quite the authority and experience which they occasionally need. This can lead to a junior doctor feeling that his or her role is sometimes being undermined, and the senior staff have to be careful to avoid this by allowing staff to exercise suitable autonomy and by including junior staff in discussions with patients and relatives. This poses a problem since such discussions are often difficult and the presence of a nurse and another doctor can be inhibiting. Yet this is also when observation may be of most value to the trainee. This conflict of interest can only be resolved by including the junior staff in discussions whenever it is reasonable to do so.

Nursing staff

The nursing approach on our unit is the "key nurse" model in which patients are assigned to an individual nurse who is responsible for their continuing care. This nurse is present at all important discussions with the patient and family, and presents the nursing report on ward rounds and at staff meetings. At an early stage we decided that nurses would not wear uniforms, but certain restrictions in daily dress proved to be essential. Denim jeans are not allowed for reasons of hygiene, and figure-hugging clothes are discouraged. Nurses make it clear to the patients that they are "a nurse first and a friend second". Defining the limits of tolerance of adolescent behaviour can be especially difficult for nurses. They have the closest contact and may be only a little older than the patients. They use the knowledge and example of the more experienced staff members, both nursing and medical.

Support for nurses come from other members of the nursing team and from other members of staff. One staff member is trained as a child psychotherapist and she has played an important part in providing advice and counselling for nursing staff as needed. The basic rule adopted by the nursing team is that problems of whatever nature are dealt with as soon as they arise. As with the medical staff, relapse and death pose intense strain on the ward but the aim is to share the burden by close communication.

The key nurse keeps in touch with the patient and family when they are at home, and helps to ensure that outpatient treatment or investigations (such as interim blood counts) are carried out according to plan. Home visits are undertaken if there are particular reasons to do so. Examples are the education of community teams on the care of Hickman lines, or bereavement visits. Visits to schools are sometimes necessary and requested by the teenager in order to explain the nature of the illness and its treatment. The nurse is in contact with community nurses responsible for the patient, and, if the patient dies, keeps in touch with the rest of the family as long as they find this helpful. The team works very closely with the Macmillan home nursing teams who most often provide practical bereavement support. Partnership is promoted, on both an inpatient and an outpatient basis, by allowing the patients to negotiate on admission times and to write their own care plan.

There is a weekly "multidisciplinary meeting" at which the progress of the patients admitted during the current week is discussed with doctors, nursing staff, the ward teacher, psychotherapist, dietitian, and social worker. Particular problems, if any, are highlighted and an agreed plan of action is formulated. This is a good forum for ensuring continuity of care and information.

Helping the patient and family

The essential concern of the unit is to provide the highest possible standard of technical medical care and to achieve the best cure rate with the least toxicity. All our patients are treated as part of national and international studies embodying the best of medical practice. Our second and equal concern is to do what we can to prevent or alleviate the associated stress. In this respect a confident, well-informed team is the major essential ingredient. The team aims to be receptive as possible, but above all to be coherent and consistent in the advice and explanation given at each stage.

A particular difficulty, which comes from placing all these patients in a single unit, is that patients know each other and so do parents. A relapse, or an amputation or a death, can produce anxiety in other patients and their families. The medical and nursing team has to recognise this and to be prepared to talk about the event as openly as can be permitted. When a metastasis develops, the patients and family are often well aware of what this can mean. This has a positive aspect since it engenders a useful realism, but there is no doubt that close proximity of this type produces additional tensions of which the unit staff must be aware.

Conclusion

Our experience over the last five years has not altered our confidence that units of this type offer considerable advantages for the care of adolescents with cancer. The work is technically and emotionally demanding and the most important requirement for care is a united and mutually supportive medical multidisciplinary team.

Index

Note: *passim* means when the discussion of a topic is scattered throughout a range of pages.
Abbreviations used: ALL, acute lymphoblastic leukaemia; AML, acute myeloid leukaemia